BEHCET'S DISEASE

Edited by **Müzeyyen Gönül**
and **Selda Pelin Kartal**

Behcet's Disease
http://dx.doi.org/10.5772/65884
Edited by Müzeyyen Gönül and Selda Pelin Kartal

Contributors

Orhan Saim Demirtürk, Alexander Fraser, Fahd Adeeb, Maria Usman Khan, Austin Stack, Feride Çoban Gül, Hülya Nazik, Yuki Nanke, Genadi Georgiev Genadiev, Stefano Camparini, Lorenzo Mortola, Roberta Arzedi, Giuseppe Deiana, Francesco Spanu, Ozge Keseroglu, Müzeyyen Gönül, Isil Deniz Oguz, Pelin Hızlı, Arzu Kilic, Esra Sahli, Ozlem Gurbuz-Koz, Yildiz Ozdemir

Published by InTech
Janeza Trdine 9, 51000 Rijeka, Croatia

Publishing Process Manager Edi Lipovic
Technical Editor SPi Global
Cover InTech Design team

First published May, 2017
Printed in Croatia
Legal deposit, Croatia: National and University Library in Zagreb

Additional hard copies can be obtained from orders@intechopen.com

Behcet's Disease, Edited by Müzeyyen Gönül and Selda Pelin Kartal
p. cm.
Print ISBN 978-953-51-3225-7
Online ISBN 978-953-51-3226-4

For EU product safety concerns:
IN TECH d.o.o., Prolaz Marije Krucifikse Kozulić 3, 51000 Rijeka, Croatia,
info@intechopen.com or visit our website at intechopen.com.

Meet the editors

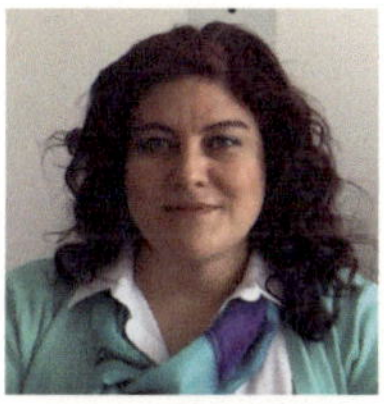

Dr. Muzeyyen Gonul graduated from Ankara University School of Medicine. Currently, she is an associate professor in the Department of Dermatology at Dişkapi Yildirim Beyazit Education and Research Hospital in Ankara, Turkey. She has coauthored over 120 published articles and supervised several master and postdoctoral students. Her research interests are psoriasis, urticaria, autoimmune bullous diseases, and Behçet's disease.

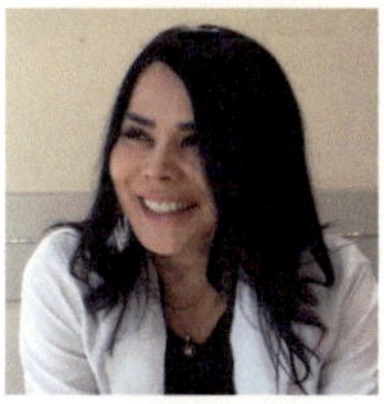

Dr. Selda Pelin Kartal graduated from Hacettepe University School of Medicine. Currently, she is an associate professor in the Department of Dermatology at Dişkapi Yildirim Beyazit Education and Research Hospital in Ankara, Turkey. She has coauthored over 100 published articles and supervised several master and postdoctoral students. Her actual interests are focused on acne, psoriasis, urticaria, autoimmune bullous diseases, Behçet's disease, and cosmetic dermatology.

Contents

Preface

Vasculitis is a specific pattern of inflammation of the blood vessels and can affect small, medium-sized, or large vessels of arterial and/or venous systems. Different types of vasculitis affect vessels of different sizes. Behçet's disease is a unique vasculitis in that vessels in all sizes are involved and can cause damage to both arteries and veins. It can manifest itself in a wide symptom spectrum in almost all organs and systems, so it concerns all areas of medicine. We aim to present information to our colleagues in different branches of medicine by discussing the various aspects of Behçet's disease in the ten chapters in this book:

- Overview of Behçet's disease
- Epidemiologic aspects of the disease worldwide
- Etiopathogenesis (genetic, immunologic, and microbial) of Behçet's disease in two chapters
- Mucocutaneous findings of the disease
- Diagnosis and activity markers of the disease
- Ocular involvement of the disease
- Joint involvement of the disease
- Cardiovascular involvement of the disease
- Surgical treatment of cardiovascular involvement

We believe that this book will be a valuable reference to students, researchers, dermatologists, and other healthcare professionals interested in Behçet's disease. I am very happy and honored to be the editor of a book about Behçet's disease defined by a Turkish dermatologist Hulusi Behçet Uz. Also, I am very grateful to all the authors for their strong effort and patience needed to bring out this book. In addition, I thank the assistance of Mr. Edi Lipović, whose guidance and encouragement were truly invaluable.

Muzeyyen Gonul, MD, Associate Professor,
Health Science University,
Dışkapı Yıldırım Beyazıt Training and Research Hospital
Dermatology Clinic, Ankara, Turkey

Dr. Selda Pelin Kartal,
Department of Dermatology,
Dişkapi Yildirim Beyazit Education and Research Hospital,
Ankara, Turkey

Section 1

General Description of Behçet's Disease

Chapter 1

Introductory Chapter: Behcet's Disease - An Overview

Müzeyyen Gönül and Selda Pelin Kartal

Additional information is available at the end of the chapter

http://dx.doi.org/10.5772/intechopen.69050

1. Introduction

Behçet's disease (BD) is a multisystem inflammatory disease with unknown etiology [1]. It may affect vascular, gastrointestinal, neurologic, articular, pulmonary, cardiac, and urogenital systems [1, 2].

2. History

The disease was first described by a Turkish dermatologist, Hulusi Behçet, in 1937 as a triple symptom complex; aphthous stomatitis, genital ulcers, and relapsing uveitis [2]. Hulusi Behçet was born in 1889 in Istanbul/Turkey. In 1910, he became a medical doctor, and in 1914, he received a dermatologist title. In 1933, he became a professor of dermatology and venereal diseases. Hulusi Behçet is the first academician with a titled professor in the history of Turkish academy. Hulusi Behçet observed aphthous symptoms in the mouth and genital area and several findings in the eye in his three patients whom he followed 21, 7 and 3 years. He believed that this was a new disease. In 1937, he reported his observations in "DermatologischeWochenschrift" and then he presented his patients in a dermatology meeting in Paris. In later times, same cases were reported from various regions of the world. In 1947, the new disease was named as "*Morbus Behçet*" in International Congress of Geneva [3].

3. Epidemiology

BD has a worldwide distribution. But it is commonly observed in the Silk Road countries between the Mediterranean Sea, including such countries Spain, Portugal, Turkey, Iran, and

Far East countries like China and Japan [4, 5]. The disease is most common in Turkey with the prevalence of 20-602 per 100.000 [6, 7]. It develops at any age, but it most appears between the second and fourth decade of life [8]. BD patients with early onset may have the more severe disease [9]. BD is uncommon in children. Patients with initial symptoms at age 16 years or younger are classified as juvenile-onset BD. The prevalence of juvenile BD is unknown. But in few series, it is reported between 3, 3 and 26% of BD patients were before age of 16 years [10]. BD affects the both gender equally [11]. The disease is more severe among male patients, and vascular disease is the major risk factor of death in male patients. It is shown that vascular disease, folliculitis, papulopustular skin lesions, positive pathergy test, and ocular disease are more common in men while erythema nodosum, genital ulcers, and joint involvement are more common among women [12, 13].

4. Etiology

Although several immunological abnormalities have been demonstrated, the real etiologic mechanism of the disease is unclear.

4.1. Infectious agents

The most probablehypothesis is that in genetically predisposed individuals some infectious agents such as *Herpes simplex virus* (HSV)-1, *Streptococcus sangiuinis* (*S. sanguinis*) or some autoantigens such as heat shock proteins (HSP) trigger the autoinflammatory reactions [1]. BD has aspects of both autoimmune disease and auto inflammatory disease. The autoimmunity indicators are the effectiveness of classical immunosuppressives such as azathioprine and cyclosporine, and the suggested role of the candidate autoantigen, human heat-shock protein 60 (HSP60). Also, the lack of significant high-titer autoantibodies or antigen-specific T-cells, strong involvement of major histocompatibility complex (MHC) class I molecules, clinical episodes of unprovoked recurrent inflammation, mainly caused by neutrophils, and the therapeutic effectiveness of colchicine, are signs of autoinflammation [14].

Infection agents have an important role in the pathogenesis of BD. Several investigations have shown the association between HSV and BD. But, in some studies, this association could not detected [1, 15, 16]. Therefore, the role of HSV at the etiopathogenesis of BD is not clear.

Several potential bacteria have been investigated but the most commonly implicated microorganism is *S. sanguinus* [17]. It was found that Bes-1 gene and HSP-65 derived from oral *S. sanguinis*, are supposed to play important roles as an extrinsic factor in BD pathogenesis. The peptides of the Bes-1 gene are highly homologous with the retinal protein Brn3b, and moreover, the Bes-1 peptides were homologous with HSP-65 derived from microorganisms in association with the counterpart human HSP-60, which appeared reactively in the BD patients. Some homologous peptides of HSP-65 were found to reduce IL-8, IL-12, and TNF-alpha in active BD patients [18]. Also, it is shown that *S. sanguinis* antigens increase IFN-γ and IL-6 secretion from the peripheral blood cell T cell of BD patients [19].

From another report, it was detected that *Streptococcus mutans (S. mutans)* colonization rate was significantly higher in BD. *S. mutans* presence in saliva was associated with oral ulcers, and it was associated with severe disease course than milder disease [20].

Heat shock protein (HSP) functions as an intracellular chaperonin of other proteins and significant sequence homology is found between mammalian HSP and microbial HSP HSP60/65 was thought to be a major cause of the skewed immune responses in patients with BD because of the molecular mimicry between human HSP and microbial HSP. HSP60 regulates Th1 cell differentiation through multiple immunologic pathways [21].

Gut microbiota compositional alteration may have an association with immune dysfunction in patients with BD. Direct comparison of the relative abundance of bacterial taxa demonstrated that the genera *Bifidobacterium* and *Eggerthella* increased significantly and the genera *Megamonas* and *Prevotella* decreased significantly in BD patients compared with normal individuals. The authors suggested that the compositional changes of gut microbes may be one type of dysbiosis (unfavorable microbiota alteration) in patients with BD. The dysbiosis may have an association with the pathophysiology of BD [22].

4.2. Genetic factors

Genetic factors play important roles in the pathogenesis of BD. Multiple studies have demonstrated that BD is strongly associated with the presence of human leukocyte antigen (HLA)-B5 and its split antigen HLA-B51 [11, 23]. The association with HLA-B5 was first described by Ohno et al. in 1973. Several studies confirmed the HLA-B51 association with BD and HLA-B51 is the strongest known genetic factor for BD [1]. The MHC region on chromosome 6p21 contains HLA and other essential genes in the immune response [14]. A meta-analysis based on 72 studies in 74 study populations revealed the moderate association of HLA-B5/-B*51 with male gender, the high prevalence of eye involvement, skin involvement, and genital ulcers, and low prevalence of gastrointestinal involvement [24]. Some of the other susceptible genes associated with BD are IL10, IL23R-IL12RB2, STAT4, TNFAIP3, CCR1-CCR3, KLRC4, FUT2, IL12A, IL23R, TLR4, MEFV, and NOD2. The genes identified are involved in both innate and adaptive immunity and support the idea that polarization in Th1/Th17 pathway plays a critical role in BD pathogenesis [14].

5. Clinical manifestations

5.1. Mucocutaneous findings

5.1.1. Oral aphthosis (ulceration)

Oral ulceration is the most detected symptom that seen over 97% of the patients. It is a painful, recurrent, round, and oval ulceration with well-defined borders and central yellowish pseudomembrane. An erythematous halo surrounds the ulcers. The most common sites are mucous membranes of the lips, buccal mucosa, tongue, and soft palate. They can be classified as minor, major or herpetiform on the basis of ulcer size and number. Oral ulcer often resolves spontaneously within 1–4 weeks. Local trauma can trigger new oral ulceration. At the differential diagnosis of oral ulcers herpes simplex, erythema multiforme, fixed drug eruption, MAGIC syndrome, Reiter's syndrome, and Sweet's syndrome, anemia due to a deficiency of iron, vitamin B12 or folic acid, inflammatory bowel diseases, and systemic lupus erythematosus must consider [1, 25, 26].

5.1.2. Genital ulcers

Genital ulcers can be seen 60–89% of the patients. Genital ulcers are similar in appearance to oral ulcers. The scrotum is the most frequently involved site in males. Ulcers can also be observed on the shaft and glans penis. In females, the ulcers most commonly occur on the labia but the vaginal mucosa and rarely the cervix can also be affected. Vaginal ulcers often cause a discharge. GU may occur in both sexes in the groin, perineal and perianal area. They usually heal within 10–30 days and deep ulcers may lead scarring. Genital herpes simplex infection, erythema multiforme, fixed drug eruption, sexually transmitted diseases such as syphilis, chancroid, lymphogranuloma Venere um and HIV infection should be considered in differential diagnosis [1, 25, 26].

5.1.3. Erythema nodosum like lesions

Erythema nodosum like lesions is mostly seen in females. They are characterized by painful multiple subcutaneous nodules that vary in size and color. They are frequently seen at the lower extremities but they can also be localized to the face, neck, forearms, and buttock. The lesions resolve spontaneously within 2–3 weeks. The histopathological features of erythema nodosum-like lesions are characterized by the presence of vasculitis or vascular reaction; different from erythema nodosum secondary to other systemic causes. The presence of the erythema nodosum like lesion may be an indicator of the mildness of Behçet's disease; and the presence of histopathological evidence of severe vasculitis, especially phlebitis, in erythema nodosum-like lesions may be an indicator of the involvement of the gastrointestinal tract in Behçet's disease [1, 26, 27].

5.1.4. Papulopustularlesions (PPL)

PPL are cutaneous, sterile, folliculitis – or acne-like lesions on an erythematous base which appear as a papule and in the course of 24–48 h become a pustule. Trunk, buttocks, and the lower limbs are the most common localizations. Differential diagnosis of PPL is difficult from acne vulgaris. In a recent study, it is suggested that in BD patients the inflammatory lesions located on the face were less than those in the acne vulgaris. Inflammatory lesions such as folliculitis on the legs were only seen, in the BD group. The papulopustular lesions of BD could not be distinguished from AV by histology [1, 25, 28].

5.1.5. Superficial thrombophlebitis

Superficial thrombophlebitis is the most frequent type of venous involvement. The patients usually present with erythematous, tender, subcutaneous nodules arranged in a linear fashion.

The small vein can be palpated as a string-like hardening of the subcutaneous tissue with reddening of the overlying skin. It is more common in males and frequently confused with erythema nodosum like lesions. Superficial thrombophlebitis is often associated with other forms of vascular disease in BD [1, 25].

5.1.6. Other cutaneous lesions

Extragenital ulcerations clinically resemble aphthous lesions of the disease. They are recurrent and usually heal with scarring. The lesions have been reported on various locations such as the legs, axillae, breast, neck, interdigital skin of the foot, inguinal region, and neck.

Sweet syndrome like lesions are characterized by painful erythematous plaques and nodules which usually localize to face, neck, and extremities. Other cutaneous vasculitic lesions include pyodermagangrenosum-like, erythema multiforme-like lesions, palpable purpura, subungual infarctions, hemorrhagic bullae, furuncles, and abscesses [1, 3, 25].

5.1.7. Skin pathergy test

Pathergy phenomenon is defined as a state of altered tissue reactivity that occurs in response to minor trauma. A papule or a sterile pustule occurs 24–48 h after an intradermal injection of the skin with a 20-gauge needle. The positivity rate of pathergy test in BD was found to vary from country to country. It is most prevalent around the silk route, which extends from the Far East to the Mediterranean Basin. Other diseases that can be seen positive pathergy test are; pyodermagangrenosum, interferon alpha-treated chronic myeloid leukemia patients, Sweet's syndrome, eosinophilic pustular folliculitis, inflammatory bowel disease and healthy individuals [26, 29].

5.2. Ocular manifestations

Ocular involvement is one of the most disabling complications of BD, causing loss of vision that may progress to blindness if left untreated. The typical form of ocular involvement is a relapsing and remitting panuveitis and retinal vasculitis. Uveitis occurs in approximately two-thirds of BD patients. A single attack will usually heal spontaneously without a sequel. But destructive and recurrent attacks, especially with the posterior segment and retina involvement, may cause irreversible ocular structural changes and permanent damage in the sensory retina, resulting in loss of vision [30, 31].

5.3. Vascular involvement

Vascular involvement in BD includes venous thrombosis, arterial occlusion, and pulmonary artery and aortic aneurysm formation [32]. Lower extremity deep venous thrombosis is the most common form of vascular involvement in BD [9]. Venous thrombosis may occur at any site of the body and any size of vessels may be affected [26]. Inferior vena cava, superior vena cava, and pulmonary artery are the other common involved vessels. Pulmonary artery involvement, the most common form of arterial involvement, manifests as aneurysms and "in situ" thrombosis. Pulmonary artery involvement and Budd-Chiari syndrome are the leading causes of increased mortality. In a vascular cluster, typically, several types of venous or arterial vascular involvement may accumulate in the same individual. Vascular involvement is more common and more severe among males [33].

5.4. Gastrointestinal involvement

Intestinal BD is characterized by ulcers on the gastrointestinal tract, usually at the ileocecal region. Patients can present with abdominal pain, diarrhea, constipation or acute abdomen due to perforation of an ulcer. To distinguish clinical symptoms of intestinal BD from inflammatory bowel disease may be difficult. Some colonoscopy and histopathological findings may help for differentiating the two disease [9, 26].

5.5. Neurologic involvement

Neurobehcet disease is a rare complication of BD. But it is an important cause of morbidity and mortality in BD. Little is known about this neuro-Behçet because there are no confirmed diagnostic criteria, and all the studies have a small number of patients. The prevalence reported normally ranges between 5 and 15% and it is more frequent amongst men between 20 and 40 years old. The typical presentations include focal parenchymal lesions, vascular thrombosis, arterial vasculitis, and aseptic meningoencephalitis [34].

5.6. Joint involvement

Joint manifestations are common in Behçet's disease. Most patients suffer from a nonerosive, nondeforming oligoarthritis typically involving the knees, ankles, and wrists [35].

6. Diagnosis

There is not a universally accepted pathognomonic test for diagnosis of BD. The diagnose is primarily based on clinical criteria and exclusion of alternative diagnosis [1]. Various criteria have been used. The mostly used one is International Study Group for Behçet's Disease criteria (ISG criteria) which formulated at 1990. According to ISG criteria, the presence of oral aphthosis was mandatory. Two of the following symptoms were required for the diagnosis of BD: Genital aphthosis, skin manifestations, ocular lesions, and positive pathergy reaction [36]. Later in 2006, a new set was proposed by the International Team for the Revision of the International Criteria for Behçet's Disease (ITR-ICBD). According to ITR-ICBD, oral aphthosis, skin manifestations, vascular manifestations, and positive pathergy reaction score one point each. Genital ulcers and ocular manifestations get two points each. The diagnosis of BD is made when three or more points are collected [37]. Then at 2013, the new criteria were revised under the name International Criteria for Behçet's disease (ICBD). In this criteria oral ulcer, genital ulcer, and ocular manifestations get each two points; skin lesions, neurological manifestations, vascular manifestations, and positive pathergy test get each one point. For the diagnosis, four points are required [38].

7. Prognosis

BD has a chronic course with unpredictable remissions and exacerbations. The diagnosis is difficult in many patients because there is not a universally accepted diagnostic criteria and the clinical symptoms may be seen in many other diseases. In a study from Germany, it was shown that because of the ethnicity, in Turkish patients, the diagnosis of BD is earlier than German patients. Because in German patients the diagnosis was later and more difficult than Turkish patients, some of the patients might be followed with the wrong diagnosis for long times. It is mentioned that the diagnosis is more difficult in non-endemic areas [39]. But recognizing the disease may permit early diagnosis and treatment. An oral ulcer is the most commonly seen clinical symptom followed by a genital ulcer, PPL, erythema nodosum like lesions and articular and ocular lesions. These clinical symptoms lead to pain and loss of function. On the other hand pulmonary especially large vessel involvement, neurological involvement, and bowel perforation are causes of mortality [1]. It is shown that male sex, arterial involvement, and a high number of BD flares were independently associated with the risk of mortality [40].

8. Conclusion

BD is a chronic inflammatory multisystem disease that affects any size of the vessels. The etiology is not clear yet. However, infectious and genetic factors are thought to act roles in the etiopathogenesis. There is no specific serological marker and the diagnosis of the disease depends on clinical criteria only. Moreover, the clinical symptoms of the disease may be seen in many diseases. So, knowing the findings, diagnostic criteria, prognosis, and complications of the disease provides the early diagnosis of the BD that is very important for the treatment of the disease, which has risks of mortality and morbidity. So, in this book, epidemiology, etiopathogenesis, cutaneous, and systemic findings and treatment of BD will be reviewed in detail.

Author details

Müzeyyen Gönül* and Selda Pelin Kartal

*Address all correspondence to: muzeyyengonul@gmail.com

University of Health Sciences, Dışkapı Yıldırım Beyazıt Training and Research Hospital, Dermatology Clinic, Ankara, Turkey

References

[1] Alpsoy E. Behçet's disease: A comprehensive review with a focus on epidemiology, etiology and clinical features, and management of mucocutaneous lesions. The Journal of Dermatology. 2016;**43**:620–632. DOI: 10.1111/1346-8138.13381

[2] Behçet H. Überrezidivierende, aphtÖsedurchein Virus verursachteGeschwüre am Mund, am auge und den Genitalien [Caused about recurrent aphtous by a virüs Ulcers of the mouth, the eyes and genitals]. DermatolMonatsschrWochenschr 1937;**105**:1152–1157

[3] Tüzün Y, Fresko İ, Mat MC, Özyazgan Y, Hamuyudan V. Behçet sendromu. In: Tüzün Y, Gürer MA, Serdaroğlu S, Oğuz O, Aksungur VL. Dermatoloji 3rd. Istanbul: Nobel; 2008.pp. 913–928

[4] Kappen JH, van Dijk EH, Baak-Dijkstra M, van Daele PL, Lam-Tse WK, van Hagen PM, van Laar JA. Behçet's disease, hospital-based prevalence and manifestations in the Rotterdam area. The Netherlands Journal of Medicine. 2015;**73**:471–477

[5] Keino H, Okada AA. Behçet's disease: Global epidemiology of an Old Silk Road disease. British Journal of Ophthalmology. 2007;**91**:1573–1574

[6] Mahr A, Maldini C. Epidemiology of Behçet's disease. La Revue de Médecine Interne. 2014;**35**:81–89

[7] Baş Y, Seçkin HY, Kalkan G, Takcı Z, Önder Y, Çıtıl R, Demir S, Şahin Ş. Investigation of Behçet's disease and recurrent aphthous stomatitis frequency: The highest prevalence in Turkey. Balkan Medical Journal. 2016;**33**:390–395. DOI: 10.5152/balkanmedj.2016.15101

[8] Onder M, GürerMA. The multiple faces of Behçet's disease and its aetiologicalfactors. Journal of the European Academy of Dermatology and Venereology. 2001;**15**:126–136

[9] Hatemi G, Seyahi E, Fresko I, Talarico R, Hamuryudan V. Behçet's syndrome: A critical digest of the 2014–2015 literature. Clinical and Experimental Rheumatology. 2015;**33**:3–14

[10] Koné-Paut I. Behçet's disease in children, an overview. Pediatric Rheumatology Online Journal. 2016;14:10. DOI: 10.1186/s12969-016-0070-z

[11] Pamuk ÖN, Çakır N. The epidemiology of Behcet's disease. Turkiye Klinikleri Journal of Medical Sciences. 2005;**1**:39

[12] Bonitsis NG, Luong Nguyen LB, LaValley MP, Papoutsis N, Altenburg A, Kötter I, Micheli C, Maldini C, Mahr A, Zouboulis CC. Gender-specific differences in Adamantiades-Behçet's disease manifestations: An analysis of the German registry and meta-analysis of data from the literature. Rheumatology (Oxford). 2015;**54**:121–133. DOI: 10.1093/rheumatology/keu247

[13] Kural-Seyahi E, Fresko I, Seyahi N, Ozyazgan Y, Mat C, Hamuryudan V, Yurdakul S, YaziciH.The long-term mortality and morbidity of Behçet syndrome: A 2-decade outcome survey of 387 patients followed at a dedicated center. Medicine (Baltimore). 2003;**82**:60–76

[14] Takeuchi M, Kastner DL, Remmers EF. Theimmunogenetics of Behçet's disease: A comprehensive review. Journal of Autoimmunity. 2015;**64**:137–148. DOI: 10.1016/j.jaut.2015.08.013

[15] Nomura Y, Kitteringham N, Shiba K, Goseki M, Kimura A, MineshitaS.Use of the highly sensitive PCR method to detect the Herpes simplex virus type 1 genome and its

expression in samples from Behçet disease patients. Journal of Medical and Dental Sciences. 1998;**45**:51–58

[16] Tojo M, Zheng X, Yanagihori H, Oyama N, Takahashi K, Nakamura K, Kaneko F.Detection of herpes virus genomes in skin lesions from patients with Behçet's disease and other related inflammatory diseases. Acta Dermato-Venereologica. 2003;**83**:124–127

[17] Houman MH, BelFeki N. [Pathophysiology of Behçet's disease]. Revue de Médecine Interne. 2014;**35**:90–96. DOI: 10.1016/j.revmed.2013.10.012

[18] Kaneko F, Oyama N, Yanagihori H, Isogai E, Yokota K, OgumaK. The role of streptococcal hypersensitivity in the pathogenesis of Behçet's disease. European Journal of Dermatology. 2008;**18**:489–498. DOi: 10.1684/ejd.2008.0484

[19] Hirohata S, Oka H, Mizushima Y. Streptococcal-related antigens stimulate production of IL6 and interferon-gamma by T cells from patients with Behcet's disease. Cellular Immunology. 1992;**140**:410–419

[20] Mumcu G, Inanc N, Aydin SZ, Ergun T, Direskeneli H. Association of salivary *S. mutans* colonisation and mannose-binding lectin deficiency with gender in Behçet's disease. Clinical and Experimental Rheumatology. 2009;**27**:32–36

[21] Shimizu J, Izumi T, Suzuki N. Aberrant activation of heat shock protein 60/65 reactive T cells in patients with Behcet's disease. Autoimmune Disorders. 2012;**2012**:105205. DOI: 10.1155/2012/105205

[22] Shimizu J, Kubota T, Takada E, Takai K, Fujiwara N, Arimitsu N, Ueda Y, Wakisaka S, Suzuki T, Suzuki N. Bifidobacteria abundance-featured gut microbiota compositional change in patients with Behcet's disease. PLoS One. 2016;**11**:e0153746. DOi: 10.1371/journal.pone.0153746

[23] Ahmed Z, Rossi ML, Yong S, Martin DK, Walayat S, Cashman M, Tsoraides S, Dhillon S. Behçet's disease departs the 'Silk Road': A case report and brief review of literature with geographical comparison. Journal of Community Hospital Internal Medicine Perspectives. 2016;**6**:30362. DOI: 10.3402/jchimp.v6.30362

[24] Maldini C, Lavalley MP, Cheminant M, de Menthon M, Mahr A. Relationships of HLA-B51 or B5 genotype with Behcet's disease clinical characteristics: Systematic review and meta-analyses of observational studies. Rheumatology (Oxford). 2012;**51**:887–900

[25] Alpsoy E, Zouboulis CC, Ehrlich GE. Mucocutaneous lesions of Behcet's disease. Yonsei Medical Journal. 2007;**48**:573–585

[26] Leonardo NM, McNeil J. Behcet's disease: Is there geographical variation? A review far from the Silk Road. International Journal of Rheumatology. 2015;**2015**:945262. DOI: 10.1155/2015/945262

[27] Misago N, Tada Y, Koarada S, Narisawa Y. Erythemanodosum-like lesions in Behçet's disease: A clinicopathological study of 26 cases. Acta Dermato-Venereologica. 2012;**92**:681–686. DOI: 10.2340/00015555-1349

[28] Kutlubay Z, Mat CM, Aydin Ö, Demirkesen C, Calay Ö, Engın B, Tüzün Y, Yazici H. Histopathological and clinical evaluation of papulopustular lesions in Behçet's disease. Clinical and Experimental Rheumatology. 2015;**33**:101–106

[29] Sequeira FF, Daryani D. The oral and skin pathergytest. Indian Journal of Dermatology, Venereology and Leprology. 2011;**77**:526–530. DOI: 10.4103/0378-6323.82399

[30] Ozyazgan Y, Ucar D, Hatemi G, Yazici Y. Ocular involvement of Behçet's syndrome: A comprehensive review. Clinical Reviews in Allergy & Immunology. 2015;**49**:298–306. DOI: 10.1007/s12016-014-8425-z

[31] Kitaichi N, Miyazaki A, Iwata D, Ohno S, Stanford MR, Chams H. Ocular features of Behcet's disease: An international collaborative study. British Journal of Ophthalmology. 2007;**91**:1579–1582

[32] Yahalom M, Bloch L, Suleiman K, Rosh B, TurgemanY. Cardiovascular involvement in Behçet disease: Cardiovascular involvement in Behçet disease. 2016;**25**:84–86. DOI: 10.1055/s-0035-1551796

[33] Seyahi E. Behçet's disease: How to diagnose and treat vascular involvement. Best Practice & Research Clinical Rheumatology. 2016;**30**:279–295. DOI: 10.1016/j.berh.2016.08.002

[34] Peño IC, De lasHeras Revilla V, Carbonell BP, Di Capua Sacoto D, Ferrer ME, García-Cobos R, González RA. Neurobehçet disease: Clinical and demographic characteristics. EuropeanJournalofNeurology.2012;**19**:1224–1227.DOI:10.1111/j.1468-1331.2012.03706.x

[35] Benamour S, Zeroual B, Alaoui FZ. Joint manifestations in Behçet's disease. A review of 340 cases. Revue du rhumatisme (English ed.). 1998;**65**:299–307

[36] Criteria for Diagnosis of Behçet's Disease. International Study Group for Behçet's disease. Lancet. 1990;**335**:1078–1080

[37] di Meo N, Bergamo S, Vidimari P, Bonin S, Trevisan G. Analysis of diagnostic criteria in adamantiades-behçet disease: A retrospective study. Indian Journal of Dermatology. 2013;**58**:275–277. DOI: 10.4103/0019-5154.113936

[38] International Team for the Revision of the International Criteria for Behçet's Disease (ITR-ICBD).The International Criteria for Behçet's Disease (ICBD): A collaborative study of 27 countries on the sensitivity and specificity of the new criteria. Journal of the European Academy of Dermatology and Venereology. 2014;**28**:338–347. DOI: 10.1111/jdv.12107

[39] Zouboulis CC, Kötter I, Djawari D, Kirch W, Kohl PK, Ochsendorf FR, Keitel W, Stadler R, Wollina U, Proksch E, Söhnchen R, Weber H, Gollnick HP, Hölzle E, Fritz K, Licht T, Orfanos CE. Epidemiological features of Adamantiades-Behçet's disease in Germany and in Europe. Yonsei Medical Journal. 1997;**38**:411–422

[40] Saadoun D, Wechsler B, Desseaux K, Le ThiHuong D, Amoura Z, Resche-Rigon M, Cacoub P. Mortality in Behçet's disease. Arthritis & Rheumatology. 2010;**62**:2806–2812. DOi: 10.1002/art.27568

Section 2

Clinical Findings and Treatments of Behçet's Disease

Chapter 2

The Epidemiology of Behçet's Disease

Işıl Deniz Oguz, Pelin Hizli and Muzeyyen Gonul

Additional information is available at the end of the chapter

http://dx.doi.org/10.5772/68055

Abstract

Behçet's disease (BD), a chronic vasculitis affecting any type of the blood vessels, was first described by a Turkish dermatologist Hulusi Behçet. Although it has a worldwide distribution, it is commonly seen in the Silk Road countries around the Mediterranean Sea. The country in which the disease is most commonly seen is Turkey with a prevalence of 20–602/100,000. The disease most appears between the second and fourth decades of the life. BD affects both genders equally. However, the gender distribution may differ among different regions.

Keywords: Behçet's disease, epidemiology, prevalence, age, pathergy, HLAB51

1. Introduction

Behçet's disease (BD) is a chronic multisystem vasculitis, which affects any type and shape of blood vessels, particularly veins [1, 2]. The disease was first described in 1937 by a Turkish dermatologist, Hulusi Behçet, as a triple symptom complex, aphthous stomatitis, genital ulcers and relapsing uveitis [3]. Most widely used classification criteria is suggested by The International Study Group (ISG) for BD in 1990 [4]. According to the ISG, the major criterion exactly required for the diagnosis is recurrent oral ulceration at least three times a year. Additionally, at least two of the minor criteria: genital ulceration, skin lesions (erythema nodosum, necrotic folliculitis, and papulopustular lesions), ocular lesions (posterior uveitis, total uveitis, and retinal vasculitis), and positive pathergy testing are required for the diagnosis [4].

2. Epidemiology

2.1. Prevalence

BD has a worldwide distribution. But it is commonly seen in the Silk Road countries around the Mediterranean Sea, including Spain, Portugal, Turkey, Iran, and Far East countries like China and Japan [5, 6]. The prevalence of the disease along the silk route is 14–20/100,000 [7]. BD is most common in Turkey with the prevalence of 20–602/100,000 [8, 9]. The other more prevalent countries are Iran, China, Tunisian, Korea, Israel, and Japan [8, 10, 11]. In North European, American, and African countries BD is less frequent [12, 13]. The prevalence of BD in some countries is shown in **Table 1** [8, 9, 12, 14–20].

Since 1982, the supported hypothesis about the etiopathogenesis of BD has been that the genetic material and the exogenous agents responsible for the disease were carried during the immigration of ancient nomadic tribes [15]. Many studies focus on immigrations so far have investigated how the genetic or environmental factors affect the development of BD. In 1997 in Germany, 218 patients with BD were investigated. Of these patients, 89 were German, 100 were Turkish, and 29 were from other nationalities. The prevalence of BD was found 0.16/100,000 in German population and 4.51/100,000 in Turkish population. The prevalence of BD in Turkish population was higher than German population. However, it was 5–18-fold lower than the prevalence found in Turkey. This study suggested that the genetic and environmental factors are both effective in the development of the disease [15]. Another similar study was performed in 2015 in the Rotterdam area of Netherland [5]. Eighty-four patients of Dutch, Turkish, or Moroccan origin with BD were identified. The prevalence of BD was found 1/100,000 in Dutch, 71/100,000 in Turkish and 39/100,000 in Moroccan population. The study mentioned that the prevalence of BD in different ethnic group was similar to that among the

Country	Prevalence (1/100,000)
Turkey [8, 9]	20–602
Israel [14, 15]	50–185
Iran [12, 16]	16.7–100
Iraq [17]	17
Japan [9]	7–13.5
China [18]	2.62
Kuwait [12]	2.1
Italy [19, 20]	4.1–15.9
Germany [21]	0.9
USA [12]	0.33

Table 1. Worldwide prevalence of Behçet's disease.

original countries of these patients. However, another study reported that no patient with BD was detected in Hawaii, where the Japan population is relatively high [11].

2.2. Age and gender

Behçet's disease can be seen at any age, but it mostly appears between the second and fourth decades of life [22]. In a study from Ankara, Turkey, the mean age of the patients with BD was found 37.2 [23]. In a study from Japan, the mean age of onset was found 36.8 [24]. The mean age of onset of BD in many countries was shown in **Table 2** [5, 13, 15, 23–34].

Regional and ethnic factors may affect the time of the diagnosis of the illness. The diagnosis of the disease is delayed in areas where the prevalence of the disease is lower [12]. In a study from Germany, it was reported that the time of diagnosis of BD in Turkish patients was earlier than in German patients. The diagnosis was later and more difficult in German patients than in Turkish patients, so that we should keep in mind that some German patients might be followed with wrong diagnosis for long times before the diagnosis of BD [15, 35].

Patients with earlier onset have more severe disease [36]. In a study from Tunisia, BD patients with onset before age of 20 and after age of 40 were compared each other. Cutaneous involvement, pseudo folliculitis, and vena cava thrombosis were more frequent in patients with earlier onset. In contrast, joint involvement was more frequent in patients with later onset [28]. Mortality in the group with earlier onset was 2.46% but no patients had died due to BD in the group with later onset [28]. Some authors reported that BD patient with earlier onset had more ophthalmic manifestations and active course of the disease [37, 38].

Country	Age of onset	Male/female
Turkey [23, 25]	37.2–38.02	0.69–1.03
Japanese [24]	36.8	0.74
Iran [26]	26.2	1.4
Israel [27]	34.9	1.22
Netherlands [5]	43	0.64
Senegal [13]	32	1.6
Tunisian [28]	29.12	2.1
Germany [15, 29]	24.5–27.4	1.51–1.38
Saudi Arabia [30]	29.3	3.4
China [31]	35.8	1.4
Italy [32]	33	1
England [33]	32	0.96
USA [34]	29.25	0.3

Table 2. Age and gender ratio distribution among countries.

BD is uncommon in children. Patients with initial symptoms at age 16 years or lower are classified as juvenile-onset BD [39]. The prevalence of juvenile BD is unknown. However, in few series, it was reported that 3.3 and 26% of the patients with BD were juvenile-onset BD [2]. The clinical symptoms are not different from adults but the diagnosis may be delayed in pediatric patients because of mild symptoms [2]. Juvenile onset patients had more familial cases compared with adult-onset patients [39]. There are some different series presenting juvenile BD. In the study of Allali et al., one-third of the patient had family history [40]. In the series of Kone-Paut et al., family history was reported as 9 and 24.4%. But in adults, family history was found as 2.2% [41–43]. The clinical features of juvenile BD in different series are seen in **Table 3** [40–42, 44–48].

BD disease affects both the gender equally [12]. But the gender distribution may differ between different regions. A few studies showed that male predominance was seen in Middle Eastern countries, while female predominance was seen in Asian countries [1]. The male/female ratios from the studies are shown in **Table 2**.

Gender affects the clinical findings and the severity of the disease as well [12]. In a long-term study performed by Kural-Seyahi et al., it was implicated that the disease is more severe in male patients, and vascular disease might be the major risk factor of death in male patients [49]. Saadoun et al. supported that male sex, arterial involvement and a high number of BD flares were independently associated with the risk of mortality [50]. In 2015, Bonitsis et al. presented a meta-analysis of the gender-specific differences in BD. They investigated both the German registry of BD and systematic literature review meta-analysis (52 other publications from Turkey, Asia, Southern Europe, Northern Europe, South America, the USA, and North Africa/Middle East) [29]. They found that vascular disease (superficial and deep venous thrombosis and heart involvement), folliculitis, papulopustular skin lesions, positive pathergy test and ocular disease are more common in males, while erythema nodosum, genital ulcers and joint involvement are more common in females [29].

Clinical features (%)	Kone-paut [42]	Kone-paut [41]	Krause [44]	Karıncaoğlu [45]	Atmaca [46]	Eldem [47]	Uziel [48]	Allali [40]
N (patients)	65	55	19	33	110	20	15	12
Oral aphthosis	96	100	100	100	100	100	100	100
Genital aphthosis	70	79	31.9	82	83	65	33	75
Cutaneous findings	92	78	89.5	52	76	35	93	16.7
Pathergy test +	–	–	41.2	37	45.5	–	40	58
Ocular signs	60	87	47.4	35	31	80	53	53
Articular findings	56	17	47.4	40	22	40	73	25
Gastrointestinal findings	14	–		36.8	–	5	46	8.3
Neurological findings	15	10	26.3	7.2	3.6	15	4	40
Vascular findings	15	21	10.5	9.6	3.6	5	0	33.3

Table 3. Clinical features of pediatric BD.

2.3. Epidemiology of clinical findings

Regional and environmental factors may affect clinical findings of BD. Prevalence of different clinical findings may differ among the patients from different regions [12]. Frequency of presence of oral aphthosis is almost same in patients from all regions with the rate of 96–100% [1, 12]. In Japan, 4.6–15% of endogen causes of uveitis are BD [13, 51]. In a study from Japan, 69% of the patients had ocular findings [52]. But uveitis is quite rare in Australia [1]. Neurological features are more common in Caucasians (23%) than Middle Eastern series (3–10%) and frequency of seizures was found to be higher than Turkish series (27 and 5%, respectively) [53]. Another study detected that Sub-Saharan African BD patients had a higher frequency of CNS involvement compared to North African and European BD patients [54]. Intestinal BD is rare in Mediterranean countries but it is more common in Japanese BD patients [12]. Clinical findings of patients from different regions are shown in **Table 4** [13, 23, 24, 28–30, 55].

2.4. Pathergy reaction

Pathergy reaction is a nonspecific skin hyper reactivity to minor trauma. Positivity is defined as occurring of a papule or pustule, 24–48 h after intradermal injection of skin with 20 gauge needle [1]. Positive pathergy test is one of the diagnosis criteria of BD [4]. The pathergy reaction is highly sensitive and specific for BD in patients from Silk Road countries like Turkey, from some Mediterranean, the Middle Eastern countries and Japan. However, it is rarely observed in patients from Northern Europe, USA and Australia [1, 56]. Although the pathergy test lost its sensitivity during the past 35 years, it is still a valuable diagnostic test [57]. Some studies from Japan and Turkey have reported a decrease in the positive pathergy reaction in BD [56]. In 1979, the skin pathergy positivity rate was found 84% in patients with BD in a study from Turkey [58]. In another study from Turkey in 1991, the rate was found 65% [59]. In a more recent study from Turkey, the rate of pathergy test positivity was

Country	Oral ulcer	Genital ulcer	Skin findings	Ocular findings	Articular findings	Vascular findings	Gastroin-testinal findings	Neurological findings	Pulmonary findings	Pathergy test +
Turkey [23]	100	73	52	40	22	9.6	1	3.5	2.6	39
Germany [29]	99.7	72.8	79.9	50.4	54.1	22.4	11.5	12.1	1.3	28.5
Senegal [13]	100	96	30	44	40	18	2	24	–	32
Japan [24]	99	72.3	88.8	61.6	52.1	8.0	12.3	10.2	–	–
Iran [55]	97.5	65.7	64.6	58.1	39.4	9.1	7	10.6	1	52.3
Saudi Arabia [30]	100	87	57	65	37	25	4	44	–	17.5
Tunisia [28]	100	85	74.4	46.5	45.7	34.9	7	32.6	–	57.7

Table 4. Clinical findings of BD among some countries.

detected as 39% [23]. The decrease of pathergy test positivity rate can be also seen in some Japanese studies. In a study from Japan in 1972 the rate of positive pathergy test was found 75%, while in an other study performed in 2011 this rate was found %50 [56]. These differences may be occurred due to different applying techniques. One of the important methods is using non-disposable/blunt needles. In 2000, it was reported that clinical evaluation of the pathergy test conducted intradermally with non-disposable/blunt needles is sufficient for both the diagnosis and determination of the activation of Behçet's disease [60]. Also it is shown that surgical cleaning of the test area before needle prick reduced the prevalence of pathergy test positivity rate [61]. This information suggests that the positive reaction might be a cutaneous response to some bacteria living on the surface of the skin. In a recent study, performed by Togashi et al. suggested that a new diagnostic pathergy test may solve the methodological problems [62]. They performed a skin prick test with filter-sterilized saliva on forearm skin. Of the patients with BD, 90% showed indurative erythema at the skin site pricked with self-saliva, and 60% of recurrent aphthous stomatitis patients showed weak reaction. They suggested that skin prick test using self-saliva can be a diagnostic test for differentiating BD from other mucocutaneous diseases [62].

The reactivity of the pathergy test is suggested to be correlated with HLA-B51 in Mediterranean countries [63]. Rates of pathergy positivity from different studies are shown in **Table 4** [13, 23, 24, 28–30, 55].

2.5. Genetic factors and epidemiology

Although familial cases were reported, a Mendelian inheritance model specific to BD is not present [12]. In the western series, familial case rates were as follows: 0.7–2.7% in Italy, 3.6% in England and 4.5% in Portugal. The familial case rates were 11.9–13.4% in the studies from Tunisia, Israel, and Korea studies [12, 15, 64]. In a study from Turkey, family history was reported as 31.2% [65]. Multiple studies have demonstrated that BD is strongly associated with the presence of HLA-B5 and its split antigen HLA-B51 [12, 66]. The association with HLA-B5 was first described by Ohno et al. in 1973 [56]. The genetic material of the BD might be carried in parallel with population movement between the Mediterranean and Asia. Supporting this content is that the distribution areas of this antigen among healthy control populations are the ancient trade route and the region in which BD is commonly seen [67]. HLA-B51 frequency is high in the Mediterranean countries but it is low in western countries like USA and England [12]. In recent studies, many new genes other than HLA-B51 (IL-10 signaling pathways, IL6–174 G/C, MMP-9, CLEC16A, NKFB1, IL-23 receptor gene, IL-18, IL-6, IL10, Vitamin D receptor, etc.) associated with BD were also identified [36]. Shigemura et al. studied on six patients over four generations with BD in 2016, and they found a common heterozygous missense mutation in A20/TNFAIP3; a gene known to regulate NF-κB signaling. Mutation in A20/TNFAIP3 was likely responsible for increased production of human inflammatory cytokines by reduced suppression of NF-κB activation. They suggested that this mutation may lead to the autosomal-dominant Mendelian mode of BD transmission in this family [68].

3. Conclusion

BD has a worldwide distribution. But it is commonly observed along the Silk Road countries between the Mediterranean Sea. It is most common in Turkey. The prevalence of the disease, the frequency of the clinical findings, and genetics may differ between different regions. The disease is more severe among males than females. Diagnosis of BD is difficult, and the disease must be recognized, because early diagnosis is important for the early treatment.

Author details

Işıl Deniz Oguz[1]*, Pelin Hizli[2] and Muzeyyen Gonul[3]

*Address all correspondence to: isildenizoguz@yahoo.com.tr

1 Department of Dermatology, Giresun University Prof. Dr. Ilhan Ozdemir Training and Research Hospital, Giresun, Turkey

2 Department of Dermatology, Giresun Kent Hospital, Giresun, Turkey

3 Department of Dermatology, Dışkapı Yıldırım Beyazıt Education and Research Hospital, Ankara, Turkey

References

[1] Leonardo NM, McNeil J. Behcet's disease: is there geographical variation? A review far from the silk road. Int J Rheumatol. 2015;2015:945262. doi:10.1155/2015/945262

[2] Koné-Paut I. Behçet's disease in children, an overview. Pediatr Rheumatol Online J. 2016 Feb 18;14:10. doi:10.1186/s12969-016-0070-z

[3] Behçet h. Überrezidivierende, aphtÖsedurchein Virus verursachteGeschwüre am Mund, am auge und den Genitalien [Caused about recurrent aphtous by a virüs Ulcers of the mouth, the eyes and genitals]. DermatolMonatsschrWochenschr 1937;105:1152–7.

[4] International Study Group for Behcet's disease. Lancet. 1990;335:1078–80.

[5] Kappen JH, van Dijk EH, Baak-Dijkstra M, van Daele PL, Lam-Tse WK, van Hagen PM, van Laar JA. Behçet's disease, hospital-based prevalence and manifestations in the Rotterdam area. Neth J Med. 2015;73:471–7.

[6] Keino H, Okada AA. Behçet's disease: global epidemiology of an Old Silk Road disease. Br J Ophthalmol. 2007;91:1573–4.

[7] Alpsoy E, Zobuboulis CC, Ehrlich CE. Mucocutaneous lesions of Behcet's disease. Yonsei Med J. 2007;48:573–585.

[8] Mahr A, Maldini C. Epidemiology of Behçet's disease. Rev Med Interne. 2014;35:81–9.

[9] Baş Y, Seçkin HY, Kalkan G, Takcı Z, Önder Y, Çıtıl R, Demir S, Şahin Ş. Investigation of Behçet's disease and recurrent aphthous stomatitis frequency: the highest prevalence in Turkey. Balkan Med J. 2016;33:390–5. doi:10.5152/balkanmedj.2016.15101

[10] Saylan T, Mat C, Fresko İ, Melikoglu M. Behcet's disease in the Middle East. Clin Dermatol. 199;17:209–23.

[11] Marshall SE, Behcet's disease. Best Prac Res Clin Rheumatol. 2004;18:291–311.

[12] Pamuk ÖN, Çakır N. [The epidemiology of Behcet's disease]. TürkiyeKlinikleri J Int Med Sci. 2005;1:39.

[13] Ndiaye M, Sow AS, Valiollah A, Diallo M, Diop A, Alaoui RA, Diatta BA, Ly F, Niang SO, Dieng MT, Kane A. Behçet's disease in black skin. A retrospective study of 50 cases in Dakar. J Dermatol Case Rep. 2015;9:98–102. doi:10.3315/jdcr.2015.1213

[14] Klein P, Weinberger A, Altmann VJ, Halabi S, Fachereldeen S, Krause I.Prevalence of Behcet's disease among adult patients consulting three major clinics in a Druze town in Israel. Clin Rheumatol. 2010;29:1163–6. doi:10.1007/s10067-010-1472-9

[15] Zouboulis CC, Kötter I, Djawari D, Kirch W, Kohl PK, Ochsendorf FR, Keitel W, Stadler R, Wollina U, Proksch E, Söhnchen R, Weber H, Gollnick HP, Hölzle E, Fritz K, Licht T, Orfanos CE. Epidemiological features of Adamantiades-Behçet's disease in Germany and in Europe. Yonsei Med J. 1997;38:411–22.

[16] Gharibdoost F, Davatchi F, Shahram F, Akbarian M, Chams C, Chams H, Mansoori P, Nadji A: Clinical manifestations of Behçet's disease in Iran. Analysis of 2176 cases. In Wechsler B, Godeau P eds. Behçet's disease. International Congress Series 1037. Amsterdam, ExcerptaMedicia, 1993,153–158.

[17] Al-Rawi ZS, Neda AH. Prevalence of Behçet's disease among Iraqis. Adv Exp Med Biol. 2003;528:37–41.

[18] Mok CC, Cheung TC, Ho CT, Lee KW, Lau CS, Wong RW. Behçet's disease in southern Chinese patients. J Rheumatol. 2002;29:1689–93.

[19] Cartella S, Filippini M, Tincani A, Airo P. Prevalence of Behçet's disease in the province of Brescia in northern Italy. Clin Exp Rheumatol. 2014;32:S176.

[20] Olivieri I, Leccese P, Padula A, Nigro A, Palazzi C, Gilio M, D'Angelo S.High prevalence of Behçet's disease in southern Italy. Clin Exp Rheumatol. 2013;31:28–31.

[21] Altenburg A, Mahr A, Maldini C, Kneifel CE, Krause L, Kötter I, Stache T, Bonitsis NG, Zouboulis CC. [Epidemiology and clinical aspects of Adamantiades-Behçet disease in Gemany. Current data]. Ophthalmologe. 2012;109:531–41. doi:10.1007/s00347-012-2601-4

[22] Onder M, Gürer MA. The multiple faces of Behçet's disease and its aetiological factors. J Eur Acad Dermatol Venereol. 2001;15:126–36.

[23] Gündüz Ö, Gürler A, TuğrulAyanoğlu B, Erdoğan FG, Alhan A. Epidemiological properties of Behçet's disease who had been followed up at Behçet's disease center. TürkiyeKlinikleri J Dermatol. 2015;25:85–91.

[24] Kirino Y, Ideguchi H, Takeno M, Suda A, Higashitani K, Kunishita Y, Takase-Minegishi K, Tamura M, Watanabe T, Asami Y, Uehara T, Yoshimi R, Yamazaki T, Sekiguchi A, Ihata A, Ohno S, Ueda A, Igarashi T, Nagaoka S, Ishigatsubo Y, Nakajima H. Continuous evolution of clinical phenotype in 578 Japanese patients with Behçet's disease: a retrospective observational study. Arthritis Res Ther. 2016;18:217.

[25] Türsen Ü, Gürler A, Boyvat A. Evaluation of clinical findings according to sex in 2313 Turkish patients with Behçet's disease. Int J Dermatol. 2003;82:60–76.

[26] Davachi F, Shahram F, Akbarian M. Behcet's disease: analysis of 3443 cases. APLAR J Rheumatol 1997;1:2–5.

[27] Krause I, Uziel Y, Guedj D. Mode of presentation and multystem involvement in Behcet's disease:the influence of sex and age of disease onset. J Rheumatol. 1998;12:1566–9.

[28] Hamzaoui A, Jaziri F, Ben Salem T, Said Imed Ben Ghorbel F, Lamloum M, Smiti Khanfir M, Houman Mohamed H. Comparison of clinical features of Behcet disease according to age in a Tunisian cohort. Acta Med Iran. 2014;52:748–51.

[29] Bonitsis NG, Luong Nguyen LB, LaValley MP, Papoutsis N, Altenburg A, Kötter I, Micheli C, Maldini C, Mahr A, Zouboulis CC. Gender-specific differences in Adamantiades-Behçet's disease manifestations: an analysis of the German registry and meta-analysis of data from the literature. Rheumatology (Oxford). 2015;54:121–33. doi:10.1093/rheumatology/keu247

[30] alDalaan AN, al Balaa SR, el Ramani K. Behcet's Disease in Saudi Arabia. J Rheumatol. 1997;21:658–61.

[31] Zhang Z1, He F, Shi Y. Behcet's disease seen in China: analysis of 334 cases. Rheumatol Int. 2013;33:645–8. doi:10.1007/s00296-012-2384-6

[32] Salvarani C, Pipitone N, Catanoso MG, Cimino L, Tumiati B, Macchioni P, Bajocchi G, Olivieri I, Boiardi L. Epidemiology and clinical course of Behçet's disease in the Reggio Emilia area of Northern Italy: a seventeen-year population-based study. Arthritis Rheum. 2007;57:171–8.

[33] Chamberlain MA. Behcet's syndrome in 32 patients in Yorkshire. Ann Rheum Dis. 1977;36:491–9.

[34] Davari P, Rogers RS, Chan B, Nagler TH, Fazel N. Clinical features of Behçet's disease: A retrospective chart review of 26 patients. J Dermatol Treat. 2016;27:70–4. doi:10.3109/09546634.2015.1054781

[35] Kötter I, Vonthein R, Müller CA, Günaydın İ, Zierhut M, Stübiger N. Behçet's disease in patients of German and Turkish origin living in Germany: a comparative analysis. J Rheumatol. 2004;31:133–9.

[36] Hatemi G, Seyahi E, Fresko I, Talarico R, Hamuryudan V. Behçet's syndrome: a critical digest of the 2014–2015 literature. Clin Exp Rheumatol. 2015;33:3–14.

[37] Bang D. Treatment of Behçet's disease. Yonsei Med J. 1997;38:401–10.

[38] Huang ZJ, Liao KH, Xu LY. Study of 310 cases of Behçets's syndrome. Chin Med J.1983;96:483–90.

[39] Karincaoglu Y, Borlu M, Toker SC, Akman A, Onder M, Gunasti S, Usta A, Kandi B, Durusoy C, Seyhan M, Utas S, Saricaoglu H, Ozden MG, Uzun S, Tursen U, Cicek D, Donmez L, Alpsoy E. Demographic and clinical properties of juvenile-onset Behçet's disease: A controlled multicenter study. J Am AcadDermatol. 2008;58:579–84.

[40] Allali F, Benomar A, Karim A. Behçet's disease in Moroccan children: a report of 12 cases. Scand J Rheumatol. 2004;33:362–3.

[41] Koné-Paut I, Gorchakoff-Molinas A, Weschler B, Touitou I. Paediatric Behçet's disease in France. Ann Rheum Dis. 2002;61:655–6.

[42] Koné-Paut I, Yurdakul S, Bahabri SA, Shafae N, Ozen S, Ozdogan H, Bernard JL. Clinical features of Behçet's disease in children: an international collaborative study of 86 cases. J Pediatr. 1998;132:721–5.

[43] Koné-Paut I, Shahram F, Darce-Bello M, Cantarini L, Cimaz R, Gattorno M, Anton J, Hofer M, Chkirate B, Bouayed K, Tugal-Tutkun I, Kuemmerle-Deschner J, Agostini H, Federici S, Arnoux A, Piedvache C, Ozen S; PEDBD group. Consensus classification criteria for paediatricBehçet's disease from a prospective observational cohort: PEDBD. Ann Rheum Dis. 2016;75:958–64. doi:10.1136/annrheumdis-2015-208491

[44] Krause I, Uziel Y, Guedj D, Mukamel M, Harel L, Molad Y, Weinberger A. Childhood Behçet's disease: clinical features and comparison with adult-onset disease. Rheumatology (Oxford). 1999;38:457–62.

[45] Karincaoglu Y, Borlu M, Toker SC, Akman A, Onder M, Gunasti S, Usta A, Kandi B, Durusoy C, Seyhan M, Utas S, Saricaoglu H, Ozden MG, Uzun S, Tursen U, Cicek D, Donmez L, Alpsoy E. Demographic and clinical properties of juvenile-onset Behçet's disease: a controlled multicenter study. J Am AcadDermatol. 2008;58:579–84.

[46] Atmaca L, Boyvat A, Yalçındağ FN, Atmaca-Sonmez P, Gurler A. Behçet disease in children. Ocul Immunol Inflamm. 2011;19:103–7. doi:10.3109/09273948.2011.555592

[47] Eldem B, Onur C, Ozen S. Clinical features of pediatric Behçet's disease. J Pediatr Ophthalmol Strabismus. 1998;35:159–61.

[48] Uziel Y, Brik R, Padeh S, Barash J, Mukamel M, Harel L, Press J, Tauber T, Rakover Y, Wolach B. Juvenile Behçet's disease in Israel. The Pediatric Rheumatology Study Group of Israel. Clin Exp Rheumatol. 1998;16:502–5.

[49] Kural-Seyahi E, Fresko I, Seyahi N, Ozyazgan Y, Mat C, Hamuryudan V, Yurdakul S, Yazici H. The long-term mortality and morbidity of Behçet syndrome: a 2-decade

outcome survey of 387 patients followed at a dedicated center. Medicine (Baltimore). 2003;82:60–76.

[50] Saadoun D, Wechsler B, Desseaux K, Le Thi Huong D, Amoura Z, Resche-Rigon M, Cacoub P. Mortality in Behçet's disease. Arthritis Rheum. 2010;62:2806–12. doi:10.1002/art.27568

[51] Nakahara H, Kaburaki T, Tanaka R, Takamoto M, Ohtomo K, Karakawa A, Komae K, Okinaga K, Matsuda J, Fujino Y. Frequency of uveitis in the Central Tokyo Area (2010–2012). Ocul Immunol Inflamm. 2016;8:1–7

[52] Nakae K, Masaki F, Hashimoto T, Inaba G, Mochizuki M, Sakane T. Recent epidemiological features of Behçet's disease in Japan. In:Goeau P, Wechsler B, (eds). Behçet's disease. Amsterdam: Excerpta Medica, 1993. pp. 145–51.

[53] Joseph FG1, Scolding NJ. Neuro-Behçet's disease in Caucasians: a study of 22 patients. Eur J Neurol. 2007;14:174–80.

[54] Savey L, Resche-Rigon M, Wechsler B, et al. Ethnicity and association with disease manifestations and mortality in Behçet's disease. Orphanet J Rare Dis. 2014;9:42. doi:10.1186/1750-1172-9-42

[55] Davatchi F, Chams-Davatchi C, Shams H, Nadji A, Faezi T, Akhlaghi M, SadeghiAbdollahi B, Ashofteh F, Ghodsi Z, Mohtasham N, Shahram F. Adult Behcet's disease in Iran: analysis of 6075 patients. Int J Rheum Dis. 2016;19:95–103. doi:10.1111/1756-185X.12691

[56] Alpsoy E. Behçet's disease: a comprehensive review with a focus on epidemiology, etiology and clinical features, and management of mucocutaneous lesions. J Dermatol. 2016;43:620–32. doi:10.1111/1346-8138.13381

[57] Davatchi F, Chams-Davatchi C, Ghodsi Z, Shahram F, Nadji A, Shams H, Akhlaghi M, Larimi R, Sadeghi-Abdolahi B. Diagnostic value of pathergy test in Behcet's disease according to the change of incidence over the time. Clin Rheumatol. 2011;30:1151–5. doi:10.1007/s10067-011-1694-5

[58] Tüzün Y, Yazici H, Pazarli H, Yalçin B, Yurdakul S, Müftüoğlu A. The usefulness of the nonspecific skin hyperreactivity (the pathergy test) in Behçet's disease in Turkey. Acta Derm Venereol. 1979;59:77–9.

[59] Ozarmagan G, Saylan T, Azizlerli G, Ovül C, Aksungur VL. Re-evaluation of the pathergy test in Behçet's disease. Acta Derm Venereol. 1991;71:75–6.

[60] Akmaz O, Erel A, Gürer MA. Comparison of histopathologic and clinical evaluations of pathergy test in Behçet's disease. Int J Dermatol. 2000;39:121–5.

[61] Fresko I, Yazici H, Bayramiçli M, Yurdakul S, Mat C. Effect of surgical cleaning of the skin on the pathergy phenomenon in Behçet's syndrome. Ann Rheum Dis. 1993;52:619–20.

[62] Togashi A, Saito S, Kaneko F, Nakamura K, Oyama N. Skin prick test with self-saliva in patients with oral aphthoses: a diagnostic pathergy for Behcet's disease and recurrent aphthosis. Inflamm Allergy Drug Targets. 2011;10:164–70.

[63] Kaneko F, Togashi A, Nomura E, Nakamura K. A New diagnostic way for Behcet's disease: skin prick with self-saliva. Genet Res Int. 2014;2014:581468. doi:10.1155/2014/581468

[64] Chang HK, Kim JW. The clinical features of Behcet's disease in Yongdong districts: analysis of a cohort followed from 1997 to 2001. J Korean Med Sci. 2002;17:784–9.

[65] Ozyurt K, Colgecen E, Baykan H. Does familial occurrence or family history of recurrent oral ulcers influence clinical characteristics of Behçet's disease? Acta Dermatovenerol Croat. 2013;21:168–73.

[66] Ahmed Z, Rossi ML, Yong S, Martin DK, Walayat S, Cashman M, Tsoraides S, Dhillon S. Behçet's disease departs the 'Silk Road': a case report and brief review of literature with geographical comparison. J Community Hosp Intern Med Perspect. 2016;6:30362. doi:10.3402/jchimp.v6.30362.eCollection2016

[67] Verity DH, Marr JE, Ohno S, Wallace GR, Stanford MR. Behçet's disease, the Silk Road and HLA-B51: historical and geographical perspectives. Tissue Antigens. 1999;54:213–20.

[68] Shigemura T, Kaneko N, Kobayashi N, Kobayashi K, Takeuchi Y, Nakano N, Masumoto J, Agematsu K. Novel heterozygous C243Y A20/TNFAIP3 gene mutation is responsible for chronic inflammation in autosomal-dominant Behçet's disease. RMD Open. 2016;2:e000223. doi:10.1136/rmdopen-2015-000223. eCollection 2016

Chapter 3

Etiology, Immunopathogenesis and Biomarkers in Behçet's disease

Fahd Adeeb, Maria Usman Khan,
Austin G. Stack and Alexander D. Fraser

Additional information is available at the end of the chapter

http://dx.doi.org/10.5772/intechopen.68342

Abstract

Behçet's disease (BD) is a type of vasculitis with many distinctive clinical manifestations and multifactorial immunopathogenesis. The cause of BD remains unknown, but it has been postulated that in a genetically predisposed or susceptible population, exogenous agents trigger the dysregulation of both autoinflammatory and autoimmune responses resulting in multisystem vasculitis. There are robust ongoing efforts across the globe to elucidate and identify signature markers to improve and assist in rapid diagnosis of the disease and to tailor the best therapy accordingly. While association of human leukocyte antigen (HLA)-B*51 (B*51:01 subtype) allele is well recognized as the strongest genetic susceptibility gene so far among genetically predisposed BD patients, further investigations using the latest technology have led to the identification of several novel single nucleotide polymorphisms (SNPs) and other associated genes involved in the pathogenesis. There are several "established" cytokines known to be involved in the pathogenesis of BD, which have been further implicated in the genome-wide association studies (GWAS)-based cytokine/receptor gene loci studies, as well as numerous "novel" cytokines, which are currently being studied and identified. This chapter offers insights into current knowledge and thoughts regarding the future of biomarkers in BD.

Keywords: Behçet's disease, Behçet's syndrome, biomarker, immunopathogenesis, immunogenetics, pathogenetics, etiopathogenesis, cytokines, HLA-B*51

1. Introduction

Behçet's disease (BD) is a type of vasculitis characterize by recurrent inflammatory attacks causing many distinctive clinical manifestations, most commonly affecting the orogenital mucosa, skin, and the eyes [1–3]. The etiology has yet to be fully established, but it has been postulated that a genetically predisposed or susceptible population, exposed to exogenous agents, may result in the dysregulation of both autoinflammatory and autoimmune responses. It is a complex disease that has been the subject of intense research and clinical interest.

In this era of precision medicine, there is a need to integrate biomarkers into clinical practice, which may serve as valuable predictive and prognostic tools to assist practicing physicians in making clinical decisions while managing complex diseases. This may also improve diagnostic capability, risk stratification, prediction of disease progression, assist in targeted therapy, and monitoring of response to treatment to improve patients' overall clinical outcome.

This review chapter will look into the most relevant articles that have defined and clarified BD over the years, as well as review the most recent publications offering new insights in order to help fill the gaps in further understanding the disease. The chapter will focus on the etiology, immunopathogenesis, recent advances in search of potential biomarkers and targets for further research.

We will examine recent advances made that have shed new light on an old disease and explore the potential genetic (including genome-wide association studies (GWAS) and next-generation DNA sequencing, looking into the human leukocyte antigen (HLA) and non-HLA genetic associations) and molecular markers (including innate immune lymphoid cells and adaptive immune cells, cytokines, chemokines, other circulating biomarkers, and signaling molecules of inflammation) and their potential correlations with disease activity and therapy.

2. The pursuit for genetic susceptibility markers in Behçet's disease

BD is a genetically complex and heterogeneous disease. The pursuit of gene discovery for causative genetic factors in BD spans over more than four decades since Professor Shigeaki Ohno first described the association of HL-A5 antigen observed in his Japanese BD cohort that was later renamed human leukocyte antigen (HLA)-B5 [4]. Other early evidence stems from the observation of familial clustering in BD families where more than one family member developed the disease [5–8], which provided further clues to a strong genetic predisposition to the disease.

2.1. The MHC I and HLA-B*51 and its association with BD

The major histocompatibility complex (MHC) has an expansive immune component including the HLA and plays a pivotal role in the genetic influences on susceptibility to autoimmunity. The ~3.5-Mb region has the highest density of genes in the human genome, the majority of which have fundamental roles in immunity [9].

A remarkably consistent body of evidence demonstrates association of HLA-B*51 (B*51:01 subtype) allele as the strongest genetic susceptibility gene so far among genetically predisposed BD patients. However, certain indigenous Amerindians have a high prevalence of HLA-B*51 but virtually no reported cases of BD. High level of recombination within the MHC is known to have occurred in these Eastern populations before their migration into Beringia and it was suggested that disruption of the genetic loci in linkage disequilibria with HLA-B*51 might be one reason for the absence of disease in these high HLA-B*51-bearing populations [10]. These findings emphasize the fundamental roles and interplay of both genetic and environmental components in the development of the disease.

There have been conflicting views, however, on whether the disease association with HLA-B*51 is attributed to a role of MHC class I variant itself or if the association is found due to its linkage disequilibrium (LD) with another variant in the region [11].

2.2. The unifying concept of MHC-I-opathy

The understanding of the pathophysiology of BD is challenging, as it is at the crossroads between autoimmune and autoinflammatory syndromes [12]. A new perspective of a unifying concept of MHC-I-opathy was proposed recently comprising of BD and several clinically distinct spondyloarthropathies (such as ankylosing spondylitis and psoriasis)—all associated with MHC Class I alleles, such as HLA-B*51, HLA-B*27, and HLA-C*0602, and epistatic endoplasmic reticulum aminopeptidase 1 (ERAP-1) interactions.

McGonagle et al. have proposed that the MHC-I-opathies share an immunopathogenetic basis including barrier dysfunction in environmentally exposed organs such as the skin and aberrant innate immune reactions at sites of mechanical stress. This they argue can often trigger secondary adaptive immune $CD8^+$ T cell responses with prominent neutrophilic inflammation that culminate in the initiation and chronicity of these diseases [13]. Further research and understanding into this unifying concept of MHC I driven inflammatory response may provide further targets for disease management.

2.3. Other MHC/HLA associations

The complexity and strong LD with the HLA-B*51 allele make it difficult to explore additional independent susceptibility loci within this region. Despite having the strongest genetic association, it remains unclear to this day whether disease susceptibility in BD is due to the HLA-B*51 itself or due to the genes located around the HLA which is in LD with it.

The MHC Class I chain-related gene A (MICA) is located in proximity and in between the HLA-B and tumor necrosis factor (TNF) genes on the short arm of chromosome 6. It has long been considered a major genetic susceptibility gene for BD and has been studied in many different populations since the first observation of a possible association by Mizuki et al. [14]. Lee et al. conducted a meta-analysis on the associations of MICA and BD and found statistically significant association in various ethnic populations [15]. However, due to its strong LD with HLA-B*51, it has been difficult to prove MICA as a primary susceptibility gene for BD. Furthermore, different GWAS did not find an independent association between MICA and BD [16–18].

Ombrello et al. performed stepwise conditional analysis and found independent genetic associations for HLA-B*15 and HLA-B*27 and risk, while HLA-B*49 and HLA-A*03 were protective

[19]. Montes-Cano et al. demonstrated HLA-B*57 as a marker for risk in the Spanish population [20], while Meguro et al. showed that HLA-A*26 is a risk marker in the Japanese population [16].

Using a custom platform (Immunochip) that includes 8572 single nucleotide polymorphisms (SNPs) in the HLA extended region, Hughes et al. demonstrated that the robust HLA-B*51 association in BD is due to a strong association signal of an SNP rs116799036 in two independent BD cohorts (Turkish and Italian) from two ancestry groups, while also identifying two additional independent genetic associations with genome-wide significance ($P < 5 \times 10^{-8}$) in the HLA region: rs12525170 and rs114854070 [21].

2.4. Genomic strategies for a complex genetic disease beyond the typical Mendelian inheritance

It was difficult to venture beyond the MHC in the past: the tools to do so were unavailable as linkage studies were only suitable for Mendelian disorders. Intriguing new techniques have surfaced in recent times accelerating the pace for gene discovery, especially for complex diseases such as BD.

2.4.1. Genome-wide association studies (GWAS)

Being a complex disease, BD does not follow the typical Mendelian law of inheritance, rather of a dichotomous nature conforming the "polygenic threshold model" where the phenotypic expression is resultant upon genetic variation at multiple rather than a single loci, with the majority of the cases occurring sporadically. This is the basis foundation for the development of GWAS, which was initially thought to be the "comprehensive" option designed to identify genetic variants associated with such complex disease [22].

The advent of GWAS earlier in this century has dramatically improved our ability to identify and map successfully susceptibility loci associated with complex diseases such as BD, usually as single nucleotide polymorphisms (SNPs). It seems that these common genetic variants contribute to polygenic disease manifestations where phenotypic variance depends on contributions from several genetic variance.

Fei et al. [23] performed the first GWAS study in BD in a relatively small Turkish population and identified several novel candidate genetic loci (KIAA1529, CPVL, LOC100129342, UBASH3B, and UBAC2) that are associated with increased susceptibility to BD. In the same year, Meguro et al. [16] found that the main susceptibility locus in BD Japanese population remains in the MHC itself, wherein reside two independent loci: HLA-B*51 and HLA-A*26. Two large GWAS conducted in Turkey and Japan followed in 2010: Remmers et al. confirmed the association of HLA-B*51, identified a second, independent association within the MHC Class I region and also found association at IL10 [17], while Mizuki et al. identified IL23R-IL12RB2 and IL10 as Behçet's disease susceptibility loci [18].

In 2012, GWAS performed by Kirino et al. identified novel susceptibility loci at chemokine receptors CCR1-CCR3, signal transducer and activator of transcription 4 (STAT4), killer cell lectin-like receptor K1 subfamily K, member 1 (KLRK-1), killer cell lectin-like receptor subfamily C, member 4 (KLRC4), and ERAP1 in a Turkish population [24], thus apparently supporting the emerging concept delineating common pathogenic mechanisms for BD, ankylosing spondylitis, and psoriasis. In the same year, Hou et al. also identified STAT4 as a novel susceptibility locus for BD in the Chinese population in their GWAS and functional studies [25].

One of the difficulties of using GWAS in cohorts of mixed ethnicity is due to the rarity and unequal distribution of disease prevalence among different ethnic background. This was overcome by novel statistical approaches, demonstrated by Kappen et al. [26] who confirmed the central role of the HLA region in the disease and validated the association of IL2A gene by meta-analysis with previous work.

2.4.2. Next-generation sequencing (NGS) and candidate gene analysis

Despite discoveries of many unimpeachable associations with GWAS, it became apparent that the approach alone could not explain the full range of heritability or genetic susceptibilities to complex diseases [27] and at best could only identify moderate proportions of genetic variants contributing to the disease heritability. Among the growing menu of techniques, targeted next-generation sequencing is the latest promising technology in search of rare genetic variants with fewer alleles (minor-allele frequency), which likely carry a greater larger impact on disease manifestations and with larger deleterious biological effects [28, 29]. Next-generation exome sequencing has the ability to generate millions of short reads of sequence, ranging from 50 to 500 bp, in parallel. It can be targeted in key regions of the genome-to make quick discoveries [29].

2.5. Non-MHC I susceptibility genes

Early data revealing the contributory influence of non-HLA susceptibility genes came from studies in the 1990s; however, some of the associations were weak or inconclusive. In 2009, Karasneh et al. published the first systematic whole genome linkage analysis from 28 Turkish BD families, which provided evidence for non-HLA susceptibility loci with the strongest evidence seen for 12p12–13 and 6p22–24 [30].

The revelation of GWAS unfolded associations with genome-wide significance ($P < 5 \times 10^{-8}$) in the interleukin 23 receptor (IL23R)-IL12RB2, IL12A, IL10, ubiquitin-associated domain containing 2 (UBAC2), STAT4, CCR1-CCR3, KLRC4, ERAP1, TNF alpha-induced protein 3 (TNFAIP3), and fucosyltransferase 2 (FUT2) loci [17, 18, 22–26]. Some of these results have been replicated since in case-control candidate gene studies from Iranian, Chinese and Spanish European populations [30–36].

Targeted next-generation sequencing revealed the additional involvement of rare non-synonymous variants in toll-like receptor 4 (TLR4), nucleotide-binding oligomerization domain-containing protein 2 (NOD2), and the Mediterranean Fever Gene (MEFV) [37]. Recently, Ognenovski et al. used whole exome sequencing in BD of European descent for the first time and identified and replicated two novel putative protein-damaging genetic variants within LIMK2 and NEIL1, which may influence cytoskeletal regulation and DNA repair [38].

The associations with ERAP1, IL23R, IL10, and MEFV variations suggest that BD may share susceptibility genes and inflammatory pathways with spondyloarthritis [39], while the TLR and FUT polymorphisms that affect response to invasive pathogens have led to an increase interest in responses to microbiomes [40].

3. Molecular markers of BD

3.1. The cytokines network of BD

The term "cytokine" was first introduced in 1974 by Cohen et al. [41] to describe a polypeptide mediator superfamily central in the immune system generation and regulation. An entwined network comprising of interleukins (ILs), interferons (IFNs), tumor necrosis factor (TNF), chemokines, and other mediators primed to regulate the immune system, however, due to several factors such as imbalance of its receptor expression and dysregulation of its functions, generates the pathologic systemic inflammatory and/or immune responses seen in various autoimmune and autoinflammatory disorders.

Pro-inflammatory and anti-inflammatory cytokines have been shown to be involved in patients with BD (as discussed in more detailed below). Several studies demonstrated elevated levels of cytokines in local lesions indicating its involvement in the disease local immune responses [42–46]. Evidence from the GWASs further implicated several cytokines underlying the pathogenesis of BD [17, 18, 22–26]. Moreover, the successful use of various anti-cytokine therapies in BD patients provides additional evidence that cytokines play a crucial role in its pathogenesis [47–64]. These overall observations highlight the fundamental role of cytokines as key players in the pathogenesis of BD.

There are several established cytokines that are known to be involved including IL1β, TNFα, IL6, IL10, and IL23. Various new promising candidate's cytokines identified to be associated with BD include IL21, IL22, IL33, IL37, and several others, all of which be described as detailed below.

3.1.1. The main pro-inflammatory cytokines

Despite the pleiotropic nature of most cytokines, this group of cytokines primarily promotes inflammation. Several pro-inflammatory cytokines have been implicated in BD.

3.1.1.1. The interleukin-1 (IL1) family: IL1β, IL18, IL33

All cells of the innate immune system express and/or are affected by IL1 family members, which play a key role in the differentiation and function of polarized innate and adaptive lymphoid cells [65]. Among the 11 cytokines in the family, IL1β is the principal pro-inflammatory cytokine, leading to the expression of many chemokines and secondary mediators of inflammation and upregulating innate immunity in response to infectious agents [66]. The levels of IL1β have been shown to be elevated in several studies [45, 46, 49, 67, 68], including in synovial fluids of BD patients [45, 46]. A proof-of-concept study by Güll et al. strongly implicated IL1β and BD with significant improvement seen especially in patients with uveitis treated with IL1β-regulating antibody [47]. Recently Tugal-Tutkun et al. demonstrated rapid control of uveitis in BD patients without the need for high-dose corticosteroid in a prospective, open-label, randomized phase II trial [48] supporting several other previous studies of the proven efficacy of IL1β to induce stable clinical remission among BD patients [49–52].

Other pro-inflammatory cytokines in the IL1 family implicated in BD especially in the last decade include IL18 [42, 69–71], an important component of polarized Th1 cell and natural killer (NK) cell responses and of the interplay between macrophages and NK cells [65]. Identified in 2005 by Schmitz et al, IL33 was noted to have the capability to activate NF-κB and MAP kinases, and induces the expression of IL-4, IL-5, and IL-13 in vivo, leading to severe pathological changes in mucosal organs [72]. In several of his studies, Hamzaoui et al. demonstrated higher levels of IL33 in sera of active BD patients compared to BD patients in remission [73–75], and this was supported by Kim et al. [76] who found elevated IL33 in BD patients with erythema nodosum (EN) and EN-like skin lesions. Surprisingly, Koca et al. found contrasting results of lower IL33 levels in active BD Turkish patients compared to the inactive patients and healthy controls (HC) but did find significantly higher levels of IL33 among BD patients with uveitis [77].

3.1.1.2. The tumor necrosis factor (TNF) superfamily

Among the 19 TNF superfamily cytokines that has so far been identified, the first member of the family, TNFα, which was the first to be discovered, is the most highly investigated. Levels have been shown to be elevated in studies from different populations [49, 69, 78–83]. Meta-analysis by Touma et al. [84] found TNF (-238A/G, -1031C/T, and -857T/C) polymorphisms are associated with susceptibility to BD, while an updated meta-analysis by Zhang et al. confirmed a significant association between the TNF–308A/G polymorphism and BD susceptibility [85]. Treatment has also been shown to be highly effective [53, 54].

There is not much information about the other members of the TNF superfamily and its association with BD, but despite the limitation, isolated studies have shown several other TNF family member to be associated with BD in different ethnic populations: Cantarini et al. found significantly higher serum soluble TNFR and soluble CD40L [86], Shaker et al. demonstrated higher levels of B cell activating factor (BAFF), A proliferation producing ligand (APRIL), and B cell maturation antigen (BCMA) in BD patients [87] and Düzgün et al. found elevated soluble CD30 levels in active BD patients compared to controls [88].

Besides TNFα, other members of the TNF superfamily may offer options as potential targets and therapeutic candidates in BD; however, more research is needed in this field to prove its efficacy and safety profile.

3.1.1.3. Interleukin-6 (IL6)

Several studies have shown higher levels of serum IL6 in active BD compared to inactive BD and HC [71, 89, 90], and interestingly in neuro-BD patients, IL6 was noted to be markedly elevated in the cerebrospinal fluid (CSF), but not in the sera [91, 92]. Blockage of IL6 signaling with tocilizumab in BD patients despite looking promising in the treatment of neuro-BD [55–58] has revealed mixed results for non-neurological manifestations [58, 59, 93, 94] and is currently undergoing further evaluation in controlled clinical trials.

3.1.2. The main anti-inflammatory cytokine: type I interferon (IFNα)

Being the oldest cytokine discovered exactly 60 years ago, interferon-α (IFNα) has been the scope of investigation in many inflammatory diseases including BD. Despite initially thought to have mainly pro-inflammatory effects, it is becoming clearer that IFNα display a more complex function and its anti-inflammatory properties have led to its use as one of the treatment modalities in BD since the mid-1980s. Different studies by Hamzaoui, Kötter, and Pay et al. in their respective Tunisian, German and Turkish populations demonstrated higher levels of IFNα among BD patients [71, 95, 96]. In 2010, Liu et al. published their in vitro experiments demonstrating the ability of IFNα to inhibit IL17 expression and increase IL10 production by PBMCs and $CD4^+$ T cells [97]. Successful uses of IFNα-2a and -2b as treatment modalities have been reported [60–62], and more recently, Lightman et al. reported the successful use of pegylated IFNα-2b in BD resulting significant reduction in corticosteroid use and improvement of quality of life [63]. The exact mechanism of IFNα, however, is still largely unknown.

3.1.3. Helper and regulatory T lymphocytes involvement in BD

There have been remarkable advances leading to our current understanding on the lineage commitment and plasticity of helper CD4+ T cells. The "naïve" $CD4^+$ T cells in the presence of its associated cytokines differentiates into distinct T helper (Th) cells populations-Th1, Th2, Th17 or Th22: tailoring their responses to address specific threats accordingly. On the other hand, $CD4^+$ $CD25^+$ regulatory T cells (Tregs), derived from the thymus or differentiation from naïve T cells, downregulate Th responses and are critical for the preservation of immune tolerance and maintaining balance in the immune system.

3.1.3.1. Th1, Th17, and Th22 cell-associated cytokines

In the early 1980s, Ohno et al. demonstrated for the first time significantly higher levels of IFNγ in Japanese BD population [98]. Ahn et al. in their case series showed that the levels of IFNγ were elevated in aqueous humor and serum in BD patients with uveitis, which was then suppressed with combined low-dose cyclosporine/prednisone treatment [99]. Many other studies similarly found elevated serum IFNγ in active BD patients [44, 71, 83, 100–106], especially in BD patients with uveitis [44, 83, 102–105].

Other Th1 cell-associated cytokines associated with BD include IL2 and IL12. Despite conflicting results for IL2 levels in the ocular fluid of active BD patients with uveitis [106, 107], it was found to be significantly elevated in the serum of BD patients [108] and in active disease [109]. The alpha-chain of the IL2R that is shed from the surface of T cells by proteolytic enzymes to form the soluble sIL2R, which retains affinity to IL2, is also found to be significantly higher in active BD [46, 79, 110–113] and specifically in BD patients with uveitis [112, 113]. Serum IL12 levels were also found to be elevated in BD patients with active uveitis [114–116] and other active manifestations [42, 117, 118].

IL23 influences Th17 cell responses but shares a common p40 subunit with IL12 [119], and like IL12 has also been shown to be elevated in BD patients with active disease [101, 105, 120, 121]. Ustekinumab, a therapeutic agent, targeting both IL12 and IL23 cytokines has been shown to be therapeutic in BD [122], and subsequently a phase 2 open-label study to evaluate the proof-of-concept of ustekinumab in BD (STELABEC) has been recently registered in France. Both IL12 and IL23 stimulates nonreceptor Janus kinase 2 (JAK2) and tyrosine kinase 2 (TYK2) activity, leading to phosphorylation of STAT family members, with IL12 particularly activating STAT4 homodimers and IL23 predominantly activating STAT3 [119, 123–125]. Tulunay et al. demonstrated that the JAK1/STAT3 signaling pathway is activated in BD, and several other studies have shown similar findings [126]. Tulunay further suggested that more direct therapies aimed at JAK/STAT-associated cytokines such as ustekinumab (anti-IL12/23) and recently the approved tofacitinib that specifically inhibits JAK1/3, may be new therapeutic options for BD [126].

Th17 and Th22 are the "newer" helper-T cell subsets that secrete pro-inflammatory cytokines IL17 and IL22, respectively. Both are also implicated in the pathogenesis of BD, and their levels were markedly increased in BD patients [97, 105, 127–133] including active uveitis [107, 127, 128]. Chi et al. in their study demonstrated that production of IL17 was successfully inhibited by treatment with cyclosporine [127]. Another interesting finding in one of the studies above is increased levels of CCL20, an essential potent chemoattractant for the recruitment of Th17 lymphocytes [129]. Sugita et al. established Th22-type T cell clones from ocular samples taken from BD patients with active uveitis, which produced large amounts of IL22 and TNFα [106]. Sugita also demonstrated that IL22 in the presence of retinal antigens were able to produce high levels of IL22 in mice with experimental autoimmune uveitis [106]. From the therapeutic point of view, Liu et al. demonstrated significantly higher levels of IL17 in active BD patients, and stimulation with IFNα significantly decreases this IL17 production [97].

IL21 is one of the more recently identified type I cytokines that has been shown to tilt the balance between Th17 cells and regulatory T cells (Tregs) [134]. Geri et al. found markedly increased IL21 in active BD patients' sera and in the CSF of active neuro-BD patients. He further demonstrated increased Th17 and Th1 differentiation and decreased frequency of Tregs cells after stimulation of $CD4^{+}$ T cells with IL21. Conversely, IL21 blockade with an IL21R-Fc restored the Th17 and Tregs homeostasis in BD patients, which might represent a potential target for novel therapy [135].

3.1.3.2. Th2 cell-associated cytokines and Tregs

The studies on Th2 cell-associated cytokines and their contribution in the pathogenesis of BD have been rather conflicting. Several studies found lower or no significant differences of the related cytokines in BD patients compared to HC [45, 106, 109, 119, 136, 137]. However, studies by Hamzaoui et al. found increased serum levels of Th2 (IL4 and IL13) cytokines, and Takeuchi et al. found elevated IL4 and IL10 in BD patients [71, 83], while studies from Raziuddin and Aridogan et al. demonstrated high levels of IL4, IL10 and IL13 in active BD patients [138, 139]. Liu et al. and Guenane et al. in separate studies found significantly higher levels of IL10 in uveitis patients with BD compared to HC and idiopathic uveitis, respectively [97, 114]. Dalghous and his colleagues observed the presence of IL4 cytokines in oral lesions only from BD patients compared to RAS patients [140], while Ben Ahmed et al. found elevated levels of IL10 comparable to the increased IFNγ levels in active lesions of BD patients [141].

The possible role of Tregs in the pathogenesis of BD has gained considerable interest in recent times. Hamzaoui and Gündüz both demonstrated decreased Tregs level in clinically active BD patients [43, 142], Nanke et al. suggested that a decreased percentage of Tregs in peripheral blood of BD patients might be a predictive marker of ocular attack [143], while Sugita et al. demonstrated that Tregs level increased significantly with infliximab therapy but not with colchicine or cyclosporine in BD patients with uveitis [144]. Another subset of Tregs expresses high levels of CD52 glycoprotein [145], and together with other CD52-bearing cells (T cells, B cells, monocytes, macrophages, NK cells, dendritic cells, and granulocytes) are molecular targets of CAMPATH-1. A humanized antibody of IgG1 CAMPATH-1H/alemtuzumab has been successfully used in BD [146, 147] including in an open trial involving 18 BD patients with complete or partial remission achieved in 84% of patients [146].

3.1.3.3. Gammadelta (γδ) T cells

Gammadelta (γδ) T cells are innate-like lymphocytes that express a unique T cell receptor (TCR) γ and δ chain. Despite constituting only a small proportion (1–5%) of lymphocytes, they are more widespread within epithelial-rich tissues, such as the skin, intestine and reproductive tract, where they can comprise up to 50% of T cells [148]. They are a unique population of T cells that have features of both innate and adaptive immunity and express characteristics of conventional T cells, natural killer cells, and myeloid antigen presenting cells [149].

The relationship between γδ T cells and BD has been noted in several studies since the early 1990s. Increased γδ T cells levels were seen in BD patients compared to HC [99, 150–155] and in active BD compared to inactive BD [99, 151, 155, 156]; however conversely, several studies did not show any significant difference with HC [157–159]. Hasan et al. postulated that these discrepancies might be due to the activation status of the disease, as a reflection of local tissue inflammation compared to peripheral blood γδ T cells and such variation might be dependent on several other factors including disease severity, usage of medications such as immunomodulatory agents, and perhaps other variables, namely, age, gender, ethnicity, and/or environmental factors [149]. Their roles in the pathogenesis and potentially as therapeutic targets remain to be elucidated.

3.1.4. Other cytokines

IL37 is part of the IL1 family (discovered in 2009 and formerly identified as IL1F7) but has emerged as an inhibitor of innate immunity [160]. It has been shown to be significantly lower in BD patients compared to HC, with pronounced inhibition in active patients, and was associated with increased production of IL1β, IL6, and TNFα in LPS-stimulated PBMCs [161, 162]. Furthermore, in vitro experiments revealed that supplementing IL37 in BD patients significantly suppresses these three pro-inflammatory cytokines [163]. There have also been suggestions of associations between BD and other cytokines such as IL15 and IL27; however, the data are still inadequate and sparse [44, 164–166].

3.1.5. Chemokines

The attraction of leukocytes to tissues is essential for inflammation and is controlled by chemokines, which are chemotactic cytokines [167]. Saruhan-Direskineli et al. observed significantly higher α-chemokine CXCL10/IP10 CSF levels in neuro-BD patients compared to patients with non-inflammatory neurological disease (NIN) and multiple sclerosis, whereas CXCL8/IL8 was increased in neuro-BD compared to NIN [168]. El-Asrar et al. found higher levels of CXCL9/MIG, CXCL10/IP10 and CXCL11 in BD patients' serum with uveitis [169], while its receptors CXCR3 expression were observed by Dalghous et al. to be higher in oral lesions biopsied form BD patients [140]. Recently, Ambrose et al. demonstrated significantly higher production of CXCL10/IP10 in blood monocytes of BD patients stimulated with IFNγ compared to HC, rheumatoid arthritis, and systemic lupus erythematosus controls [170]. There is even more robust evidence for CXCL8/IL8, a potent neutrophil chemoattractant, being implicated in BD pathogenesis, with some of the authors proposing that it could be a marker for vascular involvement and a more reliable marker for disease activity than the C-reactive protein or erythrocyte sedimentation rate [171–174].

In regard to β-chemokines, Ozer et al. found significantly elevated levels of MCP1/CCL2, MIP1α/CCL3, and RANTES/CCL5 in active BD serum than in HC [175]. Similarly, Kökçam and Kim and their respective colleagues in two separate studies demonstrated high levels of MIP1α/CCL3 [176, 177] while Kaburaki et al. and Do et al. found higher levels of MCP1/CCL2 in BD patients compared to HC [178, 179]. In CSF of neuro-BD patients, Saruhan-Direskeneli et al. and Miyagishi et al. both demonstrated significantly higher levels of MIP1α/CCL3 compared to NIN [168, 180].

The emerging evidence of a complex cytokine and chemokine network interplay involved in the pathogenesis of BD, the identification of candidate gene including cytokine polymorphisms and the proven potency of anti-cytokines treatment shed more light on the fundamental role of cytokines and chemokines in BD. Perhaps cytokine and/or chemokine gene therapy, which has been used in cancer therapy, though not extremely impressive but nonetheless promising, may offer a novel yet powerful approach in the treatment of BD in the future.

3.2. The innate immune network

3.2.1. Neutrophil hyperfunction and endothelial cell activation

Becatti et al. demonstrated significant enhancement in leukocyte reactive oxygen species (ROS) production particularly by neutrophils in BD patients and only neutrophil-derived ROS (but not lymphocyte- or monocyte-derived ROS) showed a significant correlation with fibrinogen carbonyl content, highlighting neutrophil activation as the promoter of fibrinogen oxidation and thrombus formation in BD [181] supporting similar finding in several previous studies [182, 183]. Increasing evidence supports a role for neutrophil/lymphocyte ratio (NLR) as a cheap and simple disease activity marker in BD. NLR has been proposed as a surrogate marker for endothelial dysfunction and inflammation, and several authors have proposed the use of NLR as part of evaluation for disease activity in BD [184–187].

3.2.2. Innate lymphoid cells (ILCs)

Groundbreaking studies over recent years have formally identified innate lymphoid cells (ILCs) as a distinct arm of the innate immune system, comprising of the classic cytotoxic natural killer (NK) cells, lymphoid tissue inducer cells, and non-cytotoxic ILC populations [188]. Besides controlling tissue homeostasis, it has the ability to promote inflammation at mucosal and surface barriers [188]. Yamaguchi et al. reported that NK cells are actively involved in the induction and maintenance of disease remission in BD patients, through NK2 polarization [189] while Takeno et al. from their study concluded that abnormal killer inhibitory receptor (KIR) expression of NK cells may be associated with the development of BD [190]. Furthermore, ILCs have been recently shown as an important source of cytokines production [188, 191, 192]. The recent discovery of this latest group of diverse immune cells with its many emerging diverse roles in autoimmunity and inflammation may redefine or rather perhaps reinforce our understanding of the pathogenesis of BD in the future.

3.3. Inflammasomes

The inflammasome has been shown to be a key regulator of IL1β and IL18 via direct activation of caspase-1 [173–194]. Liang et al. demonstrated production of IL-1β was significantly decreased in ocular BD patients after the Nod-like receptor protein 3 (NLRP3) inflammasome was downregulated [195] while Kim et al. showed that the basal and LPS-induced expressions of NLRP3 inflammasome components were significantly increased at both mRNA and protein levels in BD patients [196]. Conversely, Türe-Özdemir and his team were not able to find any difference in DC and neutrophils of BD patients compared to HC after stimulating caspase-1 activation [197].

3.4. Autoantibodies

There have been several studies implicating certain autoantibodies in BD, but all are neither non-specific nor sensitive and are of limited clinical significance. Among them the most described were anti-*Saccharomyces cerevisiae* antibodies (ASCAs) [198–201] and anti-endothelial cell antibodies (AECAs) [202–205]. ASCAs were linked more to gastrointestinal manifestations in BD [198–202] and their healthy relatives [201]. AECA has been implicated with vascular [202, 204] and intestinal [205] involvement in BD and several studies demonstrated that alpha-enolase is the target antigen of AECA in BD patients [203–205]. These positive results, however, were not replicated in certain other ethnic populations [206–208].

3.5. The host-microbe interaction in BD

The role of microbial triggers in BD has long been postulated since the disease was first described. Microbial heat shock proteins (HSPs) show significant homology with human mitochondrial HSP and molecular mimicry is suggested as the mechanism of pathology exacerbating BD when patients were exposed to these foreign antigens. While both streptococci and herpes simplex virus have garnered the most particular interest among researchers [209–214], evidence of exposure to other microbes such as staphylococci and mycobacteria has also been reported [215, 216]. Nonetheless, conflicting reports have been published and a specific pathogen has yet to be identified.

3.5.1. Microbiome: the rapidly re-emerging hypothesis in inflammatory disorders

Microbiome is a term first described by Lederberg in 2001 describing the microbial ecosystem [217], but it was Metchnikoff more than a centenary ago who hypothesized that the microbiota might influence the balance between pro-inflammatory and regulatory host responses and that alterations in the composition of the microbiota (a process that is known as dysbiosis) could jeopardize host immune responses [218]. Recent evidence indicates the possible contribution of the intestinal microbiota to immunological diseases outside the gut [218, 219].

The advent of the 16S ribosomal RNA (16S rRNA) sequencing technology over the past quarter century has identified a comprehensive human microbiota far more comprehensive than we ever imagined. Despite the emergence of newer application such as metagenomics [220], due to the nature of the rRNA genes that are highly conserved and evolutionarily stable but differ in their hypervariable regions enables identification of species, and owing to a confluence of methodological advancements, 16S rRNA has re-emerged as a stand-alone molecular tool [221].

BD patients seem to exhibit specific microbiome signature. Consolandi et al. compared fecal microbiota of BD patients and HC and found significantly depleted Roseburia and Subdoligranulum genera and butyrate production in BD patients [222] while Shimizu et al. also demonstrated gut dysbiosis in BD patients with significantly increased genera Bifidobacterium and Eggerthella and decreased genera Megamonas and Prevotella compared to HC [223].

Several authors also identified salivary dysbiosis among BD patients. Seoudi et al. found in BD patients an increased colonization of *Rothia dentocariosa* at non-ulcer oral sites, while the ulcer sites were highly colonized with *Strep salivarius* compared to recurrent aphthous stomatitis (RAS) patients, and with *Strep sanguinis* compared to HC, who were more highly colonized with Neisseria and Veillonella [224]. Coit et al. found significantly less diverse microbial structure in stimulated saliva samples in BD patients both with and without immunosuppressant [225].

3.6. Other possible markers

There are other possible molecular markers that have been or are still under investigations. Fecal calprotectin (FC) were demonstrated to be significantly elevated in intestinal BD in several studies [226–228], and interestingly Özşeker et al. demonstrated high fecal FC levels in asymptomatic but endoscopically proven BD patients with intestinal involvement [226]. Vascular endothelial growth factor (VEGF) levels have been observed in BD patients, particularly in active BD [229–232]. Several studies provided evidence for the increased levels of markers for endothelial activation or dysfunction such as vascular and intercellular adhesion molecules VCAM1, ICAM1, Selectins, and YKL40 in BD [233–238]. Various authors explored the association between certain genetic mutations and thrombosis in BD; however, results have been inconclusive [239–244], and current data indicate that the pathogenesis of thrombosis in BD is not due to a coagulation abnormality [245].

The immunomodulatory role of vitamin D is of increasing interest, and several in vitro studies have demonstrated downregulation of inflammation by vitamin D [246–249]. Moreover, hypovitaminosis D had been implicated in various inflammatory disorders including BD [250–255]. Further investigations from different ethnic populations may provide further insights to this potentially clinically relevant knowledge of vitamin D as a potential suppressor of inflammatory response in BD.

4. Gaps and future directions

Efforts to develop biomarkers in BD have been confounded by substantial impediments and challenges and the greatest is probably due to the rare nature of the disease, while others include the complex role of the susceptibility genes and related cytokines, chemokines and other signaling molecules, variability of duration and severity of the disease, as well as variations between different geographical areas and the limited number of patient samples.

Standardization and quality assurance are significant hurdles and collaboration between laboratories at different centers to standardize protocols and assays is essential. There are clear similarities and differences across different ethnic groups phenotypically and at a genetic or molecular level. So far, clinical data trials support the critical role of innate cytokines TNF, IL1, and IL6 in the development of inflammatory episodes of BD, and targeting T cells or B cells may provide favorable results [256]. In this era of personalized and precision medicine, collaborative efforts nationally or internationally are needed to assemble adequately powered cohorts to perform further population- or regional-based molecular and genetic studies.

One possible way to move forward is broadening the classification criteria to combine objective clinical indicators and biomarkers, but despite the emergence of these candidate markers, there is still a lack of sufficient widespread evidence to support their implementation and incorporation into the contemporary classification criteria. In the meantime, it must be noted that BD remains fundamentally a clinical diagnosis.

Many questions remain a conundrum including (1) which patients will develop a more severe form of disease, (2) who will be resistant to certain therapy, (3) which patients with recurrent aphthous ulcers will progress to develop BD, and (4) who will benefit the most from a particular therapy. The search remains a highly scientific priority, but until we find the biomarkers, likelihood is, many of these questions will remain uncertain.

5. Conclusions

It has been a long, challenging journey in search of biomarkers in Behçet's disease. There are clear genetic and molecular similarities and variability between different ethnic populations.

Collaborative efforts nationally or internationally are needed to assemble sufficiently powered sample size to perform further population- or regional-based molecular and/or genetic studies in the search for the elusive "magic bullet" as the signature marker that will revolutionize the field of BD.

Author details

Fahd Adeeb[1,3]*, Maria Usman Khan[1,3], Austin G. Stack[2,3] and Alexander D. Fraser[1,3]

*Address all correspondence to: fahd_adeeb@yahoo.com

1 Department of Rheumatology, University Hospital Limerick, Limerick, Ireland

2 Department of Nephrology, University Hospital Limerick, Limerick, Ireland

3 Graduate Entry Medical School, University of Limerick, Limerick, Ireland

References

[1] Davatchi F, Chams-Davatchi C, Shams H, Shahram F, Nadji A, Akhlaghi M, et al. Behcet's disease: Epidemiology, clinical manifestations, and diagnosis. Expert Review of Clinical Immunology. 2017;**13**:57–65

[2] Fitzgerald CW, Adeeb F, Timon CV, Shine NP, Fraser AD, Hughes JP. Significant laryngeal destruction in a northern European cohort of Behçet's disease patients. Clinical and Experimental Rheumatology. 2015;**33**(6 Suppl 94):S123–S128

[3] Emmungil H, Yaşar Bilge NŞ, Küçükşahin O, Kılıç L, Okutucu S, Gücenmez S, et al. A rare but serious manifestation of Behçet's disease: Intracardiac thrombus in 22 patients. Clinical and Experimental Rheumatology. 2014;**32**(4 Suppl 84):S87–S92

[4] Ohno S, Aoki K, Sugiura S, Nakayama E, Itakura K. Letter: HL-A5 and Behcet's disease. Lancet. 1973;**2**:1383–1384

[5] Vaiopoulos G, Sfikakis PP, Hatzinikolaou P, Stamatelos G, Kaklamanis P. Adamantiadis-Behçet's disease in sisters. Clinical Rheumatology. 1996;**15**:382–384

[6] Woodrow JC, Graham DR, Evans CC. Behçet's syndrome in HLA-identical siblings. British Journal of Rheumatology. 1990;**29**:225–227

[7] Koné-Paut I, Geisler I, Wechsler B, Ozen S, Ozdogan H, Rozenbaum M, et al. Familial aggregation in Behçet's disease: High frequency in siblings and parents of pediatric probands. Journal of Pediatrics. 1999;**135**:89–93

[8] Gül A, Inanç M, Ocal L, Aral O, Koniçe M. Familial aggregation of Behçet's disease in Turkey. Annals of the Rheumatic Diseases. 2000;**59**:622–625.

[9] Muers M. Complex disease: Ups and downs at the MHC. Nature Reviews Genetics. 2011;**12**:456–457

[10] Verity DH, Marr JE, Ohno S, Wallace GR, Stanford MR. Behçet's disease, the Silk Road and HLA-B51: Historical and geographical perspectives. Tissue Antigens. 1999;**54**:213–220

[11] Takeuchi M, Kastner DL, Remmers EF. The immunogenetics of Behçet's disease: A comprehensive review. Journal of Autoimmunity. 2015;**64**:137–148

[12] McGonagle D, McDermott MF. A proposed classification of the immunological diseases. PLoS Medicine. 2006;**3**(8):e297

[13] McGonagle D, Aydin SZ, Gül A, Mahr A, Direskeneli H. 'MHC-I-opathy'-unified concept for spondyloarthritis and Behçet disease. Nature Reviews Rheumatology. 2015;**11**:731–740

[14] Mizuki N, Ota M, Kimura M, et al. Triplet repeat polymorphism in the transmembrane region of the MIC-A gene: A strong association of six GCT repetitions with Behcet disease. Proceedings of the National Academy of Sciences of the United States of America. 1997;**94**:1298–1303

[15] Lee YH, Song GG. Associations between major histocompatibility complex class I chain-related gene A polymorphisms and susceptibility to Behcet's disease. A meta-analysis. Zeitschrift für Rheumatologie. 2015;**74**:714–721

[16] Meguro A, Inoko H, Ota M, Katsuyama Y, Oka A, Okada E, et al. Genetics of Behçet disease inside and outside the MHC. Annals of the Rheumatic Diseases. 2010;**69**:747–754

[17] Remmers EF, Cosan F, Kirino Y, Ombrello MJ, Abaci N, Satorius C, et al. Genome-wide association study identifies variants in the MHC class I, *IL10*, and *IL23R-IL12RB2* regions associated with Behçet's disease. Nature Genetics. 2010;**42**:698–702

[18] Mizuki N, Meguro A, Ota M, Ohno S, Shiota T, Kawagoe T, et al. Genome-wide association studies identify IL23R-IL12RB2 and IL10 as Behçet's disease susceptibility loci. Nature Genetics. 2010;**42**:703–706

[19] Ombrello MJ, Kirino Y, de Bakker PI, Gül A, Kastner DL, Remmers EF. Behcet disease-associated MHC class I residues implicate antigen binding and regulation of cell-mediated cytotoxicity. Proceedings of the National Academy of Sciences of the United States of America. 2014;**111**:8867–8872

[20] Montes-Cano MA, Conde-Jaldón M, García-Lozano JR, Ortiz-Fernández L, Ortego-Centeno N, Castillo-Palma MJ, et al. HLA and non-HLA genes in Behçet's disease: A multicentric study in the Spanish population. Arthritis Research & Therapy. 2013;**15**(5):R145

[21] Hughes T, Coit P, Adler A, Yilmaz V, Aksu K, Düzgün N, et al. Identification of multiple independent susceptibility loci in the HLA region in Behçet's disease. Nature Genetics. 2013;**45**:319–324

[22] Hirschhorn JN, Daly MJ. Genome-wide association studies for common diseases and complex traits. Nature Reviews Genetics. 2005;**6**:95–108

[23] Fei Y, Webb R, Cobb BL, Direskeneli H, Saruhan-Direskeneli G, Sawalha AH. Identification of novel genetic susceptibility loci for Behçet's disease using a genome-wide association study. Arthritis Research & Therapy. 2009;**11**(3):R66

[24] Kirino Y, Bertsias G, Ishigatsubo Y, Mizuki N, Tugal-Tutkun I, Seyahi E, et al. Genome-wide association analysis identifies new susceptibility loci for Behçet's disease and epistasis between HLA-B51 and ERAP1. Nature Genetics. 2013;**45**:202–207

[25] Hou S, Yang Z, Du L, Jiang Z, Shu Q, Chen Y, et al. Identification of a susceptibility locus in STAT4 for Behçet's disease in Han Chinese in a genome-wide association study. Arthritis & Rheumatology. 2012;**64**:4104–4113

[26] Kappen JH, Medina-Gomez C, Hagen PMv, Stolk L, Estrada K, Rivadeneira F, et al. Genome-wide association study in an admixed case series reveals *IL12A* as a new candidate in Behçet disease. PLoS One. 2015;**10**(3):e0119085

[27] Kilpinen H, Barrett JC. How next-generation sequencing is transforming complex disease genetics. Trends Genetics. 2013;**29**:23–30

[28] Nelson RM, Pettersson ME, Carlborg Ö. A century after Fisher: Time for a new paradigm in quantitative genetics. Trends Genetics. 2013;**29**:669–676

[29] Tennessen JA, Bigham, AW, O'Connor TD, Fu W, Kenny EE, Gravel S, et al. Evolution and functional impact of rare coding variation from deep sequencing of human exomes. Science. 2012;**337**:64–69

[30] Karasneh J, Gul A, Ollier WE, Silman AJ, Worthington J. Whole-genome screening for susceptibility genes in multicase families with Behcet's disease. Arthritis & Rheumatology. 2005;**52**:1836–1842

[31] Lee YJ, Horie Y, Wallace GR, Choi YS, Park JA, Choi JY, et al. Genome-wide association study identifies GIMAP as a novel susceptibility locus for Behcet's disease. Annals of the Rheumatic Diseases. 2013;**72**:1510–1516

[32] Xavier JM, Shahram F, Sousa I, Davatchi F, Matos M, Abdollahi BS, et al. FUT2: Filling the gap between genes and environment in Behçet's disease? Annals of the Rheumatic Diseases. 2015;**74**:618–624

[33] Wu Z, Zheng W, Xu J, Sun F, Chen H, Li P, et al. IL10 polymorphisms associated with Behcet's disease in Chinese Han. Human Immunology. 2014;**75**:271–276

[34] Xavier JM, Shahram F, Davatchi F, Rosa A, Crespo J, Abdollahi BS, et al. Association study of IL10 and IL23R–IL12RB2 in Iranian patients with Behcet's disease. Arthritis & Rheumatology. 2012;**64**:2761–2772

[35] Li H, Liu Q, Hou S, Du L, Zhou Q, Zhou Y, et al. TNFAIP3 gene polymorphisms confer risk for Behcet's disease in a Chinese Han population. Human Genetics. 2013;**132**:293–300

[36] Hou S, Shu Q, Jiang Z, Chen Y, Li F, Chen F, et al. Replication study confirms the association between UBAC2 and Behçet's disease in two independent Chinese sets of patients and controls. Arthritis Research & Therapy. 2012;**14**(2):R70

[37] Kirino Y, Zhou Q, Ishigatsubo Y, Mizuki N, Tugal-Tutkun I, Seyahi E, et al. Targeted resequencing implicates the familial Mediterranean fever gene MEFV and the toll-like receptor 4 gene TLR4 in Behçet disease. Proceedings of the National Academy of Sciences of the United States of America. 2013;**110**:8134–8139

[38] Ognenovski M, Renauer P, Gensterblum E, Kötter I, Xenitidis T, Henes JC, et al. Whole exome sequencing identifies rare protein-coding variants in Behçet's disease. Arthritis & Rheumatology. 2016;**68**:1272–1280

[39] Gül A. Genetics of Behçet's disease: Lessons learned from genomewide association studies. Current Opinion in Rheumatology. 2014;**26**:56–63

[40] Morton LT, Situnayake D, Wallace GR. Genetics of Behçet's disease. Current Opinion in Rheumatology. 2016;**28**:39–44

[41] Cohen S, Bigazzi PE, Yoshida T. Similarities of T cell function in cell-mediated immunity and antibody production. Cellular Immunology. 1974;**12**:150–159

[42] Nagafuchi H, Takeno M, Yoshikawa H, Kurokawa MS, Nara K, Takada E, Masuda C, Mizoguchi M, Suzuki N. Excessive expression of Txk, a member of the Tec family of tyrosine kinases, contributes to excessive Th1 cytokine production by T lymphocytes in patients with Behcet's disease. Clinical & Experimental Immunology. 2005;**139**:363–370

[43] Hamzaoui K, Borhani Haghighi A, Ghorbel IB, Houman H. RORC and Foxp3 axis in cerebrospinal fluid of patients with neuro-Behçet's disease. Journal of Neuroimmunology. 2011;**233**:249–253

[44] Ahn JK, Yu HG, Chung H, Park YG. Intraocular cytokine environment in active Behçet uveitis. American Journal of Ophthalmology. 2006;**142**:429–434

[45] Pay S, Erdem H, Pekel A, Simsek I, Musabak U, Sengul A, et al. Synovial proinflammatory cytokines and their correlation with matrix metalloproteinase-3 expression in Behçet's disease. Does interleukin-1beta play a major role in Behçet's synovitis? Rheumatology International. 2006;**26**:608–613

[46] Ertenli I, Kiraz S, Calgüneri M, Celik I, Erman M, Haznedaroglu IC. Synovial fluid cytokine levels in Behçet's disease. Clinical and Experimental Rheumatology. 2001;**19**(5 Suppl 24):S37–S41

[47] Gül A, Tugal-Tutkun I, Dinarello CA, Reznikov L, Esen BA, Mirza A, et al. Interleukin-1β-regulating antibody XOMA 052 (gevokizumab) in the treatment of acute exacerbations of resistant uveitis of Behcet's disease: An open-label pilot study. Annals of the Rheumatic Diseases. 2012;**71**:563–566

[48] Tugal-Tutkun I, Kadayifcilar S, Khairallah M, Lee SC, Ozdal P, Özyazgan Y, et al. Safety and efficacy of gevokizumab in Patients with Behçet's disease uveitis: Results of an exploratory phase 2 study. Ocular Immunology and Inflammation. 2016;**30**:1–9

[49] Düzgün N, Ayaşlioğlu E, Tutkak H, Aydintuğ OT. Cytokine inhibitors: Soluble tumor necrosis factor receptor 1 and interleukin-1 receptor antagonist in Behçet's disease. Rheumatology International. 2005;**25**:1–5

[50] Emmi G, Talarico R, Lopalco G, Cimaz R, Cantini F, Viapiana O, et al. Efficacy and safety profile of anti-interleukin-1 treatment in Behçet's disease: A multicenter retrospective study. Clinical Rheumatology. 2016;**35**:1281–1286

[51] Cantarini L, Vitale A, Scalini P, Dinarello CA, Rigante D, Franceschini R, et al. Anakinra treatment in drug-resistant Behçet's disease: A case series. Clin Rheumatol 2015; **34**: 1293–301

[52] Vitale A, Rigante D, Caso F, Brizi MG, Galeazzi M, Costa L, et al. Inhibition of interleukin-1 by canakinumab as a successful mono-drug strategy for the treatment of refractory Behçet's disease: A case series. Dermatology. 2014;**228**:211–214

[53] Vallet H, Riviere S, Sanna A, Deroux A, Moulis G, Addimanda O, et al. Efficacy of anti-TNF alpha in severe and/or refractory Behçet's disease: Multicenter study of 124 patients. Journal of Autoimmunity. 2015;**62**:67–74

[54] Arida A, Fragiadaki K, Giavri E, Sfikakis PP. Anti-TNF agents for Behçet's disease: Analysis of published data on 369 patients. Seminars in Arthritis & Rheumatology. 2011;**41**:61–70

[55] Addimanda O, Pipitone N, Pazzola G, Salvarani C. Tocilizumab for severe refractory neuro-Behçet: Three cases IL-6 blockade in neuro-Behçet. Seminars in Arthritis & Rheumatology. 2015;**44**:472–475

[56] Shapiro LS, Farrell J, Borhani Haghighi A. Tocilizumab treatment for neuro-Behcet's disease, the first report. Clinical Neurology and Neurosurgery. 2012;**114**:297–298

[57] Urbaniak P, Hasler P, Kretzschmar S. Refractory neuro-Behçet treated by tocilizumab: A case report. Clinical and Experimental Rheumatology. 2012;**30**(3 Suppl 72):S73–S75

[58] Deroux A, Chiquet C, Bouillet L. Tocilizumab in severe and refractory Behcet's disease: Four cases and literature review. Seminars in Arthritis & Rheumatology. 2016;**45**:733–737

[59] Calvo-Rio V, de la Hera D, Beltran-Catalan E, Blanco R, Hernandez M, Martinez-Costa L, et al. Tocilizumab in uveitis refractory to other biologic drugs: A study of 3 cases and a literature review. Clinical and Experimental Rheumatology. 2014;**32**(4 Suppl 84):S54–S57

[60] Kotter I, Zierhut M, Eckstein A, Vonthein R, Ness T, Günaydin I, et al. Human recombinant interferon-alpha2a (rhIFN alpha2a) for the treatment of Behcet's disease with sight-threatening retinal vasculitis. Advances in Experimental Medicine and Biology. 2003;**528**:521–523

[61] Alpsoy E, Durusoy C, Yilmaz E, Ozgurel Y, Ermis O, Yazar S, et al. Interferon alfa-2a in the treatment of Behcet disease: A randomized placebo-controlled and double-blind study. Archives of Dermatology. 2002;**138**:467–471

[62] Calguneri M, Ozturk MA, Ertenli I, Kiraz S, Apraş S, Ozbalkan Z, et al. Effects of interferon alpha treatment on the clinical course of refractory Behcet's disease: An open study. Annals of the Rheumatic Diseases. 2003;**62**:492–493

[63] Lightman S, Taylor SR, Bunce C, Longhurst H, Lynn W, Moots R, et al. Pegylated interferon-α-2b reduces corticosteroid requirement in patients with Behçet's disease with upregulation of circulating regulatory T cells and reduction of Th17. Annals of the Rheumatic Diseases. 2015;**74**:1138–1144

[64] Arida A, Sfikakis PP. Anti-cytokine biologic treatment beyond anti-TNF in Behçet's disease. Clinical and Experimental Rheumatology. 2014;**32**(4 Suppl 84):S149–S155

[65] Garlanda C, Dinarello CA, Mantovani A. The interleukin-1 family: Back to the future. Immunity. 2013;**39**:1003–1018

[66] Dinarello CA, van der Meer JW. Treating inflammation by blocking interleukin-1 in humans. Seminars in Immunology. 2013;**25**:469–484

[67] Yosipovitch G, Shohat B, Bshara J, Wysenbeek A, Weinberger A. Elevated serum interleukin 1 receptors and interleukin 1B in patients with Behçet's disease: Correlations with disease activity and severity. Israel Journal of Medical Sciences. 1995;**31**:345–348

[68] Hamzaoui K, Hamza M, Ayed K. Production of TNF-α and IL-1 in active Behcet's disease. Journal of Rheumatology. 1990;**17**:1428–1429

[69] Oztas MO, Onder M, Gurer MA, Bukan N, Sancak B. Serum interleukin 18 and tumour necrosis factor-alpha levels are increased in Behcet's disease. Clinical and Experimental Dermatology. 2005;**30**:61–3

[70] Musabak U, Pay S, Erdem H, Simsek I, Pekel A, Dinc A. Serum interleukin-18 levels in patients with Behçet's disease. Is its expression associated with disease activity or clinical presentations? Rheumatology International. 2006;**26**:545–550

[71] Hamzaoui K, Hamzaoui A, Guemira F, Bessioud M, Hamza M, Ayed K. Cytokine profile in Behçet's disease patients. Relationship with disease activity. Scandinavian Journal of Rheumatology. 2002;**31**:205–210

[72] Schmitz J, Owyang A, Oldham E, Song Y, Murphy E, McClanahan TK, et al. IL-33, an interleukin-1-like cytokine that signals via the IL-1 receptor-related protein ST2 and induces T helper type 2-associated cytokines. Immunity. 2005;**23**:479–490

[73] Hamzaoui K, Kaabachi W, Fazaa B, Zakraoui L, Mili Boussen I, Haj Sassi F. Serum IL-33 levels and skin mRNA expression in Behcet's disease. Clinical and Experimental Rheumatology. 2013;**31**(Suppl. 77):6–14

[74] Hamzaoui K, Bouali E, Hamzaoui A. Interleukin-33 and Behçet disease: Another cytokine among others. Human Immunology. 2015;**76**:301–306

[75] Hamzaoui K, Borhani-Haghighi A, Kaabachi W, Hamzaoui A. Increased interleukin 33 in patients with neuro-Behcet's disease: Correlation with MCP-1 and IP-10 chemokines. Cellular & Molecular Immunology. 2014;**11**:613–616

[76] Kim DJ, Baek SY, Park MK, Park KS, Lee JH, Park SH, et al. Serum level of interleukin-33 and soluble ST2 and their association with disease activity in patients with Behcet's disease. Journal of Korean Medical Science. 2013;**28**:1145–1153

[77] Koca SS, Kara M, Deniz F, Ozgen M, Demir CF, Ilhan N, et al. Serum IL-33 level and IL-33 gene polymorphisms in Behçet's disease. Rheumatology International. 2015;**35**:471–477

[78] Mege JL, Dilsen N, Sanguedolce V, Gul A, Bongrand P, Roux H, et al. Overproduction of monocyte derived tumor necrosis factor alpha, interleukin (IL) 6, IL-8 and increased neutrophil superoxide generation in Behçet's disease: A comparative study with familial Mediterranean fever and healthy subjects. Journal of Rheumatology. 1993;**20**:1544–1549

[79] Sayinalp N, Ozcebe OI, Ozdemir O, Haznedaroğlu IC, Dündar S, Kirazli S. Cytokines in Behçet's disease. Journal of Rheumatology. 1996;**23**:321–322

[80] El Menyawi M, Fawzy M, Al-Nahas Z, Edris A, Hussein H, Shaker O, et al. Serum tumor necrosis factor alpha (TNF-α) level in patients with Behçet's disease: Relation to clinical manifestations and disease activity. Egypt Rheumatologist. 2014;**36**:139–143

[81] Kwok SK, Park SH, Park MK, Cho ML, Seo SH, Ju JH, et al. Upregulation of macrophage migration inhibitory factor (MIF) production from peripheral blood mononuclear cells (PBMCs) stimulated by tumor necrosis factor (TNF)-α in patients with Behcet's syndrome. Journal of the Korean Rheumatism Association. 2007;**14**:112–117

[82] Jiang Z, Hennein L, Tao Y, Tao L. Interleukin-23 receptor gene polymorphism may enhance expression of the IL-23 receptor, IL-17, TNF-α and IL-6 in Behcet's disease. PLoS One. 2015;**10**(7):e0134632

[83] Takeuchi M, Karasawa Y, Harimoto K, Tanaka A, Shibata M, Sato T, et al. Analysis of Th cell-related cytokine production in Behçet disease patients with uveitis before and after infliximab treatment. Ocular Immunology and Inflammation. 2016;**12**:1–10

[84] Touma Z, Farra C, Hamdan A, Shamseddeen W, Uthman I, Hourani H, et al. TNF polymorphisms in patients with Behçet disease: A meta-analysis. Archives of Medical Research. 2010;**41**:142–146

[85] Zhang M, Xu WD, Wen PF, Liang Y, Liu J, Pan HF, et al. Polymorphisms in the tumor necrosis factor gene and susceptibility to Behcet's disease: An updated meta-analysis. Molecular Vision. 2013;**19**:1913–1924

[86] Cantarini L, Pucino V, Vitale A, Talarico R, Lucherini OM, Magnotti F, et al. Immunometabolic biomarkers of inflammation in Behçet's disease: Relationship with epidemiological profile, disease activity and therapeutic regimens. Clinical & Experimental Immunology. 2016;**184**:197–207

[87] Shaker OG, Tawfic SO, El-Tawdy AM, El-Komy MH, El Menyawi M, Heikal AA. Expression of TNF-α, APRIL and BCMA in Behcet's disease. Journal of Immunology Research. 2014;**2014**:380405

[88] Düzgün N, Ayaslioglu E, Tutkak H. Serum soluble CD30 levels in Behçet's disease. Clinical and Experimental Rheumatology. 2004;**22**(4 Suppl 34):S17–S20

[89] Hamzaoui K, Hamzaoui A, Kahan A, Hamza M, Chabbou A, Ayed K. Interleukin-6 in peripheral blood and inflammatory sites in Behçet's disease. Mediators of Inflammation. 1992;**1**:281–285

[90] Yamakawa Y, Sugita Y, Nagatani T, Takahashi S, Yamakawa T, Tanaka S, et al. Interleukin-6 (IL-6) in patients with Behçet's disease. Journal of Dermatological Science. 1996;**11**:189–195

[91] Hirohata S, Isshi K, Oguchi H, Ohse T, Haraoka H, Takeuchi A, et al. Cerebrospinal fluid interleukin-6 in progressive Neuro-Behçet's syndrome. Clinical Immunology and Immunopathology. 1997;**82**:12–17

[92] Akman-Demir G, Tüzün E, Içöz S, Yeşilot N, Yentür SP, Kürtüncü M, et al. Interleukin-6 in neuro-Behçet's disease: Association with disease subsets and long-term outcome. Cytokine. 2008;**44**:373–376

[93] Diamantopoulos AP, Hatemi G. Lack of efficacy of tocilizumab in mucocutaneous Behçet's syndrome: Report of two cases. Rheumatology. 2013;**52**:1923–1924

[94] Cantarini L, Lopalco G, Vitale A, Coladonato L, Rigante D, Lucherini OM, et al. Paradoxical mucocutaneous flare in a case of Behçet's disease treated with tocilizumab. Clinical Rheumatology. 2015;**34**:1141–1143

[95] Kötter I, Koch S, Vonthein R, Rückwaldt U, Amberger M, Günaydin I, et al. Cytokines, cytokine antagonists and soluble adhesion molecules in patients with ocular Behçet's disease treated with human recombinant interferon-alpha2a. Results of an open study and review of the literature. Clinical and Experimental Rheumatology. 2005;**23**(4 Suppl 38):S20–S26

[96] Pay S, Simsek I, Erdem H, Pekel A, Musabak U, Sengul A, et al. Dendritic cell subsets and type I interferon system in Behçet's disease: Does functional abnormality in plasmacytoid dendritic cells contribute to Th1 polarization? Clinical and Experimental Rheumatology. 2007;**25**(4 Suppl 45):S34–S40

[97] Liu X, Yang P, Wang C, Li F, Kijlstra A. IFN-alpha blocks IL-17 production by peripheral blood mononuclear cells in Behcet's disease. Rheumatology. 2011;**50**:293–298

[98] Ohno S, Kato F, Matsuda H, Fujii N, Minagawa T. Detection of gamma interferon in the sera of patients with Behçet's disease. Infection and Immunity. 1982;**36**:202–208

[99] Ahn JK, Seo JM, Yu J, Oh FS, Chung H, Yu HG. Down-regulation of IFN-gamma-producing CD56+ T cells after combined low-dose cyclosporine/prednisone treatment in patients with Behçet's uveitis. Investigative Ophthalmology & Visual Science. 2005;**46**:2458–2464

[100] Djaballah-Ider F, Chaib S, Belguendouz H, Talbi D, Touil-Boukoffa C. T cells activation and interferon-γ/nitric oxide production during Behçet disease: A study in Algerian patients. Ocular Immunology and Inflammation. 2012;**20**:215–217

[101] Na SY, Park MJ, Park S, Lee ES. Up-regulation of Th17 and related cytokines in Behçet's disease corresponding to disease activity. Clinical and Experimental Rheumatology. 2013;**31**(3 Suppl 77):32–40

[102] Shen H, Xia LP, Lu J. Elevated levels of interleukin-27 and effect on production of interferon-γ and interleukin-17 in patients with Behçet's disease. Scandinavian Journal of Rheumatology. 2013;**42**:48–51

[103] Belguendouz H, Messaoudène D, Lahmar K, Ahmedi L, Medjeber O, Hartani D, et al. Interferon-γ and nitric oxide production during Behçet uveitis: Immunomodulatory effect of interleukin-10. Journal of Interferon & Cytokine Research. 2011;**31**:643–651

[104] Mesquida M, Molins B, Llorenç V, Sainz de la Maza M, Hernandez MV, Espinosa G, et al. Proinflammatory cytokines and C-reactive protein in uveitis associated with Behçet's disease. Mediators of Inflammation. 2014;**2014**:396204

[105] Chi W, Zhu X, Yang P, Liu X, Lin X, Zhou H, et al. Upregulated IL-23 and IL-17 in Behçet patients with active uveitis. Investigative Ophthalmology & Visual Science. 2008;**49**:3058–3064

[106] Sugita S, Kawazoe Y, Imai A, Yamada Y, Horie S, Mochizuki M. Inhibition of Th17 differentiation by anti-TNF-alpha therapy in uveitis patients with Behçet's disease. Arthritis Research & Therapy. 2012;**14**:R99

[107] Türkçüoğlu P, Arat YO, Kan E, Kan EK, Chaudhry IA, Koca S, et al. Association of disease activity with serum and tear IL-2 levels in Behçet disease. Ocular Immunology and Inflammation. 2016;**24**:313–318

[108] Akdeniz N, Esrefoglu M, Keleş MS, Karakuzu A, Atasoy M. Serum interleukin-2, interleukin-6, tumour necrosis factor-alpha and nitric oxide levels in patients with Behcet's disease. Annals of the Academy of Medicine, Singapore. 2004;**33**:596–599.

[109] Sugi-Ikai N, Nakazawa M, Nakamura S, Ohno S, Minami M. Increased frequencies of interleukin-2- and interferon-gamma-producing T cells in patients with active Behçet's disease. Investigative Ophthalmology & Visual Science. 1998;**39**:996–1004.

[110] BenEzra D, Maftzir G, Kalichman I, Barak V. Serum levels of interleukin-2 receptor in ocular Behçet's disease. American Journal of Ophthalmology. 1993;**115**:26–30

[111] Uchio E, Matsumoto T, Tanaka SI, Ohno S. Soluble intercellular adhesion molecule-1 (ICAM-1), CD4, CD8 and interleukin-2 receptor in patients with Behçet's disease and Vogt-Koyanagi-Harada's disease. Clinical and Experimental Rheumatology. 1999;**17**:179–184

[112] Alpsoy E, Cayirli C, Er H, Yilmaz E. The levels of plasma interleukin-2 and soluble interleukin-2R in Behçet's disease: A marker of disease activity. Journal of Dermatology. 1998;**25**:513–516

[113] Evereklioglu C1, Er H, Türköz Y, Cekmen M. Serum levels of TNF-alpha, sIL-2R, IL-6, and IL-8 are increased and associated with elevated lipid peroxidation in patients with Behçet's disease. Mediators of Inflammation. 2002;**11**:87–93

[114] Guenane H, Hartani D, Chachoua L, Lahlou-Boukoffa OS, Mazari F, Touil-Boukoffa C. Production of Th1/Th2 cytokines and nitric oxide in Behçet's uveitis and idiopathic uveitis. Journal Francais D'Ophtalmologie. 2006;**29**:146–152

[115] Belguendouz H, Messaoudene D, Hartani D, Chachoua L, Ahmedi ML, Lahmar-Belguendouz K, et al. Effect of corticotherapy on interleukin-8 and -12 and nitric oxide production during Behçet and idiopathic uveitis. Journal Francais D'Ophtalmologie. 2008;**31**:387–395

[116] Ahmedi ML, Belguendouz H, Messaoudene D, Mesbah-Amroun H, Terahi M, Lahlou-Boukoffa OS, et al. Influence of steroid hormones on the production of two inflammatory markers, IL-12 and nitric oxide, in Behçet's disease. Journal Francais D'Ophtalmologie. 2016;**39**:333–340

[117] Frassanito MA, Dammacco R, Cafforio P, Dammacco F. Th1 polarization of the immune response in Behçet's disease: A putative pathogenetic role of interleukin-12. Arthritis & Rheumatology. 1999;**42**:1967–1974

[118] Turan B, Gallati H, Erdi H, Gürler A, Michel BA, Villiger PM. Systemic levels of the T cell regulatory cytokines IL-10 and IL-12 in Behçet's disease; soluble TNFR-75 as a biological marker of disease activity. Journal of Rheumatology. 1997;**24**:128–132

[119] Teng MW, Bowman EP, McElwee JJ, Smyth MJ, Casanova JL, Cooper AM, et al. IL-12 and IL-23 cytokines: from discovery to targeted therapies for immune-mediated inflammatory diseases. Nature Medicine. 2015;**21**:719–729

[120] Habibagahi Z, Habibagahi M, Heidari M. Raised concentration of soluble form of vascular endothelial cadherin and IL-23 in sera of patients with Behçet's disease. Modern Rheumatology. 2010;**20**:154–159

[121] Gheita TA, Gamal SM, Shaker I, El Fishawy HS, El Sisi R, Shaker OG, et al. Clinical significance of serum interleukin-23 and A/G gene (rs17375018) polymorphism in Behçets disease: Relation to neuro-Behçet, uveitis and disease activity. Joint Bone Spine. 2015;**82**:213–215

[122] Baerveldt EM, Kappen JH, Thio HB, van Laar JA, van Hagen PM, Prens EP. Successful long-term triple disease control by ustekinumab in a patient with Behcet's disease, psoriasis and hidradenitis suppurativa. Annals of the Rheumatic Diseases. 2013;**72**:626–627

[123] Watford, WT, Hissong BD, Bream JH, Kanno Y, Muul L, O'Shea JJ. Signaling by IL-12 and IL-23 and the immunoregulatory roles of STAT4. Immunological Reviews. 2004;**202**:139–156

[124] Trinchieri, G. Interleukin-12 and the regulation of innate resistance and adaptive immunity. Nature Reviews Immunology. 2003;**3**:133–146

[125] Parham C, Chirica M, Timans J, Vaisberg E, Travis M, Cheung J, et al. A receptor for the heterodimeric cytokine IL-23 is composed of IL-12Rβ1 and a novel cytokine receptor subunit, IL-23R. Journal of Immunology. 2002;**168**:5699–5708

[126] Tulunay A, Dozmorov MG, Ture-Ozdemir F, Yilmaz V, Eksioglu-Demiralp E, Alibaz-Oner F, et al. Activation of the JAK/STAT pathway in Behcet's disease. Genes & Immunity. 2015;**16**:176

[127] Chi W, Yang P, Zhu X, Wang Y, Chen L, Huang X, et al. Production of interleukin-17 in Behçet's disease is inhibited by cyclosporin A. Molecular Vision. 2010;**16**:880–886

[128] Cai T, Wang Q, Zhou Q, Wang C, Hou S, Qi J, et al. Increased expression of IL-22 is associated with disease activity in Behcet's disease. PLoS One. 2013;**8**:e59009

[129] Yasuoka H, Chen Z, Takeuchi T, Kuwana M. Th17 is involved in the pathogenesis of Bechet's disease via CCL20-CCR6 axis. Arthritis Research & Therapy. 2012;**14**(Suppl 1):P79

[130] Cordero-Coma M, Calleja S, Llorente M, Rodriguez E, Franco M, Ruiz de Morales JG. Serum cytokine profile in adalimumab-treated refractory uveitis patients: Decreased IL-22 correlates with clinical responses. Ocular Immunology and Inflammation. 2013;**21**:212–219

[131] Chi W, Zhou S, Yang P, Chen L. CD4+ T cells from Behcet patients produce high levels of IL-17. Eye Science. 2011;**26**:65–69

[132] Shimizu J, Takai K, Fujiwara N, Arimitsu N, Ueda Y, Wakisaka S, et al. Excessive CD4+ T cells co-expressing interleukin-17 and interferon-γ in patients with Behçet's disease. Clinical & Experimental Immunology. 2012;**168**:68–74

[133] Al-Zifzaf DS, Mokbel AN, Abdelaziz DM. Interleukin-17 in Behçet's disease: Relation with clinical picture and disease activity. Egyptian Rheumatology and Rehabilitation. 2015;**42**:34–38

[134] Nurieva R, Yang XO, Martinez G, Zhang Y, Panopoulos AD, Ma L, et al. Essential autocrine regulation by IL-21 in the generation of inflammatory T cells. Nature. 2007;**448**:480–483

[135] Geri G, Terrier B, Rosenzwajg M, Wechsler B, Touzot M, Seilhean D, et al. Critical role of IL-21 in modulating T(H)17 and regulatory T cells in Behçet disease. Journal of Allergy and Clinical Immunology. 2011;**128**:655–664

[136] Houman H, Hamzaoui A, Ben Ghorbal I, Khanfir M, Feki M, Hamzaoui K. Abnormal expression of chemokine receptors in Behçet's disease: Relationship to intracellular Th1/Th2 cytokines and to clinical manifestations. Journal of Autoimmunity. 2004;**23**:267–273

[137] Koarada S, Haruta Y, Tada Y, Ushiyama O, Morito F, Ohta A, et al. Increased entry of CD4+ T cells into the Th1 cytokine effector pathway during T cell division following stimulation in Behcet's disease. Rheumatology. 2004;**43**:843–851

[138] Raziuddin S, al-Dalaan A, Bahabri S, Siraj AK, al-Sedairy S. Divergent cytokine production profile in Behçet's disease. Altered Th1/Th2 cell cytokine pattern. Journal of Rheumatology. 1998;**25**:329–333

[139] Aridogan BC, Yildirim M, Baysal V, Inaloz HS, Baz K, Kaya S. Serum levels of IL-4, IL-10, IL-12, IL-13 and IFN-gamma in Behçet's disease. Journal of Dermatology. 2003;**30**:602–607

[140] Dalghous AM, Freysdottir J, Fortune F. Expression of cytokines, chemokines, and chemokine receptors in oral ulcers of patients with Behcet's disease (BD) and recurrent aphthous stomatitis is Th1-associated, although Th2-association is also observed in patients with BD. Scandinavian Journal of Rheumatology. 2006;**35**:472–475

[141] Ben Ahmed M, Houman H, Miled M, Dellagi K, Louzir H. Involvement of chemokines and Th1 cytokines in the pathogenesis of mucocutaneous lesions of Behçet's disease. Arthritis & Rheumatology. 2004;**50**:2291–2295

[142] Gündüz E, Teke HU, Bilge NS, Cansu DU, Bal C, Korkmaz C, et al. Regulatory T cells in Behçet's disease: Is there a correlation with disease activity? Does regulatory T cell type matter? Rheumatology International. 2013;**33**:3049–3054

[143] Nanke Y, Kotake S, Goto M, Ujihara H, Matsubara M, Kamatni N. Decreased percentages of regulatory T cells in peripheral blood of patients with Behçet's disease before ocular attack: A possible predictive marker of ocular attack. Modern Rheumatology. 2008;**18**:354–358

[144] Sugita S, Yamada Y, Kaneko S, Horie S, Mochizuki M. Induction of regulatory T cells by infliximab in Behçet's disease. Investigative Ophthalmology & Visual Science. 2011;**52**:476–484

[145] Bandala-Sanchez E, Zhang Y, Reinwald S, Dromey JA, Lee BH, Qian J, et al. T cell regulation mediated by interaction of soluble CD52 with the inhibitory receptor Siglec-10. Nature Immunology. 2013;**14**:741–748

[146] Mohammad AJ, Smith RM, Chow YW, Chaudhry AN, Jayne DR. Alemtuzumab as remission induction therapy in Behçet disease: A 20-year experience. Journal of Rheumatology. 2015;**42**:1906–1913

[147] Perez-Pampin E, Campos-Franco J, Blanco J, Mera A. Remission induction in a case of refractory Behçet disease with alemtuzumab. Journal of Clinical Rheumatology. 2013;**19**:101–103

[148] Carding SR, Egan PJ. Gammadelta T cells: Functional plasticity and heterogeneity. Nature Reviews Immunology. 2002;**2**:336–345

[149] Hasan MS, Bergmeier LA, Petrushkin H, Fortune F. Gamma delta (γδ) T cells and their involvement in Behçet's disease. Journal of Immunology Research. 2015;**2015**:705831

[150] Fortune F, Walker J, Lehner T. The expression of γδ T cell receptor and the prevalence of primed, activated and IgA-bound T cells in Behcet's syndrome. Clinical & Experimental Immunology. 1990;**82**:326–332

[151] Suzuki Y, Hoshi K, Matsuda T, Mizushima Y. Increased peripheral blood gamma delta+ T cells and natural killer cells in Behçet's disease. Journal of Rheumatology. 1992;**19**:588–592

[152] Hamzaoui K, Hamzaoui A, Hentati F, Kahan A, Ayed K, Chabbou A, et al. Phenotype and functional profile of T cells expressing gamma delta receptor from patients with active Behçet's disease. Journal of Rheumatology. 1994;**21**:2301–2306

[153] Hasan A, Fortune F, Wilson A, Warr K, Shinnick T, Mizushima Y, et al. Role of gamma delta T cells in pathogenesis and diagnosis of Behcet's disease. Lancet. 1996;**347**:789–794

[154] Freysdottir J, Lau S, Fortune F. Gammadelta T cells in Behçet's disease (BD) and recurrent aphthous stomatitis (RAS). Clinical & Experimental Immunology. 1999;**118**:451–457

[155] Bank I, Duvdevani M, Livneh A. Expansion of gammadelta T-cells in Behçet's disease: Role of disease activity and microbial flora in oral ulcers. Journal of Laboratory and Clinical Medicine. 2003;**141**:33–40

[156] Verjans GM, van Hagen PM, van der Kooi A, Osterhaus AD, Baarsma GS. Vgamma9Vdelta2 T cells recovered from eyes of patients with Behçet's disease recognize non-peptide prenyl pyrophosphate antigens. Journal of Neuroimmunology. 2002;**130**:46–54

[157] Triolo G, Accardo-Palumbo A, Dieli F, Ciccia F, Ferrante A, Giardina E, et al. Vgamma9/Vdelta2 T lymphocytes in Italian patients with Behçet's disease: Evidence for expansion, and tumour necrosis factor receptor II and interleukin-12 receptor beta1 expression in active disease. Arthritis Research & Therapy. 2003;**5**:R262–R268

[158] Clemente A, Cambra A, Munoz-Saá I, Crespí C, Pallarés L, Juan A, et al. Phenotype markers and cytokine intracellular production by CD8+ gammadelta T lymphocytes do not support a regulatory T profile in Behçet's disease patients and healthy controls. Immunology Letters. 2010;**129**:57–63

[159] Parlakgul G, Guney E, Erer B, Kılıcaslan Z, Direskeneli H, Gul A, et al. Expression of regulatory receptors on γδ T cells and their cytokine production in Behcet's disease. Arthritis Research & Therapy. 2013;**15**:R15

[160] Nold MF, Nold-Petry CA, Zepp JA, Palmer BE, Bufler P, Dinarello CA. IL-37 is a fundamental inhibitor of innate immunity. Nature Immunology. 2010;**11**:1014–1022

[161] Bouali E, Kaabachi W, Hamzaoui A, Hamzaoui K. Interleukin-37 expression is decreased in Behçet's disease and is associated with inflammation. Immunology Letters. 2015;**167**:87–94

[162] Ye Z, Wang C, Kijlstra A, Zhou X, Yang P. A possible role for interleukin 37 in the pathogenesis of Behcet's disease. Current Molecular Medicine. 2014;**14**:535–542

[163] Hamzaoui K, Hamzaoui A. The anti-inflammatory activity of interleukin-37 in Behçet's disease. Inflammation and Cell Signaling. 2016;**3**:e1452

[164] Wang C, Tian Y, Ye Z, Kijlstra A, Zhou Y, Yang P. Decreased interleukin 27 expression is associated with active uveitis in Behçet's disease. Arthritis Research & Therapy. 2014;**16**:R117

[165] Curnow SJ, Pryce K, Modi N, Knight B, Graham EM, Stewart JE, et al. Serum cytokine profiles in Behçet's disease: Is there a role for IL-15 in pathogenesis? Immunology Letters. 2008;**121**:7–12

[166] Hamzaoui K, Hamzaoui A, Ghorbel I, Khanfir M, Houman H. Levels of IL-15 in serum and cerebrospinal fluid of patients with Behçet's disease. Scandinavian Journal of Immunology. 2006;**64**:655–660

[167] Luster AD. Chemokines—Chemotactic cytokines that mediate inflammation. New England Journal of Medicine. 1998;**338**:436–445

[168] Saruhan-Direskeneli G, Yentür SP, Akman-Demir G, Işik N, Serdaroğlu P. Cytokines and chemokines in neuro-Behçet's disease compared to multiple sclerosis and other neurological diseases. Journal of Neuroimmunology. 2003;**145**:127–134

[169] El-Asrar AM, Al-Obeidan SS, Kangave D, et al. CXC chemokine expression profiles in aqueous humor of patients with different clinical entities of endogenous uveitis. Immunobiology. 2011;**216**:1004–1009

[170] Ambrose N, Khan E, Ravindran R, Lightstone L, Abraham S, Botto M, et al. The exaggerated inflammatory response in Behçet's syndrome: Identification of dysfunctional post-transcriptional regulation of the IFN-γ/CXCL10 IP-10 pathway. Clinical & Experimental Immunology. 2015;**181**:427–433

[171] Durmazlar SP, Ulkar GB, Eskioglu F, Tatlican S, Mert A, Akgul A. Significance of serum IL-8 levels in patients with Behcet's disease: High levels may indicate vascular involvement. International Journal of Dermatology. 2009;**48**:259–264

[172] Mantas C, Direskeneli H, Oz D, Yavuz S, Akoglu T. IL-8 producing cells in patients with Behçet's disease. Clinical and Experimental Rheumatology. 2000;**18**:249–251

[173] Katsantonis J, Adler Y, Orfanos CE, Zouboulis CC. Adamantiades-Behçet's disease: Serum IL-8 is a more reliable marker for disease activity than C-reactive protein and erythrocyte sedimentation rate. Dermatology. 2000;**201**:37–39

[174] Erdem H, Pay S, Serdar M, Simşek I, Dinç A, Muşabak U, et al. Different ELR (+) angiogenic CXC chemokine profiles in synovial fluid of patients with Behçet's disease, familial Mediterranean fever, rheumatoid arthritis, and osteoarthritis. Rheumatology International. 2005;**26**:162–167

[175] Ozer HT, Erken E, Gunesacar R, Kara O. Serum RANTES, MIP-1α, and MCP-1 levels in Behçet's disease. Rheumatology International. 2005;**25**:487–488

[176] Kökçam I, Turgut D, Ilhan NF, Çiçek D. The levels of serum chemokines in patients with Behçet's disease. Turkish Journal of Medical Sciences. 2012;**42**:1105–1110

[177] Kim WU, Do JH, Park KS, Cho ML, Park SH, Cho CS, et al. Enhanced production of macrophage inhibitory protein-1α in patients with Behçet's disease. Scandinavian Journal of Rheumatology. 2005;**34**:129–135.

[178] Kaburaki T, Fujino Y, Kawashima H, Merino G, Numaga J, Chen J, et al. Plasma and whole-blood chemokine levels in patients with Behcet's disease. Graefe's Archive for Clinical and Experimental Ophthalmology. 2003;**241**:353–358

[179] Do JH, Jung JH, Park CS, Ko JS, Kim SS, Choi HC, et al. Elevated monocyte chemoattractant protein-1 in patients with Behcet's disease. Korean Journal of Medicine. 2003;**65**:458–466

[180] Miyagishi R, Kikuchi S, Fukazawa T, Tashiro K. Macrophage inflammatory protein-1α in the cerebrospinal fluid of patients with multiple sclerosis and other inflammatory neurological diseases. Journal of the Neurological Sciences. 1995;**129**:223–227

[181] Becatti M, Emmi G, Silvestri E, Bruschi G, Ciucciarelli L, Squatrito D, et al. Neutrophil activation promotes fibrinogen oxidation and thrombus formation in Behçet disease. Circulation. 2016;**133**:302–311

[182] Köse K, Yazici C, Cambay N, Aşcioğlu O, Doğan P. Lipid peroxidation and erythrocyte antioxidant enzymes in patients with Behçet's disease. The Tohoku Journal of Experimental Medicine. 2002;**197**:9–16

[183] Yazici C, Köse K, Caliş M, DemIr M, Kirnap M, Ateş F. Increased advanced oxidation protein products in Behçet's disease: A new activity marker? British Journal of Dermatology. 2004;**151**:105–111

[184] Yuksel M, Yildiz A, Oylumlu M, Turkcu FM, Bilik MZ, Ekinci A, et al. Novel markers of endothelial dysfunction and inflammation in Behçet's disease patients with ocular involvement: Epicardial fat thickness, carotid intima media thickness, serum ADMA level, and neutrophil-to-lymphocyte ratio. Clinical Rheumatology. 2016;**35**:701–708

[185] Ozturk C, Balta S, Balta I, Demirkol S, Celik T, Turker T, et al. Neutrophil–lymphocyte ratio and carotid-intima media thickness in patients with Behçet disease without cardiovascular involvement. Angiology. 2015;**66**:291–296

[186] Acikgoz N. The neutrophil-lymphocyte ratio and Behcet disease. Angiology. 2016; **67**:297

[187] Rifaioglu EN, Bülbül Şen B, Ekiz Ö, Cigdem Dogramaci A. Neutrophil to lymphocyte ratio in Behçet's disease as a marker of disease activity. Acta Dermatovenerologica Alpina, Pannonica et Adriatica. 2014;**23**:65–67

[188] Artis D, Spits H. The biology of innate lymphoid cells. Nature. 2015;**517**:293–301

[189] Yamaguchi Y, Takahashi H, Satoh T, Okazaki Y, Mizuki N, Takahashi K, et al. Natural killer cells control a T-helper 1 response in patients with Behçet's disease. Arthritis Research & Therapy. 2010;**12**:R80

[190] Takeno M, Shimoyama Y, Kashiwakura J, Nagafuchi H, Sakane T, Suzuki N. Abnormal killer inhibitory receptor expression on natural killer cells in patients with Behçet's disease. Rheumatology International. 2004;**24**:212–216

[191] Diefenbach A, Colonna M, Koyasu S. Development, differentiation, and diversity of innate lymphoid cells. Immunity. 2014;**41**:354–365

[192] Walker JA, Barlow JL, McKenzie AN. Innate lymphoid cells—How did we miss them? Nature Reviews Immunology. 2013;**13**:75–87

[193] Schroder K, Tschopp, J. The inflammasomes. Cell. 2010;**140**:821–832

[194] Strowig T, Henao-Mejia J, Elinav E, Flavell R. Inflammasomes in health and disease. Nature. 2012;**481**:278–286

[195] Liang L, Tan X, Zhou Q, Zhu Y, Tian Y, Yu H, et al. IL-1β triggered by peptidoglycan and lipopolysaccharide through TLR2/4 and ROS-NLRP3 inflammasome-dependent pathways is involved in ocular Behçet's disease. Investigative Ophthalmology & Visual Science. 2013;**54**:402–414

[196] Kim EH, Park MJ, Park S, Lee ES. Increased expression of the NLRP3 inflammasome components in patients with Behçet's disease. Journal of Inflammation. 2015;**12**:41

[197] Türe-Özdemir F, Tulunay A, Elbasi MO, Tatli I, Maurer AM, Mumcu G, et al. Pro-inflammatory cytokine and caspase-1 responses to pattern recognition receptor activation of neutrophils and dendritic cells in Behcet's disease. Rheumatology. 2013;**52**:800–805

[198] Krause I, Monselise Y, Milo G, Weinberger A. Anti-Saccharomyces cerevisiae antibodies—A novel serologic marker for Behçet's disease. Clinical and Experimental Rheumatology. 2002;**20**(suppl 26):S21–S24

[199] Fresko I, Ugurlu S, Ozbakir F, Celik A, Yurdakul S, Hamuryudan V, et al. Anti-Saccharomyces cerevisiae antibodies (ASCA) in Behçet's syndrome. Clinical and Experimental Rheumatology. 2005;**23**(4 Suppl 38):S67–S70

[200] Choi CH, Kim TI, Kim BC, Shin SJ, Lee SK, Kim WH, et al. Anti-Saccharomyces cerevisiae antibody in intestinal Behçet's disease patients: Relation to clinical course. Diseases of the Colon & Rectum. 2006;49:1849–1859

[201] Monselise A, Weinberger A, Monselise Y, Fraser A, Sulkes J, Krause I. Anti-Saccharomyces cerevisiae antibodies in Behçet's disease—A familial study. Clinical and Experimental Rheumatology. 2006;**24**(5 Suppl 42):S87–S90

[202] Aydìntug AO, Tokgöz G, D'Cruz DP, Gürler A, Cervera R, Düzgün N, et al. Antibodies to endothelial cells in patients with Behcet's disease. Clinical Immunology and Immunopathology. 1993;**67**:157–162

[203] Lee KH, Chung HS, Kim HS, Oh SH, Ha MK, Baik JH, et al. Human alpha-enolase from endothelial cells as a target antigen of anti-endothelial cell antibody in Behçet's disease. Arthritis & Rheumatology. 2003;**48**:2025–2035

[204] Lee JH, Cho SB, Bang D, Oh SH, Ahn KJ, Kim J, et al. Human anti-alpha-enolase antibody in sera from patients with Behçet's disease and rheumatologic disorders. Clinical and Experimental Rheumatology. 2009;**27**(2 Suppl 53):S63–S66

[205] Shin SJ, Kim BC, Kim TI, Lee SK, Lee KH, Kim WH. Anti-alpha-enolase antibody as a serologic marker and its correlation with disease severity in intestinal Behçet's disease. Digestive Diseases and Sciences. 2011;**56**:812–818

[206] Vaiopoulos G, Lakatos PL, Papp M, Kaklamanis F, Economou E, Zevgolis V, et al. Serum anti-Saccharomyces cerevisiae antibodies in Greek patients with Behcet's disease. Yonsei Medical Journal. 2011;**52**:347–350

[207] Filik L, Biyikoglu I. Differentiation of Behcet's disease from inflammatory bowel diseases: Anti-Saccharomyces cerevisiae antibody and anti-neutrophilic cytoplasmic antibody. World Journal of Gastroenterology. 2008;**14**:7271

[208] Rhee SH, Kim YB, Lee ES. Comparison of Behcet's disease and recurrent aphthous ulcer according to characteristics of gastrointestinal symptoms. Journal of Korean Medical Science. 2005;**20**:971–976

[209] Isogai E, Ohno S, Kotake S, Isogai H, Tsurumizu T, Fujii N, et al. Chemiluminescence of neutrophils from patients with Behçet's disease and its correlation with an increased proportion of uncommon serotypes of Streptococcus sanguis in the oral flora. Archives of Oral Biology. 1990;**35**:43–8

[210] Yokota K, Hayashi S, Fujii N, et al. Antibody response to oral streptococci in Behçet's disease. Microbiology and Immunology. 1992;**36**:815–822

[211] Mumcu G, Inanc N, Aydin SZ, Ergun T, Direskeneli H. Association of salivary S. mutans colonisation and mannose-binding lectin deficiency with gender in Behçet's disease. Clinical and Experimental Rheumatology. 2009;**27**:S32–S36

[212] Hirohata S, Oka H, Mizushima Y. Streptococcal-related antigens stimulate production of IL6 and interferon-gamma by T cells from patients with Behcet's disease. Cellular Immunology. 1992;**140**:410–419

[213] Studd M, McCance DJ, Lehner T. Detection of HSV-1 DNA in patients with Behçet's syndrome and in patients with recurrent oral ulcers by the polymerase chain reaction. Medical Microbiology. 1991;**34**:39–43

[214] Kim DY, Cho S, Choi MJ, Sohn S, Lee E-S, Bang D. Immunopathogenic role of herpes simplex virus in Behçet's disease. Genetics Research International. 2013;**2013**:638273

[215] Hatemi G, Bahar H, Uysal S, Mat C, Gogus F, Masatlioglu S, et al. The pustular skin lesions in Behcet's syndrome are not sterile. Annals of the Rheumatic Diseases. 2004;**63**:1450–1452

[216] Zouboulis CC, Turnbull JR, Mühlradt PF. Association of Mycoplasma fermentans with Adamantiades-Behçet's disease. Advances in Experimental Medicine and Biology. 2003;**528**:191–194

[217] Lederberg J, McCray AT. 'Ome Sweet' omics—A genealogical treasury of words. Scientist. 2001;**15**:8

[218] Cerf-Bensussan N, Gaboriau-Routhiau V. The immune system and the gut microbiota: Friends or foes? Nature Reviews Immunology. 2010;**10**:735–744

[219] Cua DJ, Sherlock JP. Autoimmunity's collateral damage: Gut microbiota strikes 'back'. Nature Medicine. 2011;**17**:1055–1056

[220] Tringe SG, Rubin EM. Metagenomics: DNA sequencing of environmental samples. Nature Reviews Genetics. 2005;**6**:805–814

[221] Tringe SG, Hugenholtz P. A renaissance for the pioneering 16S rRNA gene. Current Opinion in Microbiology. 2008;**11**:442–446

[222] Consolandi C, Turroni S, Emmi G, Severgnini M, Fiori J, Peano C, et al. Behçet's syndrome patients exhibit specific microbiome signature. Autoimmunity Reviews. 2015;**14**:269–276

[223] Shimizu J, Kubota T, Takada E, Takai K, Fujiwara N, Arimitsu N, et al. Bifidobacteria abundance-featured gut microbiota compositional change in patients with Behcet's disease. PLoS ONE. 2016;**11**:e0153746

[224] Seoudi N, Bergmeier LA, Drobniewski F, Paster B, Fortune F. The oral mucosal and salivary microbial community of Behçet's syndrome and recurrent aphthous stomatitis. Journal of Oral Microbiology. 2015;**7**:27150

[225] Coit P, Mumcu G, Ture-Ozdemir F, Unal AU, Alpar U, Bostanci N, et al. Sequencing of 16S rRNA reveals a distinct salivary microbiome signature in Behçet's disease. Clinical Immunology. 2016;**169**:28–35

[226] Özşeker B, Şahin C, Özşeker HS, Efe SC, Kav T, Bayraktar Y. The role of fecal calprotectin in evaluating intestinal involvement of Behçet's disease. Disease Markers. 2016;**2016**:5423043

[227] Hatemi I, Hatemi G, Çelik AF. Systemic vasculitis and the gut. Current Opinion in Rheumatology. 2017;**29**:33–38

[228] Kim DH, Park Y, Kim B, Kim SW, Park SJ, Hong SP, et al. Fecal calprotectin as a non-invasive biomarker for intestinal involvement of Behçet's disease. J Gastroenterol Hepatol 2017; **32**: 595–601

[229] Bae JH, Lee SC. Effect of intravitreal methotrexate and aqueous humor cytokine levels in refractory retinal vasculitis in Behcet disease. Retina. 2012;**32**:1395–1402

[230] Ozdamar Y, Berker N, Bahar G, Soykan E, Bicer T, Ozkan SS, et al. Inflammatory mediators and posterior segment involvement in ocular Behcet disease. European Journal of Ophthalmology. 2009;**19**:998–1003

[231] Bozoglu E, Dinc A, Erdem H, Pay S, Simsek I, Kocar IH. Vascular endothelial growth factor and monocyte chemoattractant protein-1 in Behçet's patients with venous thrombosis. Clinical and Experimental Rheumatology. 2005;**23**(4 Suppl 38):S42–S48

[232] Paroli MP, Teodori C, D'Alessandro M, Mariani P, Iannucci G, Paroli M. Increased vascular endothelial growth factor levels in aqueous humor and serum of patients with quiescent uveitis. European Journal of Ophthalmology. 2007;**17**:938–942

[233] Kose O, Stewart J, Waseem A, Lalli A, Fortune F. Expression of cytokeratins, adhesion and activation molecules in oral ulcers of Behçet's disease. Clinical and Experimental Dermatology. 2008;**33**:62–69

[234] Saglam K, Yilmaz MI, Saglam A, Ulgey M, Bulucu F, Baykal Y. Levels of circulating intercellular adhesion molecule-1 in patients with Behçet's disease. Rheumatology International. 2002;**21**:146–148

[235] Haznedaroglu E, Karaaslan Y, Büyükaşik Y, Koşar A, Ozcebe O, Haznedaroglu BC, et al. Selectin adhesion molecules in Behçet's disease. Annals of the Rheumatic Diseases. 2000;**59**:61–63

[236] Sari RA, Kiziltunç A, Taysi S, Akdemir S, Gündoğdu M. Levels of soluble E-selectin in patients with active Behcet's disease. Clinical Rheumatology. 2005;**24**:55–59

[237] Seo J, Ahn Y, Zheng Z, Kim BO, Choi MJ, Bang D, et al. Clinical significance of serum YKL-40 in Behçet disease. British Journal of Dermatology. 2016;**174**:1337–1344

[238] Bilen H, Altinkaynak K, Sebin E, Aksoy H, Akcay F. Serum YKL-40 and MDA levels in Behcet disease. Journal of the Pakistan Medical Association. 2016;**66**:1299–1302

[239] Ar MC, Hatemi G, Ekizoğlu S, Bilgen H, Saçli S, Buyru AN, et al. JAK2 (V617F) mutation is not associated with thrombosis in Behcet syndrome. Clinical and Applied Thrombosis/Hemostasis. 2012;**18**:421–426

[240] Adeeb F, Tayel M, El Kaffash DM, Idris KM, Hassan MF, Fraser AD. Janus kinase 2 V617F mutation and thrombotic events in Behcet's disease: The Alexandria experience. European Journal of Rheumatology. 2016;**3**:73–74

[241] Silingardi M, Salvarani C, Boiardi L, Accardo P, Iorio A, Olivieri I, et al. Factor V Leiden and prothrombin gene G20210A mutations in Italian patients with Behçet's disease and deep vein thrombosis. Arthritis & Rheumatology. 2004;**51**:177–183

[242] Leiba M, Seligsohn U, Sidi Y, Harats D, Sela BA, Griffin JH, et al. Thrombophilic factors are not the leading cause of thrombosis in Behçet's disease. Annals of the Rheumatic Diseases. 2004;**63**:1445–1449

[243] Gurgey A, Balta G, Boyvat A. Factor V Leiden mutation and PAI-1 gene 4G/5G genotype in thrombotic patients with Behcet's disease. Blood Coagulation & Fibrinolysis. 2003;**14**:121–124

[244] Toydemir PB, Elhan AH, Tükün A, Toydemir R, Gürler A, Tüzüner A, et al. Effects of factor V gene G1691A, methylenetetrahydrofolate reductase gene C677T, and prothombin gene G20210A mutations on deep venous thrombogenesis in Behçet's disease. Journal of Rheumatology. 2000;**27**:2849–2854

[245] Seyahi E, Yurdakul S. Behçet's syndrome and thrombosis. Mediterranean Journal of Hematology and Infectious Diseases. 2011;**3**:e2011026

[246] Guillot X, Semerano L, Saidenberg-Kermanac'h N, Falgarone G, Boissier MC. Vitamin D and inflammation. Joint Bone Spine. 2010;**77**:552–557

[247] Hamzaoui K, Ben Dhifallah I, Karray E, Sassi FH, Hamzaoui A. Vitamin D modulates peripheral immunity in patients with Behçet's disease. Clinical and Experimental Rheumatology. 2010;**28**(4 Suppl 60):S50–S57

[248] Bscheider M, Butcher EC. Vitamin D immunoregulation through dendritic cells. Immunology. 2016;**148**:227–236

[249] Szymczak I, Pawliczak R. The active metabolite of vitamin D3 as a potential immunomodulator. Scandinavian Journal of Immunology. 2016;**83**:83–91

[250] Gatenby P, Lucas R, Swaminathan A. Vitamin D deficiency and risk for rheumatic diseases: An update. Current Opinion in Rheumatology. 2013;**25**:184–191

[251] Karatay S, Yildirim K, Karakuzu A, Kiziltunc A, Engin RI, Eren YB, et al. Vitamin D status in patients with Behcet's disease. Clinics (Sao Paulo) 2011;**66**:721–723

[252] Can M, Gunes M, Haliloglu OA, Haklar G, Inanç N, Yavuz DG, Direskeneli H. Effect of vitamin D deficiency and replacement on endothelial functions in Behçet's disease. Clinical and Experimental Rheumatology. 2012;**30**(3 Suppl 72):S57–S61

[253] Khabbazi A, Rashtchizadeh N, Ghorbanihaghjo A, Hajialiloo M, Ghojazadeh M, Taei R, et al. The status of serum vitamin D in patients with active Behcet's disease compared with controls. International Journal of Rheumatic Diseases. 2014;**17**:430–434

[254] Do JE, Kwon SY, Park S, Lee ES. Effects of vitamin D expression of Toll-like receptor of monocytes from patients with Behcet's disease. Rheumatology (Oxford). 2008;**47**:840–848

[255] Kechida M, Harzallah O, Hellara I, Klii R, Na eti F, Najjar MF, et al. Vitamin D status of Behcet's patients. Analysis of correlation with activity and severity of the disease as well as with the quality of life of patients. Int Arch Med 2015; **8**: 1–7

[256] Gül A. Pathogenesis of Behçet's disease: Autoinflammatory features and beyond. Seminars in Immunopathology. 2015;**37**:413–418

Chapter 4

Infectious Agents in Etiopathogenesis of Behçet's Disease

Havva Ozge Keseroglu and Müzeyyen Gönül

Additional information is available at the end of the chapter

http://dx.doi.org/10.5772/intechopen.68776

Abstract

Behçet disease (BD) is a chronic, relapsing, multisystemic vasculitis with unknown etiopathogenesis. It is widely accepted that an altered immune response triggered by an infectious agent or by an otoantigen in a genetically predisposed individual plays major role in the pathogenesis of BD. In this chapter, the role of infectious agents in the etiopathogenesis of BD was discussed.

Keywords: Behcet's disease, etiopathogenesis, infectious agent, streptococci, gut microbiota

1. Introduction

Behçet's disease (BD) is a chronic, recurrent, inflammatory, multisystemic disease characterized by oral and genital ulcerations, uveitis, and skin lesions. Although the etiopathogenesis of BD is still unknown, it is thought that the altered immune response against some environmental triggering factors in genetically susceptible individuals plays a major role in pathogenesis. It is widely accepted that endothelial injury, neutrophils, and the tendency to thrombosis also contribute to the pathogenesis of BD [1, 2]. The presence of familial cases, unusual geographical distribution of the disease, and the strong association of BD with the major histocompatibility complex (MHC), suggests that genetic factors may play a role in etiopathogenesis [1]. But, genetic factors alone are not sufficient to elucidate the etiology of BD. Today, it is believed that the disease process is triggered by an unknown infectious or environmental agent in a genetically predisposed individual [3]. The studies showing a decrease in the risk for development of BD in people who migrate from the regions with higher prevalence for BD to the regions with lower prevalence support the role of environmental factors in etiology [4]. In this chapter, possible infectious triggering factors will be discussed.

Among the environmental factors, the role of infectious agents such as bacteria (*Streptococcus, Helicobacter pylori, Mycoplasma fermentans, Mycobacteria* and *Borrelia burgdorferi*) and viruses (*Herpes simplex virus (HSV) type 1 and 2, hepatitis viruses, Cytomegalovirus, Varicella zoster virüs (VZV), Epstein-Barr virüs (EBV)* and *Parvovirus B19*) is mostly emphasized [3, 5].

A decreased positive pathergy frequency after surgical cleaning of skin before pathergy testing, the reduction of the frequency and duration of mucocutaneous findings of BD with prophylactic penicillin treatment, and the greater frequency of chronic tonsillitis and tooth decay in these patients are important findings that suggest the role of microorganisms in BD [1, 5, 6].

Oropharyngeal pathogens are the most blamed agents in pathogenesis, as almost all individuals with BD have oral aphthae [7]. After dental procedures, increased frequency of oral ulcers and activation of disease support this view [5, 8]. It has been suggested that this condition occurs as a consequence of the passage of microorganismal antigens from oral cavity into the bloodstream [5].

2. Bacteria

Because of predominancy of streptococci in oral cavity and dental infections, they are the most frequently investigated bacteria in BD. In patients with BD, it has been shown that oral hygiene is impaired and periodontal scores are high associated with disease severity [9, 10]. The proportion of *Streptococcus sanguinis* in oral flora has been found to be higher in individuals with BD than in healthy individuals [3]. Antibodies against *S. sanguinis* and *S. pyogenes* have been detected more frequently in the sera of BD patients than in the control group [5, 8]. In one study, oral ulceration had occurred after application of streptococcal antigens to the oral mucosa by prick test [5]. It has been suggested that streptococci penetrate to the oral mucosa with their enzymes such as IgA 1 protease and neuraminidase and lead to the development of hypersensitivity against streptococci in BD individuals [5]. There are studies suggesting that, in addition to *S. sanguinis* there may be an association between *S. pyogenes, Streptococcus faecalis, Streptococcus viridans, Streptococcus haemolyticus,* and *Streptococcus salivarius* with BD [5, 8].

In addition to streptococcal antigens, it was shown that a common non-peptide antigen present in many bacteria, such as *Escherichia coli, Staphylococcus aureus,* can also activate $\gamma\delta$-T cells in BD. This finding suggests that T lymphocytes of BD patients are hyperactive to bacterial antigens in general, not against a specific bacteria [3, 7, 11]. In one study, it was shown that T cells in BD patients are stimulated with staphylococcal enterotoxins even at low concentrations that could be achieved under physiological conditions and stimulate IFN-γ production much more than the control group. The increased sensitivity of patients T cells to the several bacterial antigens may explain the exacerbation of systemic symptoms of BD after infections, dental caries treatments, operations, or trauma [11].

H. pylori is another bacteria that have been investigated in relation to BD [12–14]. In some studies, the prevalence of *H. pylori* was found to be high in patients with BD, and it was suggested that there was a relationship between the presence of *H. pylori* and gastrointestinal involvement [12, 14]. Although improvement in symptoms of BD after *H. pylori* eradication treatment have been reported in some uncontrolled studies, there are studies that do not support this [5, 14].

There are reports that some other bacteria, such as *M. fermentans, Mycobacteria, Prevotella, Fusobacterium* and *B. burgdorferi,* also induce BD, but there is no strong correlation with them [3, 5].

3. Viruses

The possible etiological relationship between viral infections and BD has been first suggested by Hulusi Behçet, due to the observation of intracellular inclusion bodies in specimens taken from aphthous lesions and was investigated by many researchers [6]. The HSV-1 genome was detected in oral and genital ulcers of BD patients [3, 6]. The amount of HSV-1 DNA in leukocytes, blood and saliva samples, and the anti-HSV-1 antibodies in serum samples of BD patients were found to be significantly higher than control group [5, 6]. The presence of immunocomplexes containing HSV-1 antigen in the blood has also been reported [15]. Besides these studies supporting the role of HSV in etiology, the results of several other studies in which HSV DNA could not be demonstrated in leukocytes, oral, and genital ulcers of BD and, improvement in clinical symptoms could not be obtained with antiviral therapy against HSV virus, have lead to giving up the hypothesis that HSV plays a role in the development of BD [3, 5]. However, in the light of today's information, it is thought that the immune response to HSV infection rather than active infection with HSV may play a role in the pathogenesis of the disease [5].

Since hepatitis viruses play a role in many vasculitic diseases, their role in the etiology of BH has been investigated. Although, in one study, *Hepatitis B virus* was detected more frequently in patients with BD, *Hepatitis A, B, C, E* and *G* viruses have not been shown to be associated with BD [5].

Parvovirus B19, considered to be the causative agent in the development of numerous vasculitic diseases, has been detected more frequently in non-ulcerous lesions of BD, such as erythema nodosum, papulopustular reactions, than genital and extragenital ulcers and control skin biopsies but these results are not enough to prove the role of parvoviruses in BD [5, 16].

In addition to these viruses, it has been suggested that there may also be a relationship between *human immunodeficiency virus, VZV, Cytomegalovirus, EBV* and BD, but this relationship has not been proved [5].

Although many infectious agents have been suggested in the etiopathogenesis of BD, there is no definitely proven or isolated microorganism that plays a role in etiology. For this reason, it is now widely accepted that BD does not originate directly from infectious agents, but microorganisms alter immune response leading to autoimmune and inflammatory diseases. So, the studies have shifted on the role of the heat shock proteins (HSP), the cytokine profile changes and, the T cell hypersensitivity.

4. Heat shock proteins

The more accepted view about the role of microorganisms in the etiology of BD is that the microorganisms mentioned in the etiology carry some antigens (HSP, etc.) which are similar to the human proteins and the resulting cross-reaction is the cause of the immunological response [4, 15, 17]. HSP is a group of proteins that are synthesized by all eukaryotic and prokaryotic cells, as a result of physiological shock (heat, anoxia, trauma, etc.) and microbial stimulus, and are expressed on the cell membrane [1, 3]. These proteins protect the cells from severe damage and premature death (apoptosis) [3]. Bacterial 65-kDa HSP (HSP65), which was isolated from mycobacterium at first, exhibits a largely similar amino acid sequence with human mitochondrial 60-kDa HSP (HSP60), and it is thought that the cross-reaction between them result in immune response [4, 17]. It is postulated that human HSP60-specific autoreactive T cell clones are formed as a result of this cross-reaction and immunopathological changes of BD occur [8]. HSP60 can lead to production of proinflammatory cytokines (IL6, IL12, IL15, and TNF-a), expression of cell adhesion molecules (ICAM and VCAM) and Th1 immune response by binding to Toll-like receptors 2 and 4 [3].

5. Molecular similarity

Retinal S antigen present in the retina shows homology with HLA-B51 and HLA-B27. Immune-mediated response to retinal S antigen develops only due to retinal damage after uveitis [4]. These data suggest that Retinal S antigen may play a role in the pathogenesis of BD through molecular similarity [3].

Bes-1, a *S. sanguinis* gene, was found in the monocytes in mucocutaneous lesions of BD. The more than 60% similarity of the amino acid sequence of the *Bes-1* gene with the human intraocular ganglion peptide, Brn-3b, suggests that the uveitis in BD may occur due to molecular similarity between the microbial and host antigens [18].

6. Antimicrobial peptides

Another research topic related to environmental factors is antimicrobial peptides. Çiçek et al. found serum and saliva concentration of hepcidin, an antimicrobial peptide, in patients with BD and recurrent aphthous stomatitis are lower than in the control group and concluded that low hepcidin levels may be associated with oral aphthous lesion development [19].

7. Mannose-binding lectins

Mannose-binding lectins (MBL), part of natural immunity, bind to mannose and N-acetylglucosaminomines on the surface of many microorganisms and lead killing of them by complement activation [5]. It is thought that the low level of mannose-binding lectin detected in BD correlates with disease activity and is associated with the colonization of *S. aureus* in pustular lesions [20].

8. Gut microbiota

Recent data indicate that gut microbiota plays an important role in human health. The dysbiosis of gut microbiota has been implicated in the etiopathogenesis of many diseases. In a recent study, comparing gut microbiota of patients with BD and healthy controls, the genera Roseburia and Subdoligranulum were found to be significantly depleted in patients with BD. Also, the butyrate production was found to be significantly decreased in these patients [21].

9. Conclusion

The etiopathogenesis of BD is still unclear. Although many infectious agents have been proposed in the etiopathogenesis, there is no definitely proven or isolated microorganism that plays a role in etiology. Today, it is believed that the altered immune response against an unknown infectious triggering agent in genetically susceptible individuals may play a role in the pathogenesis of BD.

Author details

Havva Özge Keseroglu* and Müzeyyen Gönül

*Address all correspondence to: ozgederm@yahoo.com

Department of Dermatology, Ankara Dışkapı Yıldırım Beyazıt Education and Research Hospital, Ankara, Turkey

References

[1] Mendoza-Pinto C, García-Carrasco M, Jiménez-Hernández M, Jiménez Hernández C, Riebeling-Navarro C, Nava Zavala A, Vera Recabarren M, Espinosa G, Jara Quezada J, Cervera R. Etiopathogenesis of Behcet's disease. Autoimmunity Reviews. 2010;**9**:241–245. DOI: 10.1016/j.autrev.2009.10.005

[2] Garton RA, Jorizzo JL. Behçet's disease. In: Freedberg IM, Eisen AZ, Wolff K, Frank Austen K, Goldsmith LA, Katz SI, editors. Fitzpatrick's Dermatology. In: General Medicine. 6th ed. New York: McGraw-Hill Companies; 2003. pp. 1836–1840

[3] Pineton de Chambrun M, Wechsler B, Geri G, Cacoub P, Saadoun D. New insights into the pathogenesis of Behçet's disease. Autoimmunity Reviews. 2012;**11**:687–698. DOI: 10.1016/j.autrev.2011.11.026

[4] Mendes D, Correia M, Barbedo M, Vaio T, Mota M, Gonçalves O, Valente J. Behçet's disease—A contemporary review. Journal of Autoimmunity. 2009;**32**:178–188. DOI: 10.1016/j.jaut.2009.02.011

[5] Hatemi G, Yazici H. Behçet's syndrome and micro-organisms. Best Practice & Research: Clinical Rheumatology. 2011;**25**:389–406. DOI: 10.1016/j.berh.2011.05.002

[6] Onder M, Gürer MA. Behçet's disease: An enigmatic vasculitis. Clinics in Dermatology. 1999;**17**:571–576

[7] Dalvi SR, Yildirim R, Yazici Y. Behcet's Syndrome. Drugs. 2012;**72**:2223–2241. DOI: 10.2165/11641370-000000000-00000

[8] Akman A, Alpsoy E. Behcet's disease: Current aspects in the etiopathogenesis. Turkderm 2009;**43**:32–38

[9] Mumcu G, Inanc N, Ergun T, Ikiz K, Gunes M, Islek U, Yavuz S, Sur H, Atalay T, Direskeneli H. Oral health related quality of life is affected by disease activity in Behçet's disease. Oral Diseases. 2006;**12**:145–151

[10] Akman A, Kacaroglu H, Donmez L, Bacanli A, Alpsoy E. Relationship between periodontal findings and Behçet's disease: A controlled study. Journal of Clinical Periodontology. 2007;**34**:485–491

[11] Hirohata S, Hashimoto T. Abnormal T cell responses to bacterial superantigens in Behçet's disease (BD). Clinical & Experimental Immunology. 1998;**112**:317–324

[12] Hatemi G, Seyahi E, Fresko I, Talarico R, Hamuryudan V. Behçet's syndrome: A critical digest of the 2013–2014 literature. Clinical and Experimental Rheumatology. 2014;**32**: 112–122

[13] Cakmak SK, Cakmak A, Gül U, Sulaimanov M, Bingöl P, Hazinedaroğlu MS. Upper gastrointestinal abnormalities and Helicobacter pylori in Behçet's disease. International Journal of Dermatology. 2009;**48**:1174–1176. DOI: 10.1111/j.1365-4632.2009.04145

[14] Yildirim B, Oztürk MA, Unal S. The anti-Helicobacter pylori antibiotherapy for the treatment of recurrent oral aphthous ulcers in a patient with Behcet's syndrome. Rheumatology International. 2009;**29**:477–478. DOI: 10.1007/s00296-008-0709-2

[15] Direskeneli H. Behçet's disease: Infectious aetiology, new autoantigens, and HLA-B51. Annals of the Rheumatic Diseases. 2001;**60**:996–1002

[16] Baskan EB, Yilmaz E, Saricaoglu H, Alkan G, Ercan I, Mistik R, Adim SB, Goral G, Dilek K, Tunali S. Detection of parvovirus B19 DNA in the lesional skin of patients with Behçet's disease. Clinical and Experimental Dermatology. 2007;**32**:186–190

[17] Ergun T, Ince U, Ekşioğlu-Demiralp E, Direskeneli H, Gürbüz O, Gürses L, Aker F, Akoğlu T. HSP 60 expression in mucocutaneous lesions of Behçet's disease. Journal of the American Academy of Dermatology. 2001;**45**:904–909

[18] Neves FS, Spiller F. Possible mechanisms of neutrophil activation in Behçet's disease. International Immunopharmacology. 2013;**17**:1206–1210. DOI: 10.1016/j.intimp.2013.07.017

[19] Cicek D, Dağlı AF, Aydin S, Baskaya Dogan F, Dertlioğlu SB, Uçak H, Demir B. Does hepcidin play a role in the pathogenesis of aphthae in Behçet's disease and recurrent aphthous stomatitis? Journal of the European Academy of Dermatology and Venereology. 2014;**28**:1500–1506. DOI: 10.1111/jdv.12326

[20] Yurdakul S, Yazici H. Behçet's syndrome. Best Practice & Research: Clinical Rheumatology. 2008;**22**:793–809. DOI: 10.1016/j.berh.2008.08.005

[21] Consolandi C, Turroni S, Emmi G, Severgnini M, Fiori J, Peano C, Biagi E, Grassi A, Rampelli S, Silvestri E, Centanni M, Cianchi F, Gotti R, Emmi L, Brigidi P, Bizzaro N, De Bellis G, Prisco D, Candela M, D'Elios MM. Behçet's syndrome patients exhibit specific microbiome signature. Autoimmunity Reviews. 2015;**14**:269–276. DOI: 10.1016/j.autrev.2014.11.009

Chapter 5

Mucocutaneous Findings in Behçet's Disease

Arzu Kilic

Additional information is available at the end of the chapter

http://dx.doi.org/10.5772/67841

Abstract

Behçet's disease is a chronic inflammatory disease with an unpredictable course. The disease may affect almost all organ systems resulting with significant organ-threatening morbidity and mortality. Mucocutaneous lesions mostly constitute the initial symptoms of the disease and precede other manifestations. As there is yet no pathognomonic diagnostic test in Behçet's disease, the recognition of cutaneous and mucosal findings let the physician enable an earlier diagnosis and earlier treatment. Therefore, the purpose of this chapter is to emphasize the importance of the mucocutaneous manifestations of Behçet's disease and to review the mucocutaneous lesions in detail. Finally, childhood Behçet's disease, differential diagnosis and treatment of mucocutaneous manifestations will be briefly reviewed.

Keywords: Behçet's disease, mucocutaneous manifestations, oral ulcer, genital ulcer, papulopustular lesions, pathergy test

1. Introduction

Behçet's disease (BD) is a chronic, relapsing inflammatory multi-systemic disease of unknown etiology with a course of exacerbations and remissions [1–4]. Prevalence of BD is higher in countries lying along the ancient Silk Road, extending from eastern Mediterranean to East Asia [5]. Turkey probably has the highest occurrence level of the disease with prevalences of 110–420 cases per 100,000 population [6–8]. Today, due to immigrations, BD is encountered almost all over the world [9, 10].

The disease was first defined in 1937 by the Turkish dermatologist named as 'Hulusi Behçet' with the presence of 'triple symptom complex' of recurrent oral ulcers (OU), genital ulcers

(GU) and uveitis [1]. After the initial description, it now became increasingly evident that BD is a multi-systemic disease with involvement of mucocutaneous, vascular, neurological, musculoskeletal and gastrointestinal systems with significant morbidity and mortality [2, 3, 9, 11, 12]. The main histopathological finding is the vasculitis of the arteries and veins of any size or thrombophilia according to the site of involvement [13].

Although the exact etiopathogenesis of BD is still unknown, it has been hypothesized that in genetically predisposed individuals, a development of an inflammatory reaction against to an infectious, an environmental or an autoantigen and/or the presence of disturbances in molecular mechanisms in regulating immune responses may contribute to the disease [2, 3, 11, 14–17].

Today, most of the authors classify BD as a group of systemic vasculitis (under the title of variable vessel vasculitis) as a result of the consensus; '2012 Revised International Chapel Hill Consensus Conference Nomenclature of Vasculitides' [18].

The first symptoms of BD usually occur in the third and fourth decade of life [2, 4, 9, 19]. However, childhood cases have also been reported [20]. Juvenile BD was found in 7.7% and family history was found in 11.6% of the patients in the study reported by Alpsoy et al. [21]. In another study by Gurler et al., the presence of family history in the first degree relatives of patients with BD has been reported as 7.3% [22]. Male patients, a younger onset and HLA-B51 positive patients are found to have more severe kind of the disease [11, 21, 23, 24]. Contrary to these results, Davatchi et al. found no association between severe organ involvement and male gender except vascular involvement [25]. Clinical features of BD include OU, GU, ocular inflammation, cutaneous lesions, as well as articular, vascular, neurological, pulmonary, gastrointestinal, renal and genitourinary manifestations [2–4, 11]. BD may start with just one or two symptoms but other symptoms may gradually appear over the years [19, 22, 24, 26–29].

As there is no pathognomonic test, the diagnosis of BD depends on clinical criteria [3]. In 1990, the International Study Group (ISG) for BD defined new diagnostic criteria by reviewing the data of 914 patients from 12 centres in seven countries around the world. The ISG criteria for BD have a sensitivity of 92% and specificity of 97%, compared with previous sets of criteria. According to these criteria, the diagnosis of BD consists of the presence of recurrent OU in addition to two of the following features: GU, eye involvement, skin lesions and positive skin pathergy test. At minimum three episodes of oral aphthous ulcer in a year should be observed for the diagnosis of BD [30]. In order to increase the sensitivity and specificity, these criteria are re-assessed and revised [31]. Since patients may present with only OU for a long time showing a long prediagnostic duration [19, 22, 32].

Various studies from different countries have documented that mucocutaneous manifestations are the most common, and often the first signs of the disease [2, 3, 9, 11, 21, 22, 24, 26–29, 33–37]. Mucocutaneous findings are the hallmarks of the disease and recognition of them have a great importance in confirming the diagnosis, in the follow up and in preventing both the morbidity and mortality [2, 3, 19, 21, 26, 28].

http://dx.doi.org/10.5772/67841

This chapter aims not only to define the mucocutaneous lesions but also to elaborate the features of the mucosal and cutaneous lesions in detail. Furthermore, mucocutaneous lesions in paediatric BD, differential diagnoses and the management of the mucocutaneous lesions will briefly be reviewed.

2. Mucocutaneous manifestations

Mucocutaneous manifestations that are observed in the course of BD are as follows: OU, GU, erythema nodosum (EN)-like lesions, papulopustular (PPL) lesions, superficial thrombophlebitis (TFB), extragenital ulcers, Sweet's syndrome-like lesions, cutaneous vasculitic lesions, pyoderma gangrenosum (PG)-like lesions, erythema multiforme-like lesions and skin pathergy test (SPT) [2–4, 9, 32].

The above-mentioned mucocutaneous lesions may be the initial findings of BD or may be observed at any time during the course of the disease [21, 22, 24, 28, 29]. Especially, OU is the most commonly detected lesion and mostly emerges as the initial clinical finding of the disease [2, 3, 19, 21, 33–37]. OU and GU are mostly considered as the 'fingerprint lesions'. As there is yet no pathognomonic test for the diagnosis of BD, recognition of these mucocutaneous lesions let the clinician make an earlier diagnosis, which also enables an earlier treatment [2, 3].

2.1. Oral ulcers

Oral ulcers (OUs) manifest in the majority of BD patients with a ratio of 92–100% in all countries [2–4, 6, 10, 21, 22, 27, 28, 33]. The majority of the patients experience OU as the most common presenting clinical manifestation [21, 22, 24, 26, 28, 34, 37]. For the diagnosis of BD, the presence of recurrent OU is obligatory according to criteria of ISG [4, 30].

OUs are recurrent and painful ulcerations of the oral mucosa characterized by a round or oval ulceration with sharp borders surrounded by a red erythematous inflammatory area (**Figure 1**). The base of the OU is necrotic with a yellowish-white colour. The most common sites are the mucous membranes of the lips, buccal mucosae, tongue, uvula and soft palate [2, 3, 22]. Clinically, they look like similar in appearance with conventional aphthae that may be seen in several systemic diseases such as inflammatory bowel disease, Sweet syndrome, systemic lupus erythematosus or recurrent aphthous stomatitis (RAS) [2, 12, 32]. OU in BD tends to recur more frequently and to be more in number [38]. Main and Chamberlain reported that OUs in BD have a more diffuse erythematous surrounding rim, they are localized more often in soft palate and oropharynx and they are more in number when compared with the aphthae of RAS [39]. However, no difference was found in terms of frequency of OU between the two groups [39].

OUs are usually classified into three groups based on the diameter of the ulcer [2, 11]:

1. Minor aphthae are shallow mucosal ulcers with a diameter less than 10 mm. It usually spontaneously regresses in a couple of weeks without formation of scarring.

2. Major aphthae have a deeper morphology with a diameter larger than 10 mm. Healing usually occurs in 3–4 weeks with scarring.

3. Herpetiform aphthae are pinpoint shaped, very small and shallow mucosal ulcers and localized in crops.

The majority of the patients were found to have minor aphthous ulcer (75%) followed by herpetiform (20%) and major aphthae (5%) in the study of Vaiopoulos et al. [36]. Different sizes and types of OU may be seen at the same time in oral mucosa in BD [9]. A study comparing the characteristics of OU between BD and RAS was performed by Oh et al. They reported that major OUs were significantly more common in patients with BD, and initiation of OU in BD was more likely related to menstrual cycle when compared with OU in patients with RAS. In addition, they also concluded that patients with major aphthae who have accompanying articular symptoms as initial symptoms should be strictly followed for the possible development of BD [40].

Ideguchi et al. evaluated 412 BD patients' data including 16 years follow-up. The results revealed that a mean of 7.5 years has been proceeded before a definitive diagnosis of BD. In the same study, 14% of the patients had suffered from OU for more than 20 years before the diagnosis of BD [19].

In two different studies reported by Alpsoy et al., the mean duration between the OU and the fulfilment of diagnostic criteria was determined to be 4.3 ± 5.7 and 3.77 ± 4.43 years, respectively,

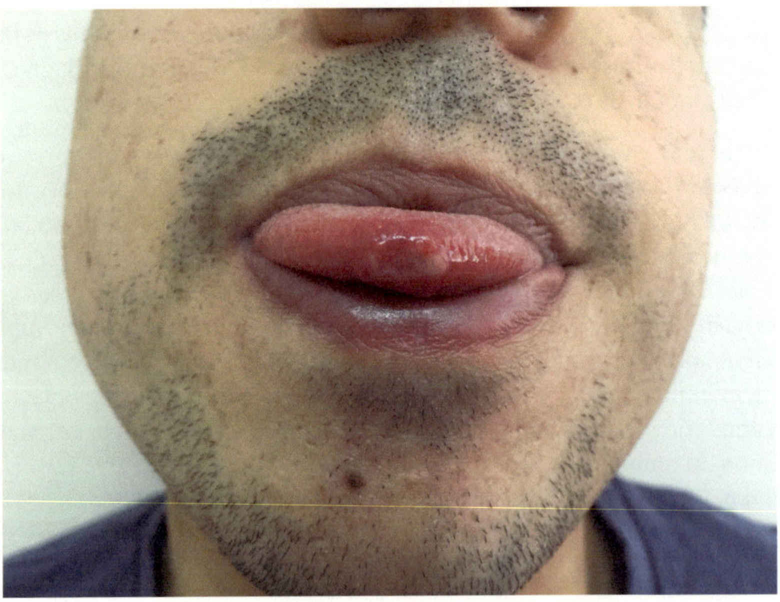

Figure 1. Aphthous ulcer on the tongue in the patient of Behçet's Disease (Courtesy of MD. Assoc. Prof. Müzeyyen Gönül).

and it has been concluded that the disease is often diagnosed with a delay of several years after the appearance of the first sign [21, 26].

Although OUs are the most common and earliest manifestation of BD, a few studies have been reported indicating a course without the presence of OU at the onset of BD [27, 41–44]. On the basis of this issue, Faezi et al. evaluated the clinical features on 175 patients with BD who do not have oral aphthosis (NOA) and compared them with the patients with OU. The results revealed that the first manifestation was uveitis with a ratio of 70.3% in the NOA group, and a pathergy test was more common in NOA group [41].

2.2. Genital ulcers

Genital ulcers (GUs) are generally the second most frequent disease manifestation [2, 9, 21, 26, 28, 45, 46]. GUs are observed in approximately 60–97% of the patients with BD at any time of the course of the disease [4, 19, 21, 22, 28, 36, 43, 47]. The lowest frequency was reported from Romania with a ratio of 55.5% [43]. As an initial symptom, GU was found in 14.2 and 7.4% of the patients with BD in two different studies from Turkey [21, 22] while in only 4% of the patients with BD in a study from Moscow [34].

GUs are usually localized on the scrotum and on the shaft of the penis in male patients while on the labium major and minor in females (**Figures 2** and **3**). They are rarely seen in the vagina and cervix in females and on the urethral orifice and glans penis in males [2, 3, 9, 11, 22]. They are usually painful or very rarely they can be asymptomatic [2]. They have mostly the same characteristic morphological features of OU. The clinical differences from oral aphthous ulcer include that GUs are larger and deeper, have more irregular borders and a longer healing duration. In addition, GU recurs less often and heal with scarring [3, 32, 48]. Therefore, in the suspicion of diagnosis of BD, scatris of GU on genital region should also be searched.

While some studies have documented higher frequency of GU among one of the genders [21, 24, 35], some did not detect any difference between the two genders [23, 25, 34]. Gender differences (Male>female) at the onset of GU have been observed in the study by Vaiopoulos et al. [36].

GU may cause severe pain, difficulty in micturition, dyspareunia and marked difficulty in physical activity. Deep ulcers located in vagina may be complicated by fistulisation to bladder, urethra or rectum [2–4, 9].

Mat et al. reported a prospective study investigating the frequency of scarring after GU. This study revealed that healing with scarring was observed in 49% of small GU while in 89% of large ulcers. They stated that ulcers on labium minors and vestibule may heal even without scar formation [48].

Faezi et al. reported 64.7% of 6935 cases with BD had GU during the course of the disease. They compared clinical and laboratory features between the patients with GU and patients who never developed GU (non-GU cases). As a result of their study, OU and other cutaneous manifestations such as pseudofolliculitis and erythema nodosum were found to be higher while eye involvement was found to be less common in the GU group [46].

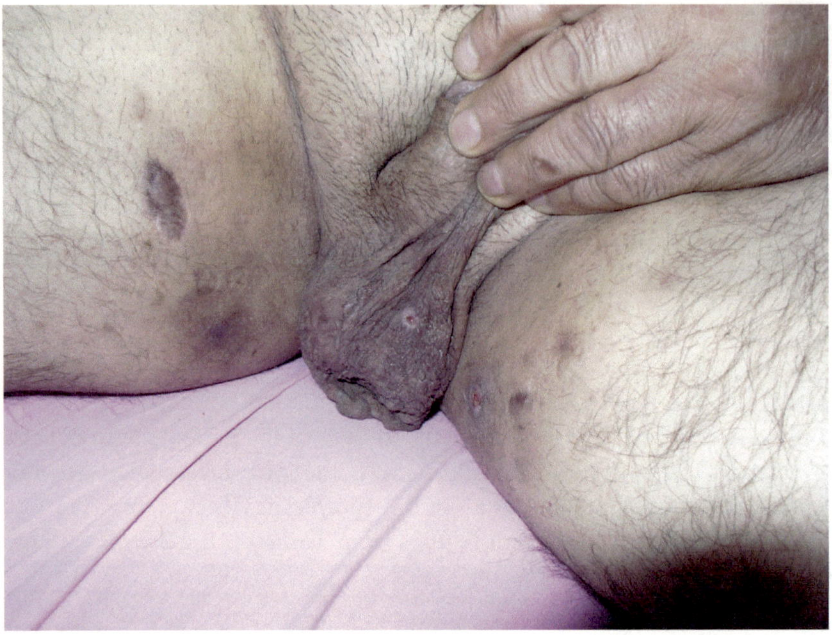

Figure 2. Genital, extragenital ulcers and their scars in male patient with Behçet's Disease (Courtesy of MD. Assoc. Prof. Müzeyyen Gönül).

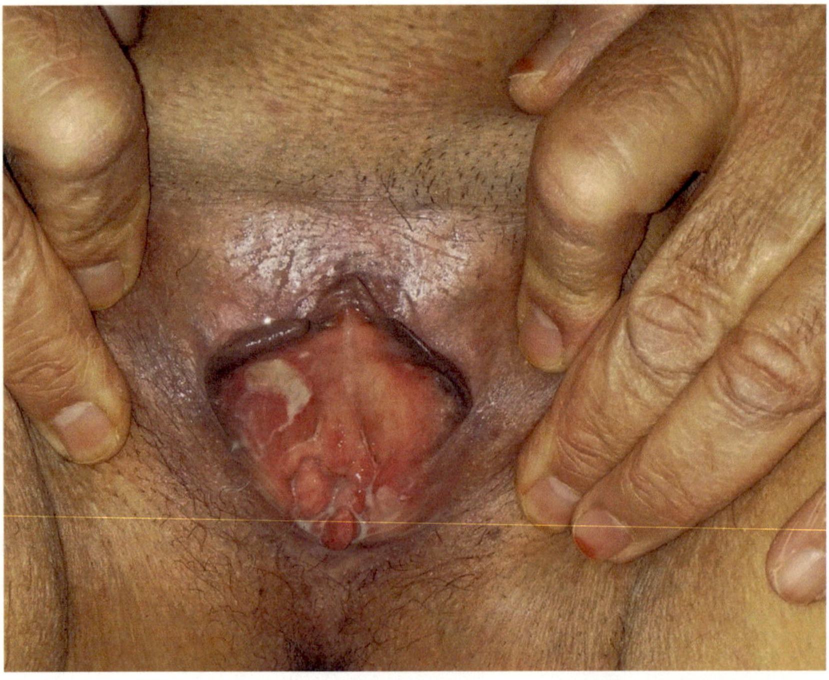

Figure 3. Genital ulcer in female patient with Behçet's Disease (Courtesy of MD. Assoc. Prof. Müzeyyen Gönül).

http://dx.doi.org/10.5772/67841

2.3. Cutaneous lesions

2.3.1. Papulopustular lesions

Papulopustular lesions (PPLs), which are also called as pseudofolliculitis or Behcet's pustulosis, are dome-shaped papules, which will convert into sterile pustule with an erythematous and edematous base [2–4]. Sometimes it can be localized around a hair follicle [9]. They are commonly seen lesions in BD [2–4]. Various studies have reported an incidence ranging between 25 and 55% [21, 22, 28, 33, 36]. PPLs have also been reported as an onset sign [22].

PPLs are usually localized on the trunk, buttocks and extremities [2, 3, 49]. However, they may be observed on any part of the body and even on palmoplantar regions [9]. In case of face and chest localization, especially in adolescence period, it may be hard to distinguish PPL from an ordinary papul/pustule of acne or folliculitis [2].

PPLs were found to occur more frequently in male patients than females in a study by Tursen et al. [35]. PPLs were found to occur more in patients with positive pathergy test [49].

Since PPLs are non-specific and resemble to ordinary acne pustules and/or folliculitis; some authors suggest that non-follicular lesions located other than face are more valuable for the diagnosis of BD [2, 27, 49] while some suggest that PPL should not be included as a diagnostic criteria [50]. It is suggested to accept PPL as a diagnostic criteria only if leukocytoclastic vasculitis or a neutrophilic reaction histopathologically is detected [2, 50].

A study by Kalkan et al. reported the histopathological evaluation of 42 biopsy specimens of papulopustular lesions of patients with BD. The results revealed leukocytoclastic vasculitis in seven specimens, lymphocytic vasculitis in three, superficial perivascular and/or interstitial infiltration in 15 and folliculitis/perifolliculitis in five. No histopathological finding of vasculitis was observed in the biopsy specimens of pustular lesions of the patients with acne vulgaris in the control group [51].

Another study by Ilknur et al. reported a statistically higher ratio of lymphocytic/leukocytoclastic vasculitis pattern in the histopathological evaluation of pustular lesions of the patients with BD compared with the control group. However, direct immunofluorescence examinations investigating the deposition of IgM, IgG, IgA, C3 or fibrinogen in dermal blood vessels revealed no difference between the two groups [52].

Chen et al. reported either lymphocytic or leukocytoclastic vasculitis of the 20 biopsy specimens performed from cutaneous lesions of BD. Eight of the 20 biopsy specimens in which vasculitis detected histopathologically was clinically compatible with PPL [53].

Contrary to these studies, Kutlubay et al. compared the number and histopathological features of PPL between patients with BD and acne vulgaris, as a result, Kutlubay et al. assessed a higher number of PPL on the back and extremities in BD group. However, histopathological interpretation was not found to be useful in differentiating PPL between two entities [54].

2.3.2. *Erythema nodosum-like lesions*

Erythema nodosum (EN)-like lesions are frequently observed skin lesions in patients with BD [9]. The incidences of EN-like lesions have been reported between 15 and 60% in various studies [21, 22, 24, 28, 55, 56]. In 2.8% of the patients with BD, EN-like lesions have been reported as an initial symptom [22]. They are more common in female patients [23, 24, 36, 55]. They are characterized by multiple painful subcutaneous nodules with different sizes. Although they are preferentially located on the lower limbs, they may also be localized on gluteal region, upper extremities and neck [2, 3, 9, 22, 55]. They heal within 10–20 days without secondary ulceration and scatris formation. The resolution generally results with residual hyperpigmentation [2, 3]. The clinical features of EN-like lesions resemble conventional EN [2, 3, 9, 11]. However, it has been noted that EN-like lesions have more erythema and oedema around the lesions than the classical EN [57]. Coskun et al. reported that the presence of EN-like lesions precede visceral involvement [55]. Faezi et al. found less common EN-like lesions among the group of BD without OA in their study in which they compared the two groups with OA and without OA [41]. Cebeci et al. compared the clinical features of two groups with and without deep vein thrombosis (DVT) in BD and found more common EN-like lesions in the group with DVT suggesting that patients with EN-like lesions should be followed up for a possible DVT [58].

The evaluation of the histopathological features of biopsy specimens performed from EN-like lesions has been reported in various studies [57, 59, 60]. Chun et al. detected focal lymphocytic vasculitis in 40% of the cases with EN-like lesions of patients with BD and suggested this finding to occur secondary to severe lymphocytic infiltration. On the rest of the cases, the histopathological changes have been found similar to conventional EN [59]. In contrary, two different studies revealed the presence of vasculitis in biopsy specimens performed from EN-like lesions of patients with BD [57, 60].

Misago evaluated the clinicopathological features of EN-like lesions in 26 patients with BD and revealed the presence of vasculitis histopathologically in 73% of the cases. In addition, they suggested that the presence of severe vasculitis, especially phlebitis, was associated with a severe disease course [57].

A study by Demirkesen et al. compared the distinguishing histopathological features of the biopsy specimens taken from EN-like lesions of BD, nodular lesions of nodular vasculitis (NV) and conventional EN. Their results revealed neutrophil-predominating infiltrate in the sub-cutis and vein involvement to be more common in EN-like lesions when compared with NV and EN [60].

2.3.3. *Superficial thrombophlebitis*

BD may affect all types of vessels [3, 11, 61]. The prevalence of vascular involvement in BD has been reported to be between 2.2 and 50% in different patient populations [4, 6, 43, 62–64]. The venous system is the major affected site [9, 11, 61–65]. Superficial thrombophlebitis (TFB) is seen in approximately 4.9–20% of the patients with BD, and it is more frequently seen in male patients [6, 28, 29]. Sarica-Kucukoglu et al. reported superficial TFB as the most common vascular symptom with a prevalence of 53.3% [62].

Superficial TFB is mostly characterized by linearly arranged erythematous subcutaneous nodules in lower extremities that migrate from day to day. The vein can be palpated as a string-like hardening showing the thrombosis and vessel sclerosis [2, 3]. EN-like lesions and migratory TFB may be thought as the differential diagnosis [2, 3]. Superficial TFB is clinically important since it is frequently associated with other forms of vascular disease in BD [2, 63].

2.3.4. *Extragenital ulcers*

Extragenital ulcer (EGU) is usually a solitary, small, round ulcer with a red rim and yellow base; however, it may have various shapes and sizes [2, 3, 32, 65]. Although observed rarely, it is the most characteristic and specific lesions of BD [2, 65]. EGU may be localized anywhere on the body such as legs, axillae, breast, interdigital skin of the foot, neck and inguinal regions. EGU may persist for a long duration, may be painful and heals usually with scarring [2, 3]. In a report of Azizlerli et al., four cases of EGU were shown to reveal vasculitis histopathologically [65].

A study reported by Ozyurt et al. detected that the patients with family history of BD had more frequent EGU than patients with negative family history of BD [66].

Few series documented common EGU in children [67, 68]. However, due to rarity of BD in childhood and few reports concerning the clinical findings in children with BD, the characteristics of the disease in this age group are not completely described [67–69].

2.3.5. *Sweet's syndrome-like lesions*

Few cases of Sweet's syndrome-like lesions have been reported in patients with BD [70–77]. Sweet's syndrome-like lesions are characterized by painful, edematous papules, plaques and nodules localized on face, neck and back [3, 70–75]. Fever and laboratory findings such as leukocytosis, elevated erythrocyte sedimentation rate and C-reactive protein accompany to the cutaneous lesions [73, 74]. Although clinical and histological overlap exists between Sweet's syndrome and BD such as the presence of OU, arthralgia, arthritis, episcleritis, pathergy positivity and neutrophilic infiltrate in the dermis in both of the diseases, there are some distinguishing features. In BD, the development of OU is more frequent, fever is rarely seen, the pattern of articular and ocular involvement is different [3]. In addition, comparing two diseases by human leucocyte antigen (HLA) typing revealed that patients with BD had higher frequencies of HLA-B51 and HLA-Dqw3, while patients with Sweet's syndrome had higher frequencies of HLA-Bw4 [77]. Sweet's syndrome-like lesions have been reported to occur in the acute phase of BD or sometimes have been thought to point a flare in BD [73].

2.3.6. *Pyoderma gangrenosum-like lesions*

Pyoderma gangrenosum (PG) is another rare neutrophilic dermatosis that may be associated with BD [78, 79]. Rare cases of PG-like lesions in patients with BD have been addressed

[78–85]. The lesion is usually characterized by large superficial ulceration localized usually on the buttock or the lower limbs; however, it may reveal vegetative or bullous variants [9, 79, 81]. Both diseases may have clinical and histopathological overlap. The patients with PG may also have OU, GU and pathergy positivity [78, 79]. However, as mentioned above, the frequency of OU and GU is higher in BD. It has been reported that PG is associated with the activation of BD [78, 79, 85]. Also, Hali et al. reported two paediatric cases of BD and PG with a fatal outcome [84].

2.3.7. *Rare cutaneous lesions*

Other rare cutaneous lesions such as palpable purpura, haemorrhagic bullae, necrotizing vasculitic lesions, Henoch Schoenlein purpura, polyarteritis nodosa-like lesions, pernio-like lesions, erythema multiforme-like lesions, acral purpuric papulonodular lesions, furoncles and abscess may also occur in the course of BD [2, 3, 70, 86–97]. It has been suggested that lesions of periarteritis nodosa appear as a marker of the severity of BD [91, 92]. These cutaneous lesions are mostly presented as case reports [86–97]. It is not clear whether these dermatological manifestations are real associations or coincidental. Therefore, it has been postulated that only lesions of 'leukocytoclastic vasculitis' detected in histopathological examination should be evaluated as a cutaneous sign of BD [2, 53, 98, 99].

2.3.8. *Rare mucosal lesions*

Conjunctival ulceration has been reported as a manifestation of BD in a few reports [100–104]. Although it is a rare finding, it has been suggested to be a specific clue for establishing the diagnosis [102, 103].

2.4. Skin pathergy test

Skin pathergy test (SPT) is a non-specific hyperreactive reaction of the skin that occurs as a response to a minor trauma such as a needle prick [2, 3]. SPT was first described by Blobner in 1937 [70, 105]. It is used as an adjunctive test in the diagnosis of BD and according to the ISG criteria for BD, a positive SPT is a criteria needed for the diagnosis of BD [2, 3, 30, 70, 105].

Positive SPT is defined as the development of erythematous, indurated papule which usually evolves into a sterile pustule at the site of the needle puncture after 24–48 hours (**Figure 4**) [70, 105]. Although the exact mechanism of the SPT is still not known, it is thought to occur as a result of enhanced non-specific inflammatory response and aberrant release of cytokines triggered by the cutaneous injury [13]. A number of studies investigating the histopathological examinations of positive SPT reaction (papule/pustule) revealed findings ranging from mononuclear cell infiltration at varying densities in perivascular or periadnexal areas to leukocytoclastic vasculitis [106–110]. Ergun et al. evaluated a chronological histopathological study of sites of SPT and observed intraepidermal pustules and polymorphonuclear infiltrate at the beginning of the inflammation [108]. Androjen receptor levels were found higher in positive SPT sites when compared with normal skin [111].

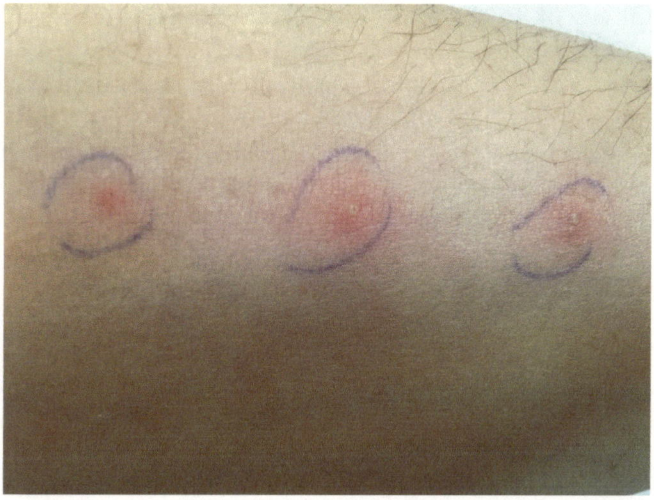

Figure 4. Pathergy positivity in Behçet's Disease (Courtesy of MD. Assoc. Prof. Müzeyyen Gönül).

Although the positivity of SPT has been accepted as a criteria in the diagnosis of BD, there is no consensus about performing a standardized method of SPT [105, 112–117]. It is usually performed under sterile conditions with a 20-gauge needle inserted intradermally into the avascular area on the forearm skin of patient with an angle of 45° [105, 112, 113]. Various techniques such as pricking with multiple needles with various applying routes including intradermal, intravenous and subcutaneous methods have been reported [9, 105, 112, 114–116]. Multiple punctures are mostly required [9, 114, 115]. Davatchi et al. suggested three intradermal punctures perpendicular or diagonally one with a 25-gauge needle with intradermal injection of one drop of normal serum saline, one with a 25-gauge needle alone (just a puncture, with no injection) and the last with a 21 gauge needle (puncture, no injection) [115]. A study by Ozdemir et al. suggested that two needle pricks are sufficient for positive SPT [114]. Another study by Ozdemir et al. analysed the changes of SPT positivity in different body areas such as flexor surfaces of the forearms, the lateral aspect of the tibial area, the scapular areas on back, and the lumbar areas of the abdominal region. They concluded that forearm was the most frequent site positive for pathergy reaction whereas abdomen was the least [113]. Akmaz et al. reported higher rate of positivity in SPT by intradermal application compared with intravenous application [117]. Dilsen et al. performed SPT with different needles including sharp and blunt needles in which they confirmed higher frequency of positivity with blunt needles [112]. Sharquie et al. demonstrated an alternative method of which they inserted the needle inside the mucous membrane of the lower lip to the sub-mucosa. However, the sensitivity of the oral pathergy test has been reported lower than of the classical pathergy test [118].

Various prevalence rates of SPT positivity in BD have been reported by several studies [21, 22, 119–123]. The positivity of SPT varies between 40 and 88% with a higher prevalence in Japan and Mediterranean countries, whereas it is lower in countries such as the United Kingdom and the United States [2, 3, 9, 22, 45, 98, 119–123]. Alpsoy et al. reported the positivity of SPT as 37.8% in their study including 661 Turkish patients with BD [21]. A study comparing the positivity of SPT between Turkish and British patients with BD revealed the positive reaction was only present among Turkish patients [119]. In a German study, SPT revealed positive results in 33.7% of patients with no significant difference between Turkish and German patients with BD [123]. The factors that may affect the rates of positivity of SPT include genetic variables, variations in ethnic origins of the patients, factors related to the method and materials used to perform the SPT and conditions of the patient and the disease [105, 112–114, 124–126].

Contrary results have been reported about the relationship between positive SPT and clinical course of BD [22, 125–128]. Chang et al. found that positive SPT was specific for BD, but not associated with clinical severity [125]. Similarly, Krause et al. found no difference in terms of clinical manifestations and severity in the comparison of pathergy positive and negative patients with BD [126]. Although Yazici et al. have found no correlation between disease severity and positive SPT, they reported that male patients with BD have stronger pathergy reaction [127]. Jorizzo et al. reported a correlation between the histopathological pathergy results and clinical severity [109]. Koç et al. detected higher positive SPT test in patients with vascular involvement compared to patients without vascular involvement [128].

It has been reported that the frequency of SPT positivity has decreased during the last years [115, 125, 129]. One of the best reasons for this issue is the use of disposable needles, which are less traumatic than non-disposable ones [105, 112, 125]. A study by Davatchi et al. investigated the sensitivity and specificity of SPT among 6607 patients followed between the years 1975 and 2010. Their results revealed that the sensitivity of pathergy test has declined, but it still preserves its specificity [115]. Moreover, positivity of SPT in many diseases other than BD has been detected. Neutrophilic dermatoses such as Sweet syndrome, PG, erythema elevatum or other diseases such as RAS, eosinophilic pustular folliculitis, inflammatory bowel diseases and spondyloarthropathies are some in which pathergy reaction positivity has been shown [70]. Despite everything, SPT has still a diagnostic value [115].

3. Childhood Behçet's disease and mucocutaneous manifestations

BD in childhood is rare, has a variable clinical course and less investigated [68, 69, 130–139]. Paediatric onset of BD was found in 5.3 and 7.6% of all the cases [130, 133]. In the study including 661 cases of BD, juvenile BD has been reported in 7.1% [21]. In paediatric cases, a family history of BD has been more frequently observed [21, 68, 130, 131, 136, 137].

The diagnosis of paediatric BD in the reported studies was based on the criteria of ISG and ICD [30, 31]. A recent classification was proposed by Kone-Paut et al., and according to this classification, the presence of any three items among recurrent oral aphthosis, GU, ocular involvement, neurological and vascular signs makes the definitive diagnosis of BD [135, 140].

http://dx.doi.org/10.5772/67841

The onset of BD has been reported at any age between 0 and 16 years [131, 136, 137]. The lowest mean age of 4.8 years old was reported by Nanthapisal et al. [134]. Similarly to clinical symptoms of adulthood BD, OU was present in most of the children and also constituted the initial symptom in most of the cases [68, 131–139]. The localization and morphology of OU in children were also similar to the characteristics of adulthood OU [136, 137, 140]. GU was detected between 55 and 94% of the paediatric cases [131, 135–138]. Distinctively from adult cases, the presence of GU has been reported significantly lesser than adults [131, 132]. However, Treudler et al. did not reveal any differences in the ratio of GU between childhood and adulthood BD [68], and Nanthapisal et al. detected recurrent GU more frequently in females [134]. The characteristics of GU were also found similar to the ones seen in adults [136, 137]. Another distinctive feature, perianal aphthosis was to be a specific feature of childhood BD [135].

Skin lesions were reported to occur between 64 and 92% of childhood BD [70, 135, 137, 138]. Kone-Paut et al. reported EN-like lesions in 40% and necrotic folliculitis in 58% [136], while Borlu et al. reported EN-like lesions in 18% and PPL in 47% of the patients [137]. Kone-Paut et al. reported necrotic folliculitis more frequently in male patients [136]. However, no gender differences were detected in terms of skin lesions in the study of Borlu et al. [137]. Erythema multiforme-like lesions and TFB have been less frequently reported [70]. Positive SPT has been reported in 37, 80 and 76% of the patients in three different studies [131, 136, 137].

Nanthapisal et al. documented skin findings in 11 (23.9%) of 46 patients: These were pustular lesions in three, skin ulceration in two, EN in two, necrotic folliculitis in two, PPL in two and positive SPT in three of the five patients [134].

The duration between the initial symptom and fulfilment of diagnosis of BD has been reported as 3.14 years in the study of Karincaoglu et al. [131], while a significant diagnostic delay up to 13.5 years has been reported in the study of Nanthapisal et al. [134]. This may be caused due to rarity and unfamiliarity of the disease in Northern Europe.

Conflicting reports have also been found in the systemic expression of BD in children [130, 132, 133]. BD was usually reported to have a less severe disease [132, 140]. Pivetti-Pezzi et al. reported similar rates of OU, GU, skin lesions in the comparison of adulthood and childhood BD. In addition, no differences were observed in the incidence of arthritis, gastrointestinal and neurological involvement except more severe ocular involvement in childhood. Another study by Sarica et al. compared the patients with mild and severe diseases. An earlier onset and more systemic involvement were found in patients with severe form of the disease [130]. More frequent neurological and gastrointestinal involvements were observed in childhood BD in the study of Karincaoglu et al. [131].

Generally, it can be interpreted that juvenile BD has a similar clinical spectrum to adulthood BD. The differences in frequency and clinical courses may reflect the geographic, ethnic and genetic variations.

4. Differential diagnosis of mucocutaneous manifestations

The differential diagnosis of mucocutaneous manifestations will not be addressed in detail as this subject does not constitute the main topic of this chapter. Only the essential differential diagnoses of OU, GU, EN-like lesions will be given below.

Oral ulcer [2, 32, 141]:

- Infectious etiology: Herpangina, primary herpetic gingivostomatitis, hand-foot and mouth disease, HIV, syphilis, tuberculosis, etc.
- Systemic diseases: Systemic lupus erythematous, Reiter's disease, Wegener's granulomatosis, blood disorders (neutropenia, leukaemia), iron deficiency, vitamin B12 deficiency, etc.
- Gastrointestinal diseases: Inflammatory bowel diseases, Celiac Disease
- Primary skin conditions: Sweet's syndrome, RAS, autoimmune bullous disorders (pemphigus vulgaris, pemphigoid, linear IgA disease, etc.)
- Medication induced: Cytotoxic agents, nicorandil, etc.
- Malign neoplasms

Genital ulcer [2, 32, 142, 143]:

- Infectious etiology: Genital herpes simplex, syphilis, chancroid, lymphogranuloma venereum, granuloma inguinale, HIV, etc.
- Non-microbial etiology: Erythema multiforme, fixed drug eruption, Lipschütz ulcers, metastatic Crohn's disease, hidradenitis suppurativa, PG, pressure ulcers, sexual trauma, psoriasis and malignancies.

Papulopustular lesions [2, 54, 144, 145]:

- Infectious etiology: Gram-positive folliculitis, Gram-negative folliculitis, Pityrosporum folliculitis, Demodicidosis, viral plane warts
- Eosinophilic pustular folliculitis
- Acne vulgaris

Erythema nodosum-like lesions [2, 70]:

- Classical EN
- Nodular vasculitis
- Panniculitis
- Cellulitis

Extragenital ulcers [146]:

- Infectious etiology: Necrotizing fasciitis (Streptococcus haemolyticus), botryomycosis (commonly *Staphylococcus aureus*), ecthyma gangrenosum (Pseudomonas aeruginosa, anthrax (Bacillus anthracis), sexually transmitted diseases (syphilis, granuloma inguinale), herpes simplex, leishmaniasis, etc.
- Autoimmune diseases: Scleroderma, rheumatoid arthritis, cutaneous lupus erythematosus, vasculitis, etc.
- Systemic disorders: Blood diseases (Polycythemia vera, sickle cell anaemia, thrombotic thrombocytopenic purpura, paraproteinemia, etc.)
- Medication-induced: Hydroxyurea, methotrexate, chemotherapeutics and immunosuppressives
- Primary skin conditions: Necrobiosis lipoidica, sarcoidosis, pyoderma gangrenosum, panniculitis, etc.
- Factitial: Dermatitis artefacta, Munchausen by proxy, etc.

5. Treatment of mucocutaneous manifestations

Oral and genital ulcers can be treated with topical and systemic treatments [3, 147–152]. In recurrent OU with or without GU, systemic colchicine (1–2 mg/day) must be started as a first choice of treatment [147–149]. Topical steroids, topical sucralfate, local anaesthetics, and tetracycline oral mouth washes are usually combined with oral colchicine treatment [147]. In case of more severe and painful OU and/or GU, a short duration of systemic steroids may be added with colchicine. Corticosteroids combined with systemic antibiotics can be used to decrease the severity of GU attacks [147–149]. In patients with severe mucocutaneous manifestations, immunosuppressive drugs such as azathioprine (AZA), methotrexate (Mtx), cyclosporine A may be used [149]. AZA has been found effective in preventing the recurrences of thrombophlebitis [147]. Thalidomide is another choice of therapy in recalcitrant OU and/or GU. However, it is not preferred due its high toxic effects [147, 149, 150]. Pentoxifylline, dapson, zinc sulphate, IFN-α and rebamipide are other alternative treatments worth for trying in OU. However, larger and well organized studies are needed in order to clarify their efficacies. In case of EN-like lesions, bed rest is usually required. Especially in female cases with GU and EN-like lesions, the combination of colchicine and benzathine penicillin is recommended [148]. This treatment combination has also been reported to decrease the frequency and duration of both OU and EN-like lesions [150]. IFN-α has been reported to decrease not only the frequency of GU and EN-like lesions but also the number of PPL [151]. Anti-TNF drugs are being used with success in patients with refractory mucocutaneous manifestations [151, 152]. Recent studies of interleukin-1 (IL-1) inhibitors (anakinra, canakinumab) have demonstrated efficacy in OU and GU resistant to conventional therapy [150]. Finally, apremilast, phosphodiesterase 4 inhibitor, has been reported to be effective in treating OU and GU [150, 152]. The treatment options can be seen more detailed in **Table 1**.

Mucocutaneous manifestation	Topical	Systemic
Oral ulcer	Topical steroids Topical sucralfate Local anaesthetics Topical amlexanox Local silver nitrate 5%	Colchicine Tetracycline Azithromycin Systemic steroids (short term) Rebamipide Dapson Immunosuppressive drugs (AZA, Mtx) Thalidomide Anti-TNF drugs IFN-α Pentoxifylline Cyclosporine A (Cyc A) Tacrolimus Apremilast Anakinra Canakinumab
Genital ulcer	Topical antibiotics Topical steroids Local anaesthetics	Colchicine Tetracycline AZA, Mtx CycA IFN-α Anti-TNF Apremilast Anakinra Canakinumab
Papulopustular lesion		Colchicine Azithromycin CycA IFN-α Thalidomide
Eryhthema nodosum-like lesions	Bed rest Wet dressings (aluminium acetat3 3–5%)	Colchicine NSAII Systemic steroids (short term) Colchicine+benzathine penicillin Dapson Anti-TNF

Table 1. Treatment options for mucocutaneous manifestations.

6. Conclusion

Mucocutaneous lesions are the most important criteria in establishing the diagnosis of BD. In case of recurrent OU, GU and other cutaneous findings mentioned above, it is important to remind the possibility of BD in the diagnosis, which will permit an earlier diagnosis and enable a decrease in mortality and morbidity.

http://dx.doi.org/10.5772/67841

Abbreviations

AZA	Azathiopurine
BD	Behçet's disease
DVT	Deep vein thromboses
EGU	Extragenital ulcer
EN	Erythema nodosum
GU	Genital ulcers
HLA	Human leucocyte antigen
IFN-α	Interferon-alpha
ISG	International study group
Mtx	Methotrexate
NV	Nodular vasculitis
PG	Pyoderma gangrenosum
PPL	Papulopustular lesions
RAS	Recurrent aphthous stomatitis
SPT	Skin pahergy test
TFB	Thrombophlebitis
OU	Oral ulcer

Author details

Arzu Kilic

Address all correspondence to: kilicarzu@gmail.com

Department of Dermatology, Balikesir University School of Medicine, Balikesir, Turkey

References

[1] Behçet H. Uber rezidivierende, apthose, durch ein Virus verursachte Geschwure am Mund, am Auge und an den Genitalien. Dermatol Wochensch. 1937;36:1152–7.

[2] Alpsoy E, Zouboulis CC, Ehrlich GE. Mucocutaneous Lesions of Behçet's disease. Yonsei Med J. 2007;48: 573–85. DOI: 10.3349/ymj.2007.48.4.573

[3] Alpsoy E. Behçet's disease: a comprehensive review with a focus on epidemiology, etiology and clinical features, and management of mucocutaneous lesions. J Dermatol. 2016;43:620–32. DOI: 10.1111/1346-8138.13381

[4] Davatchi F, Chams-Davatchi C, Shams H, Shahram F, Nadji A, Akhlaghi M, Faezi T, Ghodsi Z, Sadeghi Abdollahi B, Ashofteh F, Mohtasham N, Kavosi H, Masoumi M. Behcet's disease: epidemiology, clinical manifestations, and diagnosis. Expert Rev Clin Immunol. 2017;13:57–65. DOI: 10.1080/1744666X.2016.1205486

[5] Verity DH, MarrJE, Ohno S, Wallace GR, Stanford MR. Behcet's disease, the Silk Road and HLA-B51: historical and geographic perspectives. Tissue Antigens 1999;54:213–20.

[6] Azizlerli G(1), Köse AA, Sarica R, Gül A, Tutkun IT, Kulaç M, Tunç R, Urgancioğlu M, Dişçi R. Prevalence of Behçet's disease in Istanbul, Turkey. Int J Dermatol. 2003;42:803–6.

[7] Yurdakul S, Günaydın I, Tüzün Y. The prevalence of Behçet's syndrome in a rural area in Northern Turkey. J Rheumatol. 1988;15: 820–2.

[8] Idil A, Gurler A, Bovyat A, et al. The prevalence of Behcet's disease above the age of ten years. The results of a pilot study conducted at the Park Primary Health Care Center in Ankara, Turkey. Ophthalmic Epidemiol. 2002;9:325–31.

[9] Davatchi F, Shahram F, Chams-Davatchi C, Shams H, Nadji A, Akhlaghi M, Faezi T, Ghodsi Z, Faridar A, Ashofteh F, Sadeghi Abdollahi B. Behcet's disease: from East to West. Clin Rheumatol. 2010;29:823–33. DOI: 10.1007/s10067-010-1430-6.

[10] Mohammad A(1), Mandl T, Sturfelt G, Segelmark M. Incidence, prevalence and clinical characteristics of Behcet's disease in southern Sweden. Rheumatology (Oxford). 2013;52:304–10. DOI: 10.1093/rheumatology/kes249.

[11] Dalvi SR, Yildirim R, Yazici Y. Behcet's Syndrome. Drugs.2012;72:2223–41. DOI: 10.2165/11641370-000000000-00000.

[12] Yazici Y, Yurdakul S, Yazici H. Behçet's syndrome. Curr Rheumatol Rep. 2010;12:429–35. DOI: 10.1007/s11926-010-0132-z.

[13] Melikoglu M, Kural-Seyahi E, Tascilar K, Yazici H. The unique features of vasculitis in Behçet's syndrome. Clin Rev Allergy Immunol. 2008;35:40–6. DOI: 10.1007/s12016-007-8064-8.

[14] Akman A, Kacaroglu H, Donmez L, Bacanli A, Alpsoy E. Relationship between periodontal findings and Behcet's disease: a controled study. J Clin Periodontol. 2007;34:485–91. DOI: 10.1111/j.1600-051X.2007.01085.x

[15] Gul A. Pathogenesis of Behçet's disease: autoinflammatory features and beyond. Semin Immunopathol. 2015;37: 413–8. DOI: 10.1007/s00281-015-0502-8.

[16] Gül A. Behçet's disease as an autoinflammatory disorder. Curr Drug Targets Inflamm Allergy. 2005;4: 81–3.

[17] Pay S, Simşek I, Erdem H, Dinç A. Immunopathogenesis of Behçet's disease with special emphasize on the possible role of antigen presenting cells. Rheumatol Int. 2007;27: 417–24. DOI: 10.1007/s00296-006-0281-6

[18] Jennette JC, Falk RJ, Bacon PA, Basu N, Cid MC, Ferrario F, Flores-Suarez LF, Gross WL, Guillevin L, Hagen EC, Hoffman GS, Jayne DR, Kallenberg CG, Lamprecht P, Langford CA, Luqmani RA, Mahr AD, Matteson EL, Merkel PA, Ozen S, Pusey CD, Rasmussen N, Rees AJ, Scott DG, Specks U, Stone JH, Takahashi K, Watts RA. 2012 revised International Chapel Hill Consensus Conference Nomenclature of Vasculitides. Arthritis Rheum. 2013;65:1–11. DOI: 10.1002/art.37715.

[19] Ideguchi H, Suda A, Takeno M, Ueda A. Behçet disease: evolution of clinical manifestations. Medicine. 2011;90: 125–32. DOI: 10.1097/MD.0b013e318211bf28

[20] Koné-Paut I, Darce-Bello M, Shahram F, Gattorno M, Cimaz R, Ozen S, Cantarini L, Tugal-Tutktun I, Assaad-Khalil S, Hofer M, Kuemmerle-Deschner J, Benamour S, Al Mayouf S, Pajot C, Anton J, Faye A, Bono W, Nielsen S, Letierce A, Tran TA; PED-BD International Expert Committee. Registries in rheumatological and musculoskeletal conditions. Paediatric Behçet's disease: an international cohort study of 110 patients. One-year follow-up data. Rheumatology (Oxford). 2011; 50:184–8. DOI: 10.1093/rheumatology/keq324

[21] Alpsoy E(1), Donmez L, Onder M, Gunasti S, Usta A, Karincaoglu Y, Kandi B, Buyukkara S, Keseroglu O, Uzun S, Tursen U, Seyhan M, Akman A. Clinical features and natural course of Behçet's disease in 661 cases: a multicentre study. Br J Dermatol. 2007;157:901–6. DOI: 10.1111/j.1365-2133.2007.08116.x

[22] Gurler A, Bovyat A, Tursen U. Clinical Manifestations of Behçet's disease: an analysis of 2147 patients. Yonsei Med J. 1997;38: 423–7. DOI: 10.3349/ymj.1997.38.6.423

[23] Yazici H, Tüzün Y, Pazarli H, Yurdakul S, Ozyazgan Y, Ozdoğan H, Serdaroğlu S, Ersanli M, Ulkü BY, Müftüoğlu AU. Influence of age of onset and patient's sex on the prevalence and severity of manifestations of Behçet's syndrome. Ann Rheum Dis. 1984; 43:783–9.

[24] Balta I, Akbay G, Kalkan G, Eksioglu M. Demographic and clinical features of 521 Turkish patients with Behçet's disease. Int J Dermatol. 2014; 53: 564–9. DOI: 10.1111/j.1365-4632.2012.05756.x

[25] Davatchi F, Shahram F, Chams-Davatchi C, Sadeghi Abdollahi B, Shams H, Nadji A, Faezi T, Akhlaghi M, Ghodsi Z, Larimi R, Ashofteh F. Behcet's disease: is there a gender influence on clinical manifestations? Int J Rheum Dis. 2012;15: 306–14. DOI: 10.1111/j.1756-185X.2011.01696.x.

[26] Alpsoy E, Donmez L, Bacanli A, Apaydin C, Butun B. Review of the chronology of clinical manifestations in 60 patients with Behçet's disease. Dermatology. 2003;207:354–6. DOI: 74113

[27] Salvarani C, Pipitone N, Catanoso MG, Cimino L, Tumiati B, Macchioni P, Bajocchi G, Olivieri I, Boiardi L. Epidemiology and Clinical course of Behcet's disease in the Reggio Emilia area of Northern Italy: a seventeen-year population-based study. Arthritis Rheum. 2007;57:171–8. DOI: 10.1002/art.22500

[28] Davatchi F, Chams-Davatchi C, Shams H, Nadji A, Faezi T, Akhlaghi M, Sadeghi Abdollahi B, Ashofteh F, Ghodsi Z, Mohtasham N, Shahram F. Adult Behcet's disease in Iran: analysis of 6075 patients. Int J Rheum Dis. 2016; 19: 95–103. DOI: 10.1111/1756-185X.12691

[29] Yucel A, Marakli SS, Aksungur VL, et al. Clinical evaluation of Behçet's disease: a five year follow-up study. J Dermatol. 2005;32: 365–70.

[30] International Study Group for Behcet's disease. Criteria for diagnosis of Behçet's disease. International Study Group for Behçet's Disease. Lancet. 1990;335:1078–80.

[31] International Team for the Revision of the International Criteria for Behçet's Disease (ITR-ICBD). The International Criteria for Behçet's Disease (ICBD): a collaborative study of 27 countries on the sensitivity and specificity of the new criteria. J Eur Acad Dermatol Venereol. 2014;28: 338–47. DOI: 10.1111/jdv.12107

[32] Gunduz O. Histopathological evaluation of Behçet's disease and identification of new skin lesions. Patholog Res Int. 2012;2012:209316. DOI: 10.1155/2012/209316.

[33] Zhang Z(1), He F, Shi Y. Behcet's disease seen in China: analysis of 334 cases. Rheumatol Int. 2013;33: 645–8. DOI: 10.1007/s00296-012-2384-6.

[34] Lennikov A, Alekberova Z, Goloeva R, Kitaichi N, Denisov L, Namba K, Takeno M, Ishigatsubo Y, Mizuki N, Nasonov E, Ishida S, Ohno S. Single center study on ethnic and clinical features of Behcet's disease in Moscow, Russia. Clin Rheumatol. 2015; 34:321–7. DOI: 10.1007/s10067-013-2442-9.

[35] Tursen U, Gurler A, Boyvat A. Evaluation of clinical findings according to sex in 2313 Turkish patients with Behçet's disease. Int J Dermatol. 2003; 42:346–51.

[36] Vaiopoulos G, Konstantopoulou P, Evangelatos N, Kaklamanis PH. The spectrum of mucocutaneous manifestations in Adamantiades-Behçet's disease in Greece. J Eur Acad Dermatol Venereol. 2010; 24: 434–8. DOI: 10.1111/j.1468-3083.2009.03435.x.

[37] Rodríguez-Carballeira M, Alba MA, Solans-Laqué R, Castillo MJ, Ríos-Fernández R, Larrañaga JR, Martínez-Berriotxoa A, Espinosa G; REGEB investigators. Registry of the Spanish network of Behçet's disease: a descriptive analysis of 496 patients. Clin Exp Rheumatol. 2014;32:S33–9.

[38] Krause I, Rosen Y, Kaplan I, Milo G, Guedj D, Molad Y, Weinberger A. Recurrent apthous stomatitis in Behçet's disease. Clinical features and correlation with systemic disease expression and severity. J Oral Pathol Med. 1999; 28:193–6.

[39] Main DM, Chamberlain MA. Clinical differentiation of oral ulceration in Behçet's disease. Br J Rheumatol. 1992; 31:767–70.

[40] Oh SH, Han EC, Lee JH, Bang D. Comparison of the clinical features of recurrent aphthous stomatitis and Behçet's disease. Clin Exp Dermatol. 2009;34:e208–12. DOI: 10.1111/j.1365-2230.2009.03384.x

[41] Faezi ST, Paragomi P, Shahram F, Shams H, Shams-Davatchi C, Ghodsi Z, Nadji A, Akhlaghi M, Davatchi F. Clinical features of Behcet's disease in patients without oral aphthosis. Mod Rheumatol. 2014; 24: 637–9. DOI: 10.3109/14397595.2013.844400.

[42] Bang D, Lee JH, Lee ES, Lee S, Choi JS, Kim YK, Cho BK, Koh JK, Won YH, Kim NI, Park SD, Ahn HJ, Lee YW, Wang HY, Lee WW, Eun HC, Song ES, Lee SW, Lee CW, Lee CJ, Park JH, Song YW, Kim ST, Kim CY, Park JK, Kwon KS. Epidemiologic and clinical survey of Behcet's disease in Korea: the first multicenter study. J Korean Med Sci. 2001;16: 615–8.

[43] Tanasenau St, Pompilian V, Cojocaru I, et al. Clinical particularities in a Romanian series of Behcet's disease patients. Clin Exp Rheumatol. 2004;22:Suppl S84.

[44] Dilsen N. The implications of nonaphthous beginning of Behçet's disease. Adv Exp Med Biol. 2003;528: 73–6.

[45] Davari P, Rogers RS, Chan B, Nagler TH, Fazel N. Clinical features of Behçet's disease: A retrospective chart review of 26 patients. J Dermatolog Treat. 2016; 27:70–4. doi: 10.3109/09546634.2015.1054781

[46] Faezi ST, Chams-Davatchi C, Ghodsi SZ, Shahram F, Nadji A, Akhlaghi M, Moradi K, Paragomi P, Ghazizadeh Esslami G, Sadeghi Abdollahi B, Ashofteh F, Davatchi F. Genital aphthosis in Behçet's disease: is it associated with less eye involvement? Rheumatol Int. 2014;34:1581–7. DOI: 10.1007/s00296-014-3011-5.

[47] al-Dalaan AN, al Balaa SR, el Ramahi K, et al. Behçet's disease in Saudi Arabia. J Rheumatol 1994;21: 658–61.

[48] Mat Cem. The frequency of scarring after genital ulcers in Behçet's syndrome: a prospective study. Int J Dermatol. 2006;45: 554–6. DOI:10.1111/j.1365-4632.2006.02859.x

[49] Alpsoy E, Aktekin M, Er H, Durusoy C, Yilmaz E. A randomized, controlled and blinded study of papulopustular lesions in Turkish Behçet's patients. Int J Dermatol. 1998;37: 839–4.

[50] Jorizzo JL, Abernethy JL, White WL, Mangelsdorf HC, Zouboulis CC, Sarica R, Gaffney K, Mat C, Yazici H, al Ialaan A, et al. Mucocutaneous criteria for the diagnosis of Behçet's disease: an analysis of clinicopathologic data from multiple international centers. J Am Acad Dermatol. 1995;32:968–76.

[51] Kalkan G, Karadag AS, Astarci HM, Akbay G, Ustun H, Eksioglu M. A histopathological approach: when papulopustular lesions should be in the diagnostic criteria of Behçet's disease? J Eur Acad Dermatol Venereol. 2009 Sep;23:1056–60. DOI:10.1111/j.1468-3083.2009.03256.x.

[52] Ilknur T, Pabuççuoglu U, Akin C, Lebe B, Gunes AT. Histopathologic and direct immunofluorescence findings of the papulopustular lesions in Behçet's disease. Eur J Dermatol. 2006;16:146–50.

[53] Chen KR, Kawahara Y, Miyakawa S, Nishikawa T. Cutaneous vasculitis in Behçet's disease: a clinical and histopathologic study of 20 patients. J Am Acad Dermatol. 1997;36:689–96.

[54] Kutlubay Z, Mat CM, Aydin Ö, Demirkesen C, Calay Ö, Engin B,Tüzün Y, Yazici H. Histopathological and clinical evaluation of papulopustular lesions in Behçet's disease. Clin Exp Rheumatol. 2015;33:S101–6.

[55] Coskun B, Ozturk P, Saral Y. Are erythema nodosum-like lesions and superficial thrombophlebitis prodromal in terms of visceral involvement in Behçet's disease. Int J Clin Pract. 2005; 59:69–71. DOI: 10.1111/j.1742-1241.2005.00286.x

[56] Ajose OA, Adelowo O, Oderinlo O. Clinical presentations of Behçet's disease among Nigerians: a 4-year prospective study. Int J Dermatol. 2015; 54:889–97. DOI: 10.1111/ijd.12554

[57] Misago N, Tada Y, Koarada S, Narisawa Y. Erythema nodosum-like lesions in Behçet's disease: a clinicopathological study of 26 cases. Acta Derm Venereol. 2012; 92:681–6. DOI: 10.2340/00015555-1349

[58] Cebeci F, Onsun N, Ulusal HA, Inan B. The relationship between deep vein thrombosis and erythema nodosum in male patients with Behçet's disease. Eur Rev Med Pharmacol Sci. 2014; 18:3145–8.

[59] Chun SI, Su WP, Lee S, Rogers RS 3rd. Erythema nodosum-like lesions in Behçet's syndrome: a histopathological study of 30 cases. J Cutan Pathol. 1989; 16:259–65.

[60] Demirkesen C, Tuzuner N, Mat C, Senocak M, Buyukbabani N, Tuzun Y, Yazici H. Clinicopathological evaluation of nodular cutaneous lesions of Behçet syndrome. Am J Clin Pathol. 2001;116:341–6. DOI: 10.1309/GCTH-0060-55K8-XCTT

[61] Davatchi F, Shahram F, Chams-Davatchi C, Shams H, Nadji A, Akhlaghi M, Faezi T, Sadeghi Abdollahi B. How to deal with Behçet's disease in daily practice. Int J Rheum Dis. 2010; 13: 105–16.

[62] Sarica-Kucukoglu R, Akdag-Kose A, KayabalI M, Yazganoglu KD, Disci R, Erzengin D, Azizlerli G. Vascular involvement in Behçet's disease: a retrospective analysis of 2319 cases. Int J Dermatol. 2006;45:919–21. DOI: 10.1111/j.1365-4632.2006.02832.x

[63] Düzgün N, Ateş A, Aydintuğ OT, Demir O, Olmez U. Characteristics of vascular involvement in Behçet's disease. Scand J Rheumatol. 2006; 35:65–8. DOI: 10.1080/03009740500255761

[64] Hamdan A, Mansour W, Uthman I, Masri AF, Nasr F, Arayssi T. Behçet's disease in Lebanon: clinical profile, severity and two-decade comparison. Clin Rheumatol. 2006;25:364–7. DOI: 10.1007/s10067-005-0058-4

[65] Azizlerli G, Ozarmağan G, Ovül C, Sarica R, Mustafa SO. A new kind of skin lesion in Behçet's disease: extragenital ulcerations. Acta Derm Venereol. 1992;72:286.

[66] Ozyurt K, Colgecen E, Baykan H. Does familial occurrence or family history of recurrent oral ulcers influence clinical characteristics of Behçet's disease? Acta Dermatovenerol Croat. 2013;21:168–73.

[67] Krüger K, Fritz K, Daniel V, Zouboulis CC. Juvenile Adamantiades-Behçet disease in decreased stimulation with anti-CD3 monoclonal antibody.[Article in German] Hautarzt. 1997; 48:258–61.

[68] Treudler R, Orfanos CE, Zouboulis CC. Twenty-eight cases of juvenile-onset Adamantiades-Behçet disease in Germany. Dermatology. 1999; 199: 15–9. DOI: 18197

[69] de Carvalho VO, Abagge KT, Giraldi S, Kamoi TO, Assahide MK, Fillus Neto J,Marinoni LP. Behçet disease in a child—emphasis on cutaneous manifestations. Pediatr Dermatol. 2007;24:E57–62. DOI: 10.1111/j.1525-1470.2007.00442.x

[70] Lee ES, Bang D, Lee S. Dermatologic manifestation of Behcet's disease. Yonsei Med J. 1997;38: 380–9. DOI: 10.3349/ymj.1997.38.6.380

[71] Oguz O, Serdaroglu S, Tuzun Y, Erdogan N, Yazici H, Savaskan H. Acute febrile neutrophilic dermatosis (Sweet's syndrome) associated with Behcet's disease. Int J Dermatol. 1992; 31:645–6.

[72] Cho KH, Shin KS, Sohn SJ, Choi SJ, Lee YS. Behcet's disease with Sweet's syndrome-like presentation-a report of six cases. Clin Exp Dermatol. 1989;14: 20–4.

[73] Wu F, Luo X, Yuan G. Sweet's syndrome representing a flare of Behçet's disease. Clin Exp Rheumatol. 2009;27:S88–90.

[74] Lee MS, Barnetson RS. Sweet's syndrome associated with Behçet's disease. Australas J Dermatol. 1996;37: 99–101.

[75] Uysal H, Vahaboğlu H, Inan L, Vahaboğlu G. Acute febrile neutrophilic dermatosis (Sweet's syndrome) in neuro-Behçet's disease. Clin Neurol Neurosurg. 1993;95:319–22.

[76] Karadoğan SK, Başkan EB, Alkan G, Saricaoğlu H, Tunali S. Generalized Sweet syndrome lesions associated with Behçet disease: a true association or simply co-morbidity? Am J Clin Dermatol. 2009;10:331–5. DOI: 10.2165/11310790-000000000-00000.

[77] Mizoguchi M, Matsuki K, Mochizuki M, Watanabe R, Ogawa K, Harada S, Hino H,Amagai M, Juji T.Human leukocyte antigen in Sweet's syndrome and its relationship to Behçet's disease. Arch Dermatol. 1988;124:1069–73.

[78] Ozuguz P, Kacar SD, Manav V, Karaca S, Aktepe F, Ulu S. Genital ulcerative pyoderma gangrenosum in Behçet's Disease: a case report and review of the literature. Indian J Dermatol. 2015;60:105. DOI: 10.4103/0019-5154.147866.

[79] Kim JW, Park JH, Lee D, Hwang SW, Park SW. Vegetative pyoderma gangrenosum in Behçet's disease. Acta Derm Venereol. 2007;87:365–7. DOI: 10.2340/00015555-0221

[80] Chams-Davatchi C, Shizarpour M, Davatchi F, Shahram F, Chams H, Nadji A,Jamshidi AR. Extensive pyoderma gangrenosum-like lesion in two cases of Behçet's disease responding only to cyclosporin. Adv Exp Med Biol. 2003;528:337–8.

[81] Singh G, Sethi A, Okade R, Harish MR. Bullous pyoderma gangrenosum: a presentation of childhood Behcet's disease. Int J Dermatol. 2005;44:257–8.

[82] Joshi A, Mamta. Behçet's syndrome with pyoderma-gangrenosum-like lesions treated successfully with dapsone monotherapy. J Dermatol. 2004;31: 806–10.

[83] Rustin MH, Gilkes JJ, Robinson TW. Pyoderma gangrenosum associated with Behçet's disease: treatment with thalidomide. J Am Acad Dermatol. 1990;23:941–4.

[84] Hali F, Khadir K, Chiheb S, Bouayad K, Mikou N, Benchikhi H. [Pyoderma gangrenosum and Behçet's disease: a study of two pediatric cases]. [Article in French]. Arch Pediatr. 2011;18:1320–3. DOI: 10.1016/j.arcped.2011.09.007.

[85] Nakamura T, Yagi H, Kurachi K, Suzuki S, Konno H. Intestinal Behcet's disease with pyoderma gangrenosum: a case report. World J Gastroenterol. 2006; 12:979–81.

[86] Cantini F, Salvarani C, Niccoli L, Senesi C, Truglia MC, Padula A, Olivieri I. Behçet's disease with unusual cutaneous lesions. J Rheumatol. 1998;25:2469–72.

[87] Ates A, Karaaslan Y, Aslar Zo. A case of Behçet's disease associated with necrotizing small vessel vasculitis. Rheumatol Int. 2006; 27:91–3. DOI: 10.1007/s00296-006-0155-y

[88] Cornelis F, Sigal-Nahum M, Gaulier A, Bleichner G, Sigal S. Behçet's disease with severe cutaneous necrotizing vasculitis: response to plasma exchange--report of a case. J Am Acad Dermatol. 1989;21:576–9.

[89] Lee SH, Chung KY, Lee WS, Lee S. Behçet's syndrome associated with bullous necrotizing vasculitis. J Am Acad Dermatol. 1989;21:327–30.

[90] Park YW, Park JJ, Lee JB, Lee SS. Development of Henoch-Schönlein purpura in a patient with Behçet's disease presenting with recurrent deep vein thrombosis. Clin Exp Rheumatol. 2007;25:S96–8.

[91] Vikas A, Atul S, Singh R, Sarbmeet L, Mohan H. Behçet's disease with relapsing cutaneous polyarteritis-nodosa-like lesions responsive to oral cyclosporine therapy. Dermatol Online J. 2003;9:9.

[92] Serra-Guillén C, Llombart B, Alfaro-Rubio A, Hueso L, Martorell-Calatayud A,Requena C, Nagore E, Botella-Estrada R, Sanmartín O, Guillén C. Behçet's disease and periarteritis nodosa with cutaneous lesions. [Article in Spanish]. Actas Dermosifiliogr. 2007;98:217–8.

[93] Azuma N, Natsuaki M, Yamanishi K, Kondo N, Iwasaki T, Morimoto M, Nishioka A, Sekiguchi M, Kitano M, Hashimoto N, Matsui K, Sano H. [Cutaneous necrotizing vasculitis in a patient with Behcet's disease; mimicking polyarteritis nodosa]. [Article in Japanese]. Nihon Rinsho Meneki Gakkai Kaishi. 2010;33:149–53.

[94] Liao YH, Hsiao GH, Hsiao CH. Behçet's disease with cutaneous changes resembling polyarteritis nodosa. Br J Dermatol. 1999;140:368–9.

[95] Trad S,Saadoun D, Barete S, Frances Piette CJ, Wechsler B. Necrotizing folliculitis in Behcet's disease. Rev Med Interne. 2009;30:268–270. DOI: 10.1016/j.revmed.2008.06.007

[96] King R, Crowson AN, Murray E, Magro CM. Acral purpuric papulonodular lesions as a manifestation of Behçet's disease. Int J Dermatol. 1995;34:190–2.

[97] Jefferson JA, Pollack RB. Behcet's disease with recurrent erythema multiforme in a 20 year-old African American male. J S C Med Assoc. 2011;107:40–1.

[98] Sula B, Batmaz I, Ucmak D, Yolbas I, Akdeniz S. Demographical and Clinical Characteristics of Behcet's Disease in Southeastern Turkey. J Clin Med Res. 2014;6:476–81. DOI: 10.14740/jocmr1952w.

[99] Schreiner DT, Jorizzo JL. Behçet's disease and complex aphthosis. Dermatol Clin. 1987;5:769–78.

[100] Shenoy R. Conjunctival ulcer—mucocutaneous or ocular manifestation of Behçet's disease? A case report. Eur J Ophthalmol 2002;12:435–6.

[101] Merle H, Donnio A, Richer R, Dubreuil F, Arfi S. Isolated conjunctival ulcerations as the first sign of Behçet's disease. Eur J Ophthalmol. 2006;16:751–2.

[102] Zamir E, Bodaghi B, Tugal-Tutkun I, See RF, Charlotte F, Wang RC, Wechsler B, LeHoang P, Anteby I, Rao NA. Conjunctival ulcers in Behçet's disease. Ophthalmology. 2003;110:1137–41. DOI: 10.1016/S0161-6420(03)00265-3

[103] Fabian ID, Vishnevskia-Dai V. Conjunctival ulceration in Behçet disease: a case report. BMJ Case Rep. 2009;2009. pii: bcr08.2008.0616. DOI: 10.1136/bcr.08.2008.0616

[104] Matsuo T, Itami M, Nakagawa H, Nagayama M. The incidence and pathology of conjunctival ulceration in Behçet's syndrome. Br J Ophthalmol. 2002;86:140–3.

[105] Sequeira FF, Daryani D. The oral and skin pathergy test. Indian J Dermatol Venereol Leprol. 2011;77:526–30. DOI:10.4103/0378-6323.82399.

[106] Jorizzo JL, Solomon AR, Cavallo T. Behçet's syndrome. Immunopathologic and histopathologic assessment of pathergy lesions is useful in diagnosis and follow-up. Arch Pathol Lab Med. 1985;109:747–51.

[107] Gul A, Esin S, Dilsen N, Koniçe M, Wigzell H, Biberfeld P. Immunohistology of skin pathergy reaction in Behçet's disease. Br J Dermatol. 1995;132:901–7.

[108] Ergun T, Gürbüz O, Harvell J, Jorizzo J, White W. The histopathology of pathergy: a chronologic study of skin hyperreactivity in Behçet's disease. Int J Dermatol. 1998;37:929–33.

[109] Ozluk E, Balta I, Akoguz O, Kalkan G, Astarci M, Akbay G, Eksioglu M. Histopathologic study of pathergy test in Behçet's Disease. Indian J Dermatol. 2014;59:630. DOI: 10.4103/0019-5154.143568.

[110] Inaloz HS, Evereklioglu C, Unal B, Kirtak N, Eralp Ai Inaloz SS. The significance of immunohistochemistry in the skin pathergy reaction of patients with Behcet's syndrome. J Eur Acad Dermatol Venereol. 2004;18:56–61.

[111] Alpsoy E, Elpek GO, Yilmaz F, Ciftcioglu MA, Akman A, Uzun S, Karakuzu A. Androgen receptor levels of oral and genital ulcers and skin pathergy test in patients with Behçet's disease. Dermatology. 2005;210:31–5. DOI: 10.1159/000081480

[112] Dilsen N, Konice M, Aral O, Ocal L, Inanc M, Gul A. Comparative study of the skin pathergy test with blunt and sharp needles in Behçet's disease: confirmed specifity but decreased sensitivity with sharp needles. Ann Rheum Dis. 1993;52:823–5.

[113] Ozdemir M, Balevi S, Deniz F, Mevlitoğlu I. Pathergy reaction in different body areas in Behçet's disease. Clin Exp Dermatol. 2007;32:85–7. DOI: 10.1111/j.1365-2230.2006.02284.x

[114] Ozdemir M, Bodur S, Engin B, Baysal I. Evaluation of application of multiple needle pricks on the pathergy reaction. Int J Dermatol. 2008;47:335–8. DOI: 10.1111/j.1365-4632.2008.03568.x.

[115] Davatchi F, Chams-Davatchi C, Ghodsi Z, Shahram F, Nadji A, Shams H, Akhlaghi M, Larimi R, Sadeghi-Abdolahi B. Diagnostic value of pathergy test in Behcet's disease according to the change of incidence over the time. Clin Rheumatol. 2011;30:1151–5. DOI: 10.1007/s10067-011-1694-5

[116] Ozden MG, Bek Y, Aydin F, Senturk N, Canturk T, Turanli AY. Different applications techniques of pathergy testing among dermatologists. J Eur Acad Dermatol Venereol 2010;24:1240–42. DOI: 10.1111/j.1468-3083.2010.03622.x

[117] Akmaz O, Erel A, Gürer MA. Comparison of histopathologic and clinical evaluations of pathergy test in Behçet's disease. Int J Dermatol. 2000;39:121–5.

[118] Sharquie KE, Al-Araji A, Hatem A. Oral pathergy test in Behçet's disease. Br J Dermatol. 2002;146:168–9.

[119] Yazici H, Chamberlain MA, Tuzun Y, et al. A comparative study of the pathergy reaction among Turkish and British patients with Behcet's disease. Ann Rheum Dis. 1984;43: 74–5.

[120] Dogan B, Taskapan O, Harmanyeri Y. Prevalence of pathergy test positivity in Behçet's disease in Turkey. J Eur Acad Dermatol Venereol. 2003;17:227–9.

[121] Askari A, Al-Aboosi M, Sawalha A. Evaluation of pathergy test in North Jordan. Clin Rheumatol. 2000;19:241–51.

[122] Davies PG, Fordham JN, Kirwan JR, Barnes CG, Dinning WJ. The pathergy test and Behçet's syndrome in Britain. Ann Rheum Dis. 1984;43: 70–3.

[123] Altenburg A, Papoutsis N, Orawa H, Martus P, Krause L, Zouboulis CC. Epidemiology and clinical manifestations of Adamantiades-Behcet disease in German-current pathogenetic concepts and therapeutic possibilities. J Dtsch Dermatol Ges. 2006; 4:49–64. DOI: 10.1111/j.1610-0387.2006.05841.x

[124] Fresko I, Yazici H, Bayramicli M, Yurdakul S, Mat C. Effect of surgical cleaning of the skin on the pathergy phenomenon in Behçet's syndrome. Ann Rheum Dis. 1993;52:619–20.

[125] Chang HK, Cheon KS. The clinical significance of a pathergy reaction in patients with Behcet's disease. J Korean Med Sci. 2002;17:371–4. DOI: 10.3346/jkms.2002.17.3.371

[126] Krause I, Molad Y, Mitrani M, Weinberger A. Pathergy reaction in Behçet's disease: lack of correlation with mucocutaneous manifestations and systemic disease expression. Clin Exp Rheumatol. 2000;18:71–4.

[127] Yazici H, Tüzün Y, Tanman AB, Yurdakul S, Serdaroglu S, Pazarli H, Müftüoglu A. Male patients with Behçet's syndrome have stronger pathergy reactions. Clin Exp Rheumatol. 1985;3:137–41.

[128] Koç Y, Güllü I, Akpek G, Akpolat T, Kansu E, Kiraz S, Batman F, Kansu T, Balkanci F, Akkaya S, et al. Vascular involvement in Behçet's disease. J Rheumatol. 1992;19:402–10.

[129] Varol A, Seifert O, Anderson CD. The skin pathergy test: innately useful? Arch Dermatol Res. 2010;302:155–68. DOI: 10.1007/s00403-009-1008-9. Epub 2009 Dec 12.

[130] Sarica R, Azizlerli G, Köse A, Dişçi R, Ovül C, Kural Z. Juvenile Behçet's disease among 1784 Turkish Behçet's patients. Int J Dermatol. 1996;35:109–11.

[131] Karincaoglu Y, Borlu M, Toker SC, Akman A, Onder M, Gunasti S, Usta A, Kandi B, Durusoy C, Seyhan M, Utas S, Saricaoglu H, Ozden MG, Uzun S, Tursen U, Cicek D, Donmez L, Alpsoy E. Demographic and clinical properties of juvenile-onset Behçet's disease: a controlled multicenter study. J Am Acad Dermatol. 2008;58:579–84. DOI: 10.1016/j.jaad.2007.10.452

[132] Krause I, Uziel Y, Guedj D, Mukamel M, Harel L, Molad Y, Weinberger A. Childhood Behçet's disease: clinical features and comparison with adult-onset disease. Rheumatology (Oxford). 1999; 38:457–62.

[133] Pivetti-Pezzi P, Accorinti M, Abdulaziz MA, La Cava M, Torella M, Riso D. Behçets disease in children. Jpn J Ophthalmol. 1995;39:309–14.

[134] Nanthapisal S, Klein NJ, Ambrose N, Eleftheriou D, Brogan PA. Paediatric Behçet's disease: a UK tertiary centre experience. Clin Rheumatol. 2016; 35:2509–16. DOI: 10.1007/s10067-016-3187-z.

[135] Koné-Paut I. Behçet's disease in children, an overview. Pediatr Rheumatol Online J. 2016;14:10. DOI: 10.1186/s12969-016-0070-z.

[136] Koné-Paut I, Yurdakul S, Bahabri SA, Shafae N, Ozen S, Ozdogan H, Bernard JL. Clinical features of Behçet's disease in children: an international collaborative study of 86 cases. J Pediatr. 1998;132:721–5.

[137] Borlu M, Ukşal U, Ferahbaş A, Evereklioglu C. Clinical features of Behçet's disease in children. Int J Dermatol. 2006;45:713–6. DOI: 10.1111/j.1365-4632.2006.02754.x

[138] Vaiopoulos AG, Kanakis MA, Kapsimali V, Vaiopoulos G, Kaklamanis PG, Zouboulis CC. Juvenile Adamantiades-Behçet Disease. Dermatology. 2016;232:129–36. DOI: 10.1159/000442667

[139] Johnson EF, Hawkins DM, Gifford LK, Smidt AC. Recurrent oral and genital ulcers in an infant: neonatal presentation of pediatric Behçet Disease. Pediatr Dermatol. 2015; 32:714–7. DOI: 10.1111/pde.12512.

[140] Koné-Paut I, Shahram F, Darce-Bello M, Cantarini L, Cimaz R, Gattorno M, Anton J, Hofer M, Chkirate B, Bouayed K, Tugal-Tutkun I, Kuemmerle-Deschner J, Agostini H, Federici S, Arnoux A,Piedvache C, Ozen S; PEDBD group. Consensus classification criteria for paediatric Behçet's disease from a prospective observational cohort: PEDBD. Ann Rheum Dis. 2016;75:958–64. DOI: 10.1136/annrheumdis-2015-208491.

[141] Scully C, Shotts R. ABC of oral health. Mouth ulcers and other causes of orofacial soreness and pain. BMJ. 2000;321:162–5.

[142] Roett MA, Mayor MT, Uduhiri KA. Diagnosis and management of genital ulcers. Am Fam Physician. 2012;85:254–62.

[143] Kirshen C, Edwards L(2). Noninfectious genital ulcers. Semin Cutan Med Surg. 2015; 34:187–91. DOI: 10.12788/j.sder.2015.0168.

[144] Fujiyama T, Tokura Y. Clinical and histopathological differential diagnosis of eosinophilic pustular folliculitis. J Dermatol. 2013;40:419–23. DOI: 10.1111/1346-8138.12125.

[145] Del Rosso JQ, Silverberg N, Zeichner JA. When acne is not acne. Dermatol Clin. 2016; 34:225–8. DOI: 10.1016/j.det.2015.12.002.

[146] Morton LM, Phillips TJ.Wound healing and treating wounds: Differential diagnosis and evaluation of chronic wounds. J Am Acad Dermatol. 2016; 74:589–605; quiz 605-6. DOI:10.1016/j.jaad.2015.08.068.

[147] Alpsoy E. Behçet's disease: treatment of mucocutaneous lesions. Clin Exp Rheumatol. 2005;23:532–9.

[148] Alpsoy E, Akman A. Behçet's disease: an algorithmic approach to its treatment. Arch Dermatol Res. 2009;301:693–702. DOI: 10.1007/s00403-009-0990-2.

[149] Alexoudi I, Kapsimali V, Vaiopoulos A, Kanakis M, Vaiopoulos G. Evaluation of current therapeutic strategies in Behçet's disease. Clin Rheumatol. 2011;30:157–63. DOI: 10.1007/s10067-010-1566-4.

[150] Rotondo C, Lopalco G, Iannone F, Vitale A, Talarico R, Galeazzi M, Lapadula G, Cantarini L. Mucocutaneous involvement in Behçet's Disease: how systemic treatment has changed in the last decades and future perspectives. Mediators Inflamm. 2015;2015:451675. DOI: 10.1155/2015/451675.

[151] Sfikakis PP, Markomichelakis N, Alpsoy E, Assaad-Khalil S, Bodaghi B, Gul A, Ohno S, Pipitone N, Schirmer M, Stanford M, Wechsler B, Zouboulis C, Kaklamanis P, Yazici H. Anti-TNF therapy in the management of Behcet's disease--review and basis for recommendations. Rheumatology (Oxford). 2007;46:736–41.

[152] Comarmond C, Wechsler B, Bodaghi B, Cacoub P, Saadoun D. Biotherapies in Behçet's disease. Autoimmun Rev. 2014;13: 762–9. DOI: 10.1016/j.autrev.2014.01.056. Epub 2014 Jan 26.

Chapter 6

Activity Criteria in Behçet's Disease

Feride Coban Gul, Hulya Nazik, Demet Cicek and
Betul Demir

Additional information is available at the end of the chapter

http://dx.doi.org/10.5772/68079

Abstract

Behçet's disease is a complex disease characterized by remission and activation periods of unknown duration. It has an unpredictable course. Behçet's disease shows a heterogeneous pattern of organ involvement that occurs in recurrent episodes of acute inflammation throughout the course of the disease. Disease activity in Behçet's disease is difficult to define because of its fluctuating course, lack of laboratory tests reflecting overall disease activity, absence of a standardized form to report the severity of Behcet's disease manifestations and also trying to develop new diagnostic criteria. This led to the development of standardized disease activity index. To be useful, a measurement of disease activity must be valid, reliable, and simple enough to use in routine clinical practice. We will try to explain what the situation is in terms of Behçet's disease activity index.

Keywords: Behçet, activity, disease, criteria, remission, activation

1. Introduction

As with many inflammatory diseases, Behçet's disease has a course including periods of remissions and exacerbations. Exacerbation periods are unknown, and it is difficult to predict the duration of attacks. In addition, the severity of disease varies from one patient to another, and for a given patient, it varies from one period to another [1]. The disease has an unpredictable course.

There are no laboratory markers compliant with the clinical findings in Behçet's disease. Therefore, disease activity is evaluated based on the clinical history. The reliability of the patients' answers to retrospective questions decreases as the time interval increases. Since the disease characteristics such as exacerbation, remission, severity of the attack, and duration of the attack are not known, the disease is refractory. It is also difficult to identify whether the remission in disease findings is due to the response to treatment or to the disease course. Therefore, during the treatment period, clinicians frequently rely on clinical findings of exacerbation and quality of life scales. However, since these parameters have not been standardized yet, they are not reliable in the evaluation of the response to treatment. In addition, clinical drug researches are far from measuring the treatment efficacy with sufficient sensitivity. In conclusion, it is difficult to define the disease activity in Behçet's disease, as:

(1) the disease has a fluctuant course;

(2) there is not an established laboratory test which would represent all the disease findings;

(3) there is not a standard test to explain the severity of disease symptoms; and

(4) new diagnosis criteria are being developed, which cause diagnostic difficulties [2].

Activity scales and laboratory findings in the evaluation of Behçet's disease are, however, important in understanding the treatment and course of the disease. An ideal activity scale for Behçet's disease should have the following properties:

(1) It should be sensitive to clinical changes.

(2) It should be authentic.

(3) It should be able to evaluate all the organs and systems involved.

(4) It should be sensitive to different effects on morbidity and life quality caused by different organ and system involvements.

(5) It should be able to evaluate the fluctuations in the natural course of the disease.

(6) It should be understandable and easily applicable.

(7) It should not be time consuming.

(8) It should be valid for different communities.

(9) It should not be affected by the differences in practitioners [3].

In addition, there are two kinds of activity scales in Behçet's disease. While the first one evaluates the specific organ activity, the other one is a general activity scale.

The Composite Index for the oral ulcer activity, which is used for aphthous stomatitis, measures the pain intensity and functional response. In the Composite Index, the presence of active oral aphthous stomatitis within the past month, pain caused by the lesion and, in addition, eating, masticatory, gustatory, and speech disorders are scored. However, it is not specific to Behçet's disease and can be used in other diseases with a course of aphthous stomatitis [4]. The Disease Activity Index for Behçet's disease has been developed to evaluate the intestinal activity of Behçet's disease, although its use is limited, except in Korea where it was developed [3, 5].

Yazici et al. developed Turkish Behçet's Disease Activity Index, and later performed activity index studies for Iranian Behçet's Disease and European Behçet's Disease [6, 7]. Finally, in Behçet's Disease meeting in Leeds, UK in 1994, both studies were combined, redefined, and evaluated as Behçet's disease current activity form by Bhakta [8].

First activation criteria were defined by Yazici et al. in Turkey. The body parts affected by Behçet's disease were classified into five groups and scored based on the level of the impact. Based on these criteria, the eyes, the skin, involvement of the vascular bed, arthritis, and neurological involvement were considered. This form evaluates the findings at the time of patient's admission, and retrospective evaluation cannot be performed (**Table 1**) [6].

The Iranian Behçet's Disease Activation Form (IBDDAM) was defined by Davatchi et al. in 1991. It evaluates 18 clinical symptoms and pathergy test within the past 4 months [7]. Activity within the past 12 months can be evaluated and a mean activity score is obtained. Each 5 aphthous stomatitides, each 1 of the genital ulcers, each 10 folliculitis, each 1 of the erythema nodosum, superficial thrombophlebitis, and positive pathergy test gets 1 point. Eye involvement is evaluated based on the severities of anterior and posterior uveitis and retinal vasculitis, and uveitis is multiplied by the constant 2 and retinal vasculitis is multiplied by the constant 3. Gastrointestinal system is scored between 3 and 6, central nervous system between 1 and 6, and arthritis between 1 and 3. An additional 2 points is added for deep veins, 6 for large veins, and 2 for the presence of epididymitis. If these findings are being observed for more than 1 month, scores equivalent to the total sum of scores are added for each month (**Table 2**).

Involvement	Evaluation
Eye	0 – normal
	1 – only vitreous or anterior chamber inflammation
	2 – visual acuity 0.5
	3 – visual acuity 0.3
	4 – a few meters finger count
	5 – blindness
Skin	1 – oral ulcer
	1 – erythema nodosum
	1 – genital ulcer
Vascular involvement	5 – vena cava superior or inferior thrombosis and/or arterial occlusion
	4 – vena cava superior or inferior thrombosis
	3 – calf vein thrombosis or superficial thrombophlebitis requiring rest
	2 – bilateral calf vein thrombosis and/or superficial thrombophlebitis
	1 – unilateral calf vein thrombosis and/or superficial thrombophlebitis
Arthritis	1 – each joint
Neurological involvement	2 – intracranial hypertension
	3 – multiple sclerosis like syndrome
	4 – pyramidal and/or cerebellar involvement

Table 1. Turkish Behçet activity criteria.

Oral ulcer	Every 5 ulcer 1 point
Genital ulcer	Each lesion 1 point
Skin lesion	Every 10 papulopustulosis 1 point, every 5 erythema nodosum 1 point
Eye	Anterior uveitis: 1–4 points (cell, hypopyon, precipitate) Posterior uveitis: 1–4 points (posterior cell, snowball, snowbank) Retinal vasculitis: 1–4 points (papil edema, macular edema, papillitis, arthritis)
Arthritis	Arthralgia 1 point (irrespective of the number of joints) Monoarthritis 2 points Polyarthritis 3 points
Central nervous system	Isolated lesion 1 point Mild involvement 3 points Severe involvement 6 points
Thrombosis	Superficial thrombophlebitis 1 point Thrombophlebitis in deep venules 2 points Large vein involvement 6 points
Gastrointestinal involvement	Mild symptom 3 points (chronic diarrhea, rectal hemorrhage) Severe symptom 6 points
Epididymitis	2 points
Pathergy test (+)	1 point

Table 2. Iranian's Behçet activity criteria.

The European Behçet's Disease Index was defined in 1993. Oral ulcer, genital ulcer, skin, and joint symptoms are evaluated based on the past month. In the eye, gastrointestinal system, central nervous system involvement, scoring is based on symptoms and findings. Eye involvement is scored between 0 and 47, involvement of any other organs except the eye is scored between 0 and 5 [9].

The aforementioned indices were found insufficient due to their inability to evaluate all organs and systems, not being easily applicable, and inability to be tested for validity for different communities. Following the consensus meeting in 1994, Behçet's disease current activity index was defined to eliminate the disadvantages in other indices. Ten symptoms frequently observed in Behçet's disease were evaluated. Among these symptoms, fatigue, headache, oral ulcers, genital ulcers, erythema nodosum or superficial thrombophlebitis, papulopustular eruption, arthralgia, arthritis, nausea, vomiting or abdominal pain, and bloody diarrhea are evaluated for the past 4 weeks with scores between 0 and 4. The eye, large veins, and central nervous system, the other three organ systems, are evaluated with two different variables. The patient's feelings about the disease activity within the past 4 weeks are questioned and marked on two visual Likert-type scales with seven different facial expressions. Similar visual score is used by the clinician to evaluate total disease activity. The patient does not have a self-evaluation form and clinical appointment and the decision of the clinician are required (**Table 3**).

Japanese Behçet's disease activity phase classification was performed in 2003 [10]. In the active phase, presence of subcutaneous venous thrombosis, skin findings (i.e., erythema nodosum and genital ulcer), arthralgia, gastrointestinal ulcer, central nervous system lesions, vasculitis, or epididymitis, and serum CRP, cerebrospinal fluid, colonoscopy in the clinical examination including ophthalmologic examination, and other clinical laboratory findings are evaluated. In this evaluation, presence of a score of two or more for oral aphthous stomatitis, genital ulcer, skin and eye symptoms, or presence of the defined symptoms of Behçet's disease, are defined as active phase. In addition, for the activation phase, there are some information which are advised to be taken into consideration:

ISBD
International Society for Behçet's Disease

BEHÇET'S DISEASE CURRENT ACTIVITY FORM 2006

Date:	Name:	Sex: M/F
Centre:	Telephone	Date of birth:
Country:		
Clinician:	Address:	

All scoring depends on the symptoms present over the **4 weeks** prior to assessment.
Only clinical features that the **clinician feels are due to Behçet's Disease** should be scored.

PATIENT'S PERCEPTION OF DISEASE ACTIVITY
(Ask the patient the following question:)

"Thinking about your Behçet's disease only, which of these faces expresses how you have been feeling over the last four weeks? "(Tick one face)

☺ ☺ ☺ ☺ ☺ ☹ ☹ ☹

HEADACHE, MOUTH ULCERS, GENITAL ULCERS, SKIN LESIONS, JOINT INVOLVEMENT AND GASTROINTESTINAL SYMPTOMS

Ask the patient the following questions and fill in the related boxes **"Over the past 4 weeks have you had?"**

(please tick one box per line)

	not at all	Present for up to 4 weeks
Headache		
Mouth Ulceration		
Genital Ulceration		
Erythema		
Skin Pustules		
Joints - Arthralgia		
Joints - Arthritis		
Nausea/vomiting/abdominal pain		
Diarrhoea+altered/frank blood per rectum		

EYE INVOLVEMENT
(Ask questions below)

(please circle)

"Over the last 4 weeks have you had?"		Right Eye		Left Eye	
	a red eye	No	Yes	No	Yes
	a painful eye	No	Yes	No	Yes
	blurred or reduced vision	No	Yes	No	Yes

If any of the above is present: "Is this new"? No Yes
(circle the correct answer)

NERVOUS SYSTEM INVOLVEMENT (include intracranial vascular disease)

New Symptoms in nervous system and major vessel involvement are defined as those not previously documented or reported by the patient
(Ask questions below)

Over the last 4 weeks have you had any of the following?	*please circle*		tick if new
blackouts	No	Yes	
difficulty with speech	No	Yes	
difficulty with hearing	No	Yes	
blurring of/double vision	No	Yes	
weakness/loss of feeling of face	No	Yes	
weakness/loss of feeling of arm	No	Yes	
weakness/loss of feeling of leg	No	Yes	
memory loss	No	Yes	
loss of balance	No	Yes	
Is there any evidence of new active nervous system involvement?		No	Yes

MAJOR VESSEL INVOLVEMENT(exclude intracranial vascular disease)
(Ask question below)

"Over the last 4 weeks have you had any of the following?"	*please circle*		tick if new
had chest pain	No	Yes	
had breathlessness	No	Yes	
coughed up blood	No	Yes	
had pain/swelling/discolouration of the face	No	Yes	
had pain/swelling/discolouration of the arm	No	Yes	
had pain/swelling/discolouration of the leg	No	Yes	
Is there evidence of new active major vessel inflammation?		No	Yes

CLINICIAN'S OVERALL PERCEPTION OF DISEASE ACTIVITY

Tick one face that expresses how you feel the patient's disease has been over the last 4 weeks.

BEHÇET'S DISEASE ACTIVITY INDEX

Add up all the scores which are highlighted in blue (front page items, one tick = score of 1 on index, all other items score 'yes' = 1. You should now have a score out of 12 which is the patient's Behçet's Disease Activity Index Score.

SCORE

Patients index score	0	1	2	3	4	5	6	7	8	9	10	11	12
Transformed index score on interval scale	0	3	5	7	8	9	10	11	12	13	15	17	20

Table 3. Behçet's disease current activity form.

(1) Increasing the drug dose, changes in or addition to the medication must be done, if the findings are indicating the active phase.

(2) Since they are not good criteria for the disease activity, only in the presence of oral aphthous stomatitis and papulopustular eruption, other suggested symptoms and past findings should be considered (number, width, changes in the frequency, and length of the recovery).

(3) In cases with distinct attacks, such as uveitis, active phase is concordant with the attack duration and usually regresses within 2 weeks. However, if distinct inflammatory findings last longer than 2 weeks, it is assumed that active phase continues.

(4) Cases in inactive phase can suddenly become active.

(5) Inactive phase, which is defined as the stable phase (remission), means 0 activity index for more than 1 year [10].

The activity index is presented in **Table 4**.

Other than these activity indices, there are indices mostly used in their country of development and have a more limited use. The Behçet's Disease Activity Index by Yossipovitch in 1993 (**Tables 5** and **6**), the index prepared by Krause et al. to measure the activity of Behçet's disease in their publication in 1999 (**Table 7**), clinical activity scoring defined by Chang et al. in 2002 (**Table 8**), and the index defined in Korea in 2003 can be used to measure the activity of Behçet's disease [11–14].

Behçet's disease does not have any parameters or tests which may be indicative of specific activity. However, there are some laboratory parameters that can lead to further investigation in the clinically relevant area.

Erythrocyte sedimentation rate (ESR) and C-reactive protein (CRP) levels have been shown to be unrelated to disease activity [15]. ESR and CRP levels may be elevated when the disease is inactive, or there may be no elevation of specific organ involvement in the active phase. Higher levels are considered a clue for further research [8]. Human leukocyte antigen (HLA)-B51 is still known as the strongest genetic susceptibility factor. The T-helper 17 and interleukin (IL)-17 pathways are active, as well as play an important role, particularly in acute attacks of Behçet's disease. Neutrophil activity is increased in Behçet's disease, and the affected organs show a significant neutrophil and lymphocyte infiltration. HLA-B51 association and increased IL-17 response are thought to play a role in neutrophil activation [16]. Human mitochondrial heat shock protein (HSP) is highly homologous with microbial HSP and provokes proliferation of autologous T cells in Behçet's disease patients [10]. The HSP 60/65 plays an important role in Behçet's disease mucocutaneous lesions [10]. The Serum IL-12 levels correlate with disease activity and higher levels of soluble TNFR-75 are presented in active Behçet's disease [17].

In the active phase of Behcet's disease, oxidation protein products which can be considered as acute phase proteins, such as neopterin, anti-streptolysin, rheumatoid factor, amyloid-A, α1-antitripsin, β2-microglobulin, myeloperoxidase, and malondialdehyde levels, were found to increase [18–21]. On the other hand, a decreasing tendency in antioxidant enzyme levels, such as superoxide dismutase, catalase, and glutathione peroxidase, can be detected [22]. There was an increment in the presence of IgA, IgM, sometimes IgD, IgG-containing immunocomplexes in patients with Behçet's disease [23]. It has been also shown that an increase is observed in salivary IgA levels during oral aft activation [24]. P-selectin, I-selectin, and L-selectin among the adhesion molecules during the activation period in Behcet's disease and increases in the expression of sICAM-1 during uveitis episodes have been detected [25–27]. The increased E-selectin levels were associated with Behçet's disease particularly the eye, central nervous system involvement, and thrombosis activation [28]. Increases in homocysteine levels have been demonstrated in Behcet;'s disease patients in which thrombosis has developed, and it has been suggested that the level is more related to endothelin and nitric oxide [29, 30]. Plasminogen activator inhibitor-1 levels were increased in thrombosis and arthritis attacks in Behçet's disease [31].

Active phase	One of the following symptoms is found: uveitis, subcutaneous venous thrombosis, skin lesion such as erythema nodosum, genital ulcers (those relating to the female sexual cycle should be excluded), arthralgia, intestinal ulceration, progressive central nervous system lesions, progressive vasculitis, and epididymitis
	Inflammatory findings are also evident from clinical examination (including ophthalmological findings) and/or clinical laboratory findings (serum CRP, findings in cerebral fluid, findings by colonic fiberscopy, and others)
	As for oral aphthous ulcers, skin/genital ulcers, and ocular symptoms, cases with a score of 2 or above are defined as BD in the active phase
Non-active phase	Cases excluded by the above definition for active phase
	1 – Dosage up, change or addition of therapeutic reagents is generally required in the active phase
	2 – As for cases with only oral aphthous ulcers or follicular papules, careful diagnosis is recommended taking into account other symptoms or past symptoms, since these symptoms are not good criteria for disease activity
	3 – In cases of lesions in which attack is obvious, for example, uveitis, active phase corresponds to the attack phase and the lesions continue for no longer than 2 weeks in general. However, if obvious inflammatory findings continue for more than 2 weeks, cases can be diagnosed as in the active phase at present
	4 – One should consider that it is possible that cases in the inactive phase suddenly move into the active phase
	5 – Stable phase (remission) is defined as the inactive phase with the activity index of 0 for more than 1 year
Oral ulcer	0 – none
	1 – less than 2 weeks in the last 4 weeks
	2 – more than 2 weeks or more than 2 weeks in the last 4 weeks
	3 – lesion last 4 weeks
Skin lesion	0 – none
	1 – less than 2 weeks in the last 4 weeks
	2 – more than 2 weeks or more than 2 weeks in the last 4 weeks
	3 – lesion last 4 weeks
Eye	0 – none
	1 – 1 episode in the last 4 weeks
	2 – 2 episodes in the last 4 weeks
	3 – 3 episodes in the last 4 weeks
Arthritis	Arthritis, walking difficulty, deformity
Gastrointestinal involvement	Acute/chronic abdominal pain, melena
Epididymitis	Pain, swelling
Vascular involvement	Cardiac/aortic disease, middle or small vein occlusion, thrombophlebitis
Central nervous system involvement	Headache, dizziness, paralysis

Table 4. Japan's Behçet activity criteria.

Mild İnvolvement	Minor oral aphthous and genital ulcer
	Skin symptoms
	Arthritis less than two joints
Severe involvement	Major oral ulcer and genital ulcer
	Arthritis more than two joints
	Eye symptoms
	Neurological symptoms
	Big vessels involvement

Table 5. Yossipovitch's activity form.

Mild involvement	Oral ulcer
	Genital ulcer
	Skin symptoms
Moderate involvement	Arthritis less than three joints
	Recurrent genital ulcers
	Mild anterior uveitis
Severe involvement	Anterior and posterior uveitis
	Big vessel involvement
	Arterial aneurysm
	Arthritis more than three joints

Table 6. Yossipovitch's activity form.

Mild (each one 1 point)	Oral ulcer
	Genital ulcer
	Skin lesion
	Arthritis
	Recurrent headache
	Epididymitis
	Mild gastrointestinal disease (chronic diarrhea, abdominal pain, etc.)
	Superficial vein thrombosis
	Chest pain
Moderate (each one 2 points)	Arthritis
	Deep vein thrombosis
	Anterior uveitis
	Gastrointestinal bleeding
Severe (each one 3 points)	Posterior or panuveitis, retinal vasculitis
	Arterial thrombosis or aneurysm
	Big vein thrombosis (vena cava, hepatic vein, etc.)
	Neurological involvement
	Bowel perforation

Table 7. Krause's activity form.

1 point	Oral ulcer
	Genital ulcer
	Skin lesion (erythema nodosum-like lesion, pp eruption)
	Superficial thrombophlebitis
2 points	Arthritis more than two joints
	Gastrointestinal ulcer with complication
	Small or medium diameter vascular involvement is not related to the vital organ
3 points	Uveitis
	Gastrointestinal tract involvement with perforation or bleeding
	Big vessels involvement
	Vital organ involvement (brain, lung, heart, etc.)

Table 8. Chang's activity form.

2. Pathergy test

The skin pathergy reaction is highly specific for Behçet's disease; there is considerable variation in the rate of positivity in patients from different geographical areas, which limits its clinical usefulness. A positive pathergy reaction is common in patients from Iran, Turkey, and Japan, but rare in those from the UK, the USA, and France [8].

Correlation studies with the disease activity of the pathergy test are insufficient. It has also been suggested that the pathergy test may be a positive relationship for the formation of oral aphthae, genital ulcer, arthritis, papulopustular eruption, and erythema nodosum, and a negative relationship to the presence of uveitis and venous thrombosis [32, 33]. Generally, there was no correlation between the severity of the disease and the pathergy test and it was stated that the positivity ratio could be increased by using nondisposable blunt needle [34]. It has been reported that the group defining the IBDDAM criteria may be able to detect positivity when the pathergy test is used periodically and that negative and positive phases may be detected during the disease. Pathergy test is one of the IBDDAM criteria. It has been reported that the pathergy test can be used to assess drug treatment efficacy [7].

3. Conclusion

Behçet's disease is a chronic inflammatory disease. Behçet's disease is characterized by remissions and exacerbations. The determination of whether the disease is in the active phase is important in terms of treatment and prognosis. Therefore, the parameters that determine the active phase are important. Although a change in laboratory parameters was detected during the course of Behçet's disease, no specific marker was detected. For this reason, disease activity index have been started to be developed on the basis of clinical history in order to detect disease activity. The activity index based on the story of clinical features appears to be more useful following the disease activity and treatment.

Author details

Feride Coban Gul[1]*, Hulya Nazik[2], Demet Cicek[3] and Betul Demir[3]

*Address all correspondence to: feridecobangul@gmail.com

1 Elazig Research and Education Hospital, Turkey

2 Bingol State Hospital, Turkey

3 Firat University Hospital, Turkey

References

[1] Yazıcı H. Behçet's syndrome. Current Opinion Rheumatology. 1999;11:53–57.

[2] Neves FS, Moraes JC, Kowalski SC, Goldenstein-Schainberg C, Lage LV, Gonçalves CR. Cross-cultural adaptation of the Behçet's Disease Current Activity Form (BDCAF) to Brazilian Portuguese language. Clinical Rheumatology. 2007;26:1263–1267.

[3] Ergun T. Activation criteria. Turkiye Klinikleri Journals. 2011;4:10–14.

[4] Mumcu G, Sur H, Inanc N, Karacaylı U, Cimilli H, Sisman N, et al. A composite index for determining the impact of oral ulcer activity in Behcet's disease and recurrent aphthous stomatitis. Journal of Oral Pathology and Medicine. 2009;38:785–791. DOI: 10.1111/j.1600-0714.2009.00803.x

[5] Cheon JH, Han DS, Park JY, Ye BD, Jun SA, Kim YS, et al. Inflammatory Bowel Disease. 2011;17:605–613. DOI: 10.1002/ibd.21313.

[6] Yazici H, Tüzün Y, Pazarli H, Yurdakul S, Ozyazgan Y, Ozdoğan H, et al. Influence of age of onset and patient's sex on the prevalence and severity of manifestations of Behçet's syndrome. Annals of the Rheumatic Disease. 1984;43:783–789.

[7] Davatchi F, Akbaran M, Shahram F, Jamshidi A, Gharibdoost F, Chams C. Iran Behçet's Disease Dynamic Activity Measure. Abstracts of the XIIth European Congress of Rheumatology. Hung Rheumatology. 1991;32:10–100.

[8] Bhakta BB, Brennan P, James TE, Chamberlain MA, Noble BA, Silman AJ. Behçet's disease: evaluation of a new instrument to measure clinical activity. Rheumatology. 1999;38:728–733.

[9] Bhakta B, Hamuryudan V, Brennan P, Chamberlain MA, Barnes C, Silman AJ. Assessment of disease activity in Behçet's disease. In: Wechsler B, Godeau P, eds. Excerpta Medica Int Congress Series 1037, 611. Amsterdam: Elsevier Science Publishers BV; 1993. pp. 235–240.

[10] Kurokawa MS, Suzuki N. Behcet's disease. Clinical and Experimental Medicine. 2004;3: 10–20.

[11] Yosipovitch G, Shohat B, Bshara J, Wysenbeek A, Weinberger A. Elevated serum interleukin 1 receptors and interleukin 1B in patients with Behçet's disease: correlations with disease activity and severity. Israel Journal of Medical Science. 1995;31:345–348.

[12] Krause I, Rosen Y, Kaplan I, Milo G, Guedj D, Molad Y, Weinberger A. Recurrent aphthous stomatitis in Behçet's disease: clinical features and correlation with systemic disease expression and severity. Journal of Oral Pathology and Medicine. 1999;28:193–196.

[13] Chang HK, Cheon KS. The clinical significance of a pathergy reaction in patients with Behcet's disease. Journal of Korean Medical Science. 2002;17:371–374. DOI: 10.3346/jkms.2002.17.3.371

[14] Lee ES, Kim HS, Bang D, Yu HG, Chung H, Shin DH, et al. Development of clinical activity form for Korean patients with Behçet's disease. Advance in Experimental Medicine and Biology. 2003;528:153–156.

[15] Türsen U. Activation Markers in Behcet Disease. Turkderm 2009;43:74–86.

[16] Alpsoy E. Behçet's disease: A comprehensive review with a focus on epidemiology, etiology and clinical features, and management of mucocutaneous lesions. Journal of Dermatology. 2016;43:620–632. DOI: 10.1111/1346-8138.13381.

[17] Turan B, Gallati H, Erdi H, Gürler A, Michel BA, Villiger PM. Systemic levels of the T cell regulatory cytokines IL-10 and IL-12 in Bechçet's disease; soluble TNFR-75 as a biological marker of disease activity. Journal of Rheumatology. 1997;24:128–132.

[18] Evereklioglu C. Current concepts in the etiology and treatment of Behcet disease. Survey of Ophthalmology. 2005;50:297–350.

[19] Bang D, Kim HS, Lee ES, Lee S. The significance of laboratory tests in evaluating the clinical activity of Behcet's disease. In: Bang D, Lee ES, Lee S, eds. Behcet's Disease, 9th International Conference on Behcet's Disease, Seoul, Korea; 2000. pp. 125–1277.

[20] Köse O, Arca E, Akgül O, Erbil K. The levels of serum neopterin in Behçet's disease – objective marker of disease activity. Journal of Dermatological Science. 2006;42:128–130.

[21] Aygunduz M, Bavbek N, Ozturk M, Kaftan O, Koflar A, Kirazli S. Serum beta 2-microglobulin reflects disease activity in Behcet's disease. Rheumatology International. 2002; 22:5–8.

[22] Erkiliç K, Evereklioglu C, Cekmen M, Ozkiris A, Duygulu F, Dogan H. Adenosine deaminase enzyme activity is increased and negatively correlates with catalase, superoxide dismutase and glutathione peroxidase in patients with Behçet's disease: original contributions/clinical and laboratory investigations. Mediators Inflammation. 2003;12:107–116.

[23] Sunakawa M, Ohshio G. Serum secretory IgA levels in patients with Behçet disease. Metabolic, Pediatric and Systemic Ophthalmology. 1989;12:110–112.

[24] Scully C, Boyle P, Yap PL. Immunoglobulins G, M, A, D and E in Behcet's syndrome. Clinical Chimica Acta. 1982;120:237–242.

[25] Assaad-Khalil SH, Abou-Seif M, Youssef I, Farahat N. L-selectin expression on leukocytes of patients with Behçet's disease. Advance in Experimental Medicine and Biology. 2003;528:273–278. DOI: 10.1007/0-306-48382-3_55

[26] Haznedaroglu E, Karaaslan Y, Büyükaflik Y, Koflar A, Ozcebe O, Haznedaroglu C, et al. Selectin adhesion molecules in Behçet's disease. Annals of Rheumatic Diseases. 2000;59:61–63.

[27] Uchio E, Matsumoto T, Tanaka SI, Ohno S. Soluble intercellular adhesion molecule-1 (ICAM-1), CD4, CD8 and interleukin-2 receptor in patients with Behçet's disease and Vogt-Koyanagi-Harada's disease. Clinical and Experimental Rheumatology. 1999;17: 179–184.

[28] Sari RA, Kiziltunç A, Taysi S, Akdemir S, Gündoğdu M. Levels of soluble E-selectin in patients with active Behcet's disease. Clinical Rheumatology. 2005;24:55–59. DOI: 10.1007/s10067-004-0982-8

[29] Ates A, Aydintug O, Olmez U, Duzgun N, Duman M. Serum homocysteine level is higher in Behçet's disease with vascular involvement. Rheumatology Intenational. 2005;25:42–44. DOI: 10.1007/s00296-003-0398-9

[30] Er H, Evereklioglu C, Cumurcu T, Türköz Y, Ozerol E, Sahin K, Doganay S. Serum homocysteine level is increased and correlated with endothelin-1 and nitric oxide in Behçet's disease. British Journal of Ophthalmology. 2002;86:653–657.

[31] Ozturk MA, Ertenli I, Kiraz S, Haznedaroglu CI, Celik I, Kirazli S, Calguneri M. Plasminogen activator inhibitor-1 as a link between pathological fibrinolysis and arthritis of Behcet's disease. Rheumatology International. 2004;24:98–102. DOI: 10.1007/s00296-003-0324-1

[32] Mansoori P, Chams C, Davatchi F, Shahram F, Akbarian M, Gharipdoost F, et al. Relationship of pathergy phenomenon and Behçet's disease manifestations. In: Wechsler B, Godeau P, eds. Behçet's Disease, Proceedings of the 6th International Conference on Behçet's Disease. Amsterdam: Excerpta Medica; 1993. pp. 367–369.

[33] Azizleri G. Behçet hastalığında deri bulgulari. Aktüel Tip Dergisi.1997;2:94.

[34] Dilsen N, Koniçe M, Aral O, Ocal L, Inanç M, Gül A. Comparative study of the skin pathergy test with blunt and sharp needles in Behçet's disease: confirmed specificity but decreased sensitivity with sharp needles. Annals of the Rheumatic Disease. 1993;52:823–825.

Chapter 7

Ocular Manifestations of Behçet's Disease

Esra Sahli and Ozlem Gurbuz-Koz

Additional information is available at the end of the chapter

http://dx.doi.org/10.5772/intechopen.69049

Abstract

Behçet's disease (BD) is a multisystemic autoimmune inflammatory disorder characterized by oral aphthous lesions, genital ulcerations, iridocyclitis with hypopyon, and skin lesions. While ocular manifestations occur in nearly 50% of the patients with Behçet's disease, ocular involvement is the initial manifestation in only less than 20% of the patients. Ocular Behçet's disease clinically presents iridocyclitis with or without hypopyon, vitritis, retinitis, occlusive retinal vasculitis, and cystoid macular edema. However, anterior uveitis is usually the only initial ocular manifestation; the most common form is panuveitis. The usual course of the disease is characterized by recurrent inflammatory periods. Recurrent inflammatory attacks may result in irreversible damage and significant visual loss. Early and effective treatment is required to prevent ocular morbidity. Recent developments in the treatment of ocular Behçet's disease like biological agents are promising with a rapid effect and high remission rates.

Keywords: behçet's disease, iridocyclitis, retinal vasculitis, retinitis, immunosuppressants, biological agents

1. Introduction

Behçet's disease (BD) is a multisystemic autoimmune inflammatory disorder characterized by oral aphthous lesions, genital ulcerations, iridocyclitis with hypopyon, and skin lesions. It often involves the central nervous system, cardiovascular system, gastrointestinal system, and joints as well. An enhanced or dysregulated immune response triggered by environmental factors in immunogenetically susceptible individuals plays a major role in etiopathogenesis of the disease [1].

The prevalence of BD is higher in Eastern Mediterranean and Eastern Asia countries than in Northern European countries and the USA. The highest disease incidence has been reported in Turkey as 20–421 per 100,000 people [2]. The prevalence rate in Japan is reported as 1/10,000 [3]. Studies from Iran, Greece, and the USA indicate 16–100 per 100,000 people, 6 per 100,000 people, and 4 per 1,000,000 people, respectively [4–6].

BD is an obliterative and necrotizing systemic vasculitis that involves different organ systems. Occlusive vasculitis is a characteristic of BD that is not typically seen in other forms of uveitis. It affects both arteries and veins. Its histopathological appearance is characterized by non-granulomatous inflammation with perivascular T lymphocytes and neutrophil infiltration and increased expression of adhesion molecules. Local expression of proinflammatory cytokines including tumor necrosis factor-alpha (TNF-α), interleukin-1-beta (IL-1β), and interleukin-8 (IL-8); increased circulating immune complexes; endothelial dysfunction; and abnormal coagulation system play role in the pathogenesis of BD-associated vasculitis [7].

Diagnosing BD can be challenging since there are no specific laboratory tests or pathognomonic findings. The diagnosis relies mainly on clinical findings. Positive skin pathergy test and positive of HLA-B51 values can help verify the diagnosis, but these are not used exclusively for BD diagnosis. The most commonly used diagnostic criterion is defined by the International Study Group for BD. Recurrent oral ulcer that occurs at least three times a year, is mandatory for the diagnosis. In addition, two of the four major symptoms, including eye lesion, recurrent genital ulcers, skin lesions, and a positive pathergy test, are sufficient for the diagnosis of BD [8]. According to Behçet's Disease Research Committee of Japan, there are four major and five minor criteria. The major criteria include recurrent aphthous ulcers, skin findings (similar of those erythema nodosum or acne and a pathergy test), genital ulcers, and ocular involvement. The minor criteria include arthritis, intestinal ulcers, epididymitis, vascular disease, and neuropsychiatric involvement. This diagnostic system requires only one major symptom in addition to typical ocular symptoms for the diagnosis of ocular BD [9, 10].

2. Ocular involvements of Behçet's disease

BD has wide range of clinical manifestations. While ocular manifestations occur in nearly 50% of the patients with BD (50–70% of affected men and 20–30% of affected women), ocular involvement is the initial manifestation in less than 20% of the patients [11]. BD has been reported as the most common diagnosis (32.2%) among patients with uveitis in Turkey and the third most common cause of noninfectious uveitis, following sarcoidosis and Vogt-Koyanagi-Harada disease, in Japan [12, 13].

Ocular findings generally occur within the first 2–4 years of the disease. In 80% of the patients, the manifestations are bilateral [14]. According to a study with a large patient group, the ratio of bilaterality was found 80% among men and 64% among women in the beginning of the disease. However, at the end of a 20-year follow-up, the ratio increased to 87% among men and 71% among women [15].

The gender seems to affect the clinical manifestations and prognosis. The disease usually has a more severe course in men with a younger age of onset. Isolated anterior uveitis has a higher frequency in females than in males. Males have greater visual morbidity because of the higher incidence of vitritis, retinitis, retinal vasculitis (RV), and retinal hemorrhages than females. The course of BD may also vary due to geographical ethnic factors and individual characteristics [14]. Although several familial cases and a pair of monozygotic twins correspondent for BD have been reported, no consistent inheritance pattern has been confirmed [16].

The most common form of BD is panuveitis. The usual course of the disease is characterized by recurrent inflammatory periods. Early recognition of ocular involvement is important, as uveitis management differs from extraocular involvements with high ocular morbidity. Despite modern treatment modalities, the disease still carries poor visual prognosis.

The ocular symptoms are usually first manifested during the third or fourth decade of life. The primary manifestation can be unilateral in 50–87% of patients and occurs usually as an anterior uveitis. Later in nearly two-thirds of the cases, it changes to bilateral panuveitis with a chronic relapsing course. Panuveitis is seen significantly more often in men than in women [3, 16, 17].

The diagnosis of ocular BD is done based on clinical findings obtained from slit-lamp biomicroscopy and ophthalmoscopy. In addition, fluorescein angiography (FA) and indocyanine green angiography (ICGA) examinations are seen to be helpful in the diagnosis [17].

Ocular BD clinically presents iridocyclitis with or without hypopyon, vitritis, retinitis, occlusive RV, and cystoid macular edema (CME). Band keratopathy, glaucoma, vitreoretinal hemorrhage, posterior vitreous detachment, macular degeneration, epiretinal membrane, vein occlusion, and phthisis of the eye may also be observed as complications of ocular BD [18].

During acute inflammation, diffuse infiltration of neutrophils and lymphocytes in the iris, ciliary body, and choroid is seen. After recurrences, increased collagen can lead to iris atrophy, posterior synechiae, cyclitic membrane formation, and the thickening of the choroid. In the retina, infiltration of leukocytes and plasma cells in and around blood vessels and into retinal tissue appears, histopathologically. Veins are more affected than arteries. During the inflammation, retinal vascular endothelial cells become swollen; neutrophil migration and thrombus formation are also seen. In more advance cases, fibrosis of blood vessels and complete vascular obliteration may be present. Rods and cones get destroyed. Fibrosis of the inner nuclear layer appears; however, the destruction of retinal pigment epithelium is minimal. The optic nerve vessels can be affected and can result in optic neuritis, ischemia, and finally optic atrophy [16].

In addition, recurrences are very common, and the recurrent attacks of ocular inflammation may result in severe ocular damage. BD may produce permanent vision loss in up to 20% of affected individuals. The poor long-term visual outcome is usually related to glaucoma, cataract, and RV [15].

Uveitis in BD may involve the anterior and/or the posterior segment of the eye. The location of the inflammation is important both therapeutically and prognostically. If the lesions affect the posterior segment, vision loss is usually permanent and significant. The most common presentation of BD is bilateral non-granulomatous panuveitis with RV.

3. Anterior segment involvement

Anterior uveitis is usually the only initial ocular manifestation in patients with BD, and it can occur as an isolated finding in about 10% of the patients. This presentation is more common in females. Anterior uveitis, also known as iridocyclitis, is limited to the iris and the vitreous. The inflammatory response in the anterior chamber is of non-granulomatous nature. Although ocular BD is characterized by explosive acute hypopyon uveitis, a more common presentation is iridocyclitis without hypopyon, which is seen in two-thirds of the cases [17, 19].

Patients' complaints are often redness, pain in the globe, photophobia, tearing, and blurred vision. Slit-lamp biomicroscopic examination reveals conjunctival injection, perilimbal flush, cells and flare in the anterior chamber, keratic precipitates, and hypopyon. Disruption of the blood-aqueous barrier results in aqueous flare and cells, which are the two inflammatory parameters of anterior chamber inflammation. Cells in the aqueous humor can be detected as particles identified by backscattering light from the incoming beam with slit-lamp biomicroscopy. Grading systems have been developed to standardize quantification of cells and flare in the anterior chamber, based on slit-lamp examination. Increased protein content of the aqueous humor produces flare. It can be measured by laser flare photometry, which is an objective quantitative method. Yalcindag et al. reported that flare levels in the aqueous humor were correlated with fluorescein leakage on FA and suggested that higher flare values were associated with poor vision [20]. Keratic precipitate is an inflammatory cellular deposit seen usually on the lower part of the corneal endothelium. These precipitates are composed of the aggregation of polymorphonuclear cells and lymphocytes. They are fine, irregular, and almost always nonpigmented. Hypopyon is formed by the accumulation of cells and fibrin in the lower part of the anterior chamber of the eye. It is seen as a whitish or grayish fluid (**Figure 1**). Hypopyon includes mostly polymorphonuclear cells. Hypopyon typically freely moves and slowly shifts with gravity according to head position within minutes as opposed to the sticky hypopyon of HLA-B27-associated uveitis. The presence of hypopyon without ciliary injection is called

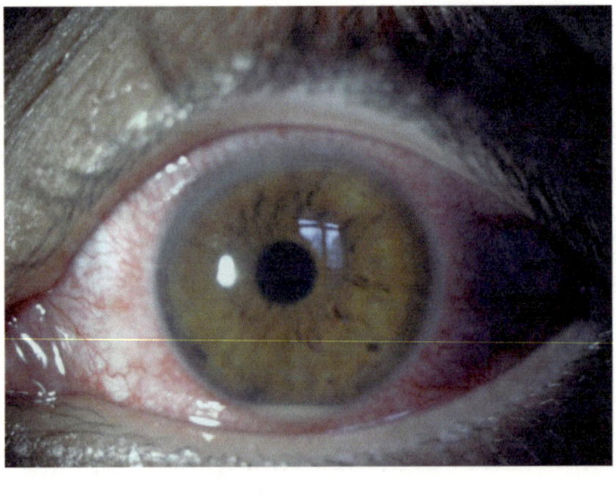

Figure 1. Hypopyon in a patient with Behçet's disease.

"cold hypopyon." A small layer of leucocytes can be observed in the anterior chamber angle by gonioscopy and is called angle hypopyon. The eye can be seen white despite inflammatory reaction in the anterior chamber. The hypopyon can be overlooked during the eye examination because this finding is transient. At the same time, hypopyon nowadays is less commonly seen because of earlier and more aggressive treatments. In the convalescent period of uveitis with hypopyon, slightly thickened pigment particles presenting as multiple dark brown spots can be seen in the inferior angle [17, 21].

The anterior uveitis appears very rapidly; its nature is explosive. It may get resolved spontaneously within 2–3 weeks even if it is not treated. Almost all nonpermanent inflammatory findings may disappear after each attack. Recurrent inflammatory attacks can result in structural changes of the anterior segment of the eye including posterior synechiae, iris atrophy, and peripheral anterior synechiae. Posterior synechiae are the adhesion between the posterior iris and the anterior lens surface. Pigment epithelial cells can be seen on the lens surface when the pupil is dilated (**Figure 2**). Mydriatic agents and topical corticosteroids are useful in breaking and preventing the formation of posterior synechiae. Posterior synechiae may be segmental or annular. Seclusio pupillae, 360° adhesions of pupillary margin to anterior capsule of the lens, and occlusio pupillae, the presence of a fibrovascular membrane across the pupil, may also be seen (**Figure 3**). Peripheral anterior synechiae, adhesion between the anterior iris and cornea, may be seen in result of the dense inflammation. Peripheral anterior synechiae and iris bombe formation associated with seclusion of pupilla may cause secondary glaucoma. Neovascularization of the iris may be seen secondary to occlusive RV.

The other anterior segment changes include episcleritis, scleritis, conjunctivitis, conjunctival ulcerations, and subconjunctival hemorrhages, keratitis, and rarely extraocular muscle paralysis.

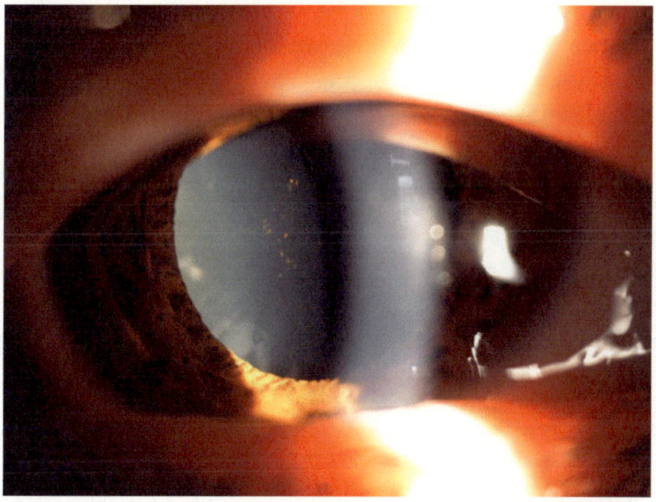

Figure 2. Pigment epithelial cells on the lens surface when pupil is dilated in a patient with Behçet's disease.

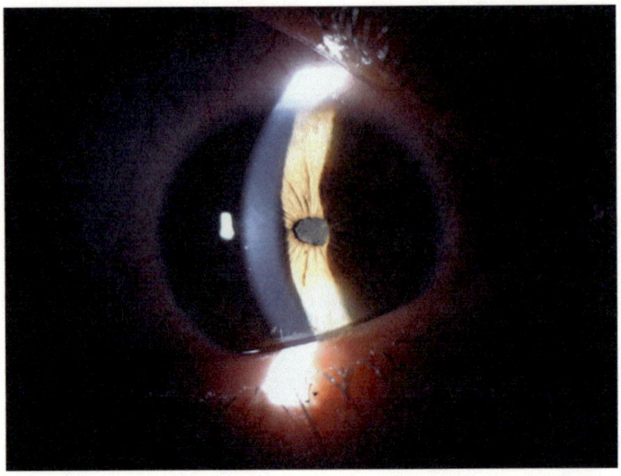

Figure 3. Posterior synechiae formation secondary to anterior uveitis in a patient with Behçet's disease.

4. Posterior segment involvement

The most common posterior segment findings are vitritis and RV. They are found in nearly 90% of Behçet patients with uveitis. However, an isolated vitritis, white cell infiltration of the vitreous body, is not a characteristic of BD. Increased vascular permeability of the retina, choroid, and ciliary body vessels results in cells in the vitreous and vitreous haze. White cell infiltration in the vitreous ranges from variable number of cells suspended in the vitreous fibrils to a dense plasmoid reaction in the acute phase. Vitreous haze is usually a proteinous material. It is important to follow up because it demonstrates the posterior segment activation. Even though the presence of vitreous cells is considered as the evidence of activation, they may also be seen as the persistent opacities in the vitreous cavity. They can be displaced by movements of the head easily and can be evaluated with slit-lamp biomicroscopy. Vitritis may last in a chronic smoldering course. In most cases, posterior vitreous detachment occurs at an early stage of ocular disease (92%) [22].

The essential manifestation of the posterior segment in patients with ocular BD is an occlusive and necrotizing RV. RV is defined as a disruption in the blood-retinal barrier and results in retinal vascular leakage on FA and perivascular infiltrates on dilated fundus examination in addition to the presence of other signs of intraocular inflammation such as cell infiltration into the vitreous, anterior chamber, retina, or choroid [23]. RV occurs as recurrent vaso-occlusive episodes that lasts for weeks. Active periods are then followed by periods of relative quiescence.

In most patients, RV mainly affects the retinal veins, which is pathognomonic for BD. In addition to this, BD is the only systemic vasculitis affecting small- and medium-sized arteries and also veins. Venous and capillary dilatation with engorgement may also be seen (**Figure 4**) [21].

Retinal vasculitis can be concluded as a finding such as an intraretinal hemorrhage or cotton wool exudate. Intraretinal hemorrhage indicates an abnormality of retinal vessel wall. Cotton wool

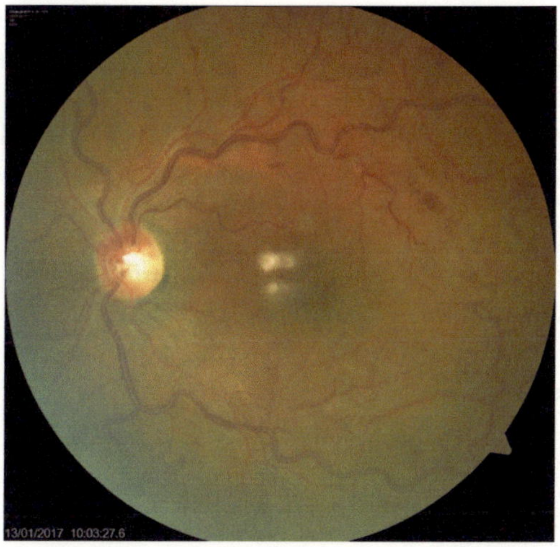

Figure 4. Fundus photograph of a patient with Behçet's disease showing diffuse retinal vasculitis.

exudates indicate local retinal ischemia caused by occlusive vasculitis. In BD with RV, patchy perivascular sheathing and whitish yellow exudates surrounding retinal hemorrhages are often observed. Severe RV can result in ischemic changes due to vascular occlusion. Choroidal vascular involvement also occurs, and choroidal infarcts can also be seen [14, 16, 24].

Based on necrotizing obliterative vasculitis, neovascularization of the optic disc and peripheral retina can cause retinal detachment with or without vitreous hemorrhage. The process could be summarized as follows: vascular occlusion causes retinal hypoxia, which stimulates the neovascularization of the optic disc and elsewhere. Both of them can rupture and cause vitreous hemorrhage. Vitreous hemorrhage may organize with transvitreal membrane formation, which may exert traction on the retina. This traction may lead to rhegmatogenous or combined tractional-rhegmatogenous retinal detachment [1, 15].

Retinitis is the next most common posterior segment manifestation. Retinitis is evidenced by soft infiltrates. These soft exudates resolve spontaneously in a few weeks, but diffuse vitreous opacity may stay for a few months [1].

Inflammatory cell infiltrations that affect the superficial and deep layers of the retina and hemorrhages coexisting with infiltration appear in occasional cases. In the acute disease transient, superficial white infiltrates that heal without scarring may be observed. Exudative retinal detachment may also appear after acute retinitis. Retinal atrophy can occur following the resolution of retinal exudates and hemorrhage [1].

Retinal edema is present in 20–75% of cases especially in the macula. Cystoid or diffuse macular edema caused by vascular leakage is one of the most important findings [15]. Optical coherence tomography (OCT) imaging reveals retinal thickening and is useful for follow-up. Thrombosis of the central retinal vein or its branches may be seen, but they are the less common findings. Occlusion of the central retinal artery is extremely rare. Bilateral retinal vein thromboses and bilateral posterior ischemic optic neuropathy have been reported [25, 26].

The optic nerve is affected in at least one-fourth of patients with BD. This condition may either present as an isolated papillitis or as a finding of sagittal sinus thrombosis due to neurological involvement of BD. Papillitis with optic disc hyperemia and blurring of the margins is the most common involvement of the optic nerve. Optic disc edema may occur as a result of the microvasculitis of the arterioles supplying the optic disc. While it is not seen very often, it can lead to progressive optic atrophy [15].

End-stage disease is characterized by optic atrophy, gliosis and sheathing, and attenuation of retinal vessels and ghost vessels. Destructive and recurrent attacks of uveitis especially with posterior segment involvement may result in permanent damage in the sensory retina, causing irreversible loss of vision.

5. Complementary imaging modalities and laboratory tests

Fluorescein angiography is essential and gold standard in evaluating the activity and the extent of the vasculitis in Behçet patients. FA demonstrates fluorescein staining on the vessel wall and/or fluorescein leakage from the vessel, which shows increased vascular permeability caused by the breakdown of the inner blood-retinal barrier, in RV.

If the posterior segment of the eye is involved, FA may reveal macular hyperfluorescence or perivascular staining with dye leakage from the dilated retinal capillaries even before retinal perivasculitis can be detected ophthalmoscopically [17]. FA provides a significant contribution in detecting vascular leakage, demonstrating the presence of macular edema, capillary non-perfusion, occlusion of the retinal vessels, collateral formation, and neovascularization in BD (**Figure 5**). Atmaca reported that FA revealed fluorescein leakage from retinal vessels in 6.3% of Behçet patients who had no vision loss or no abnormal findings on fundus examination, in 1989 [27].

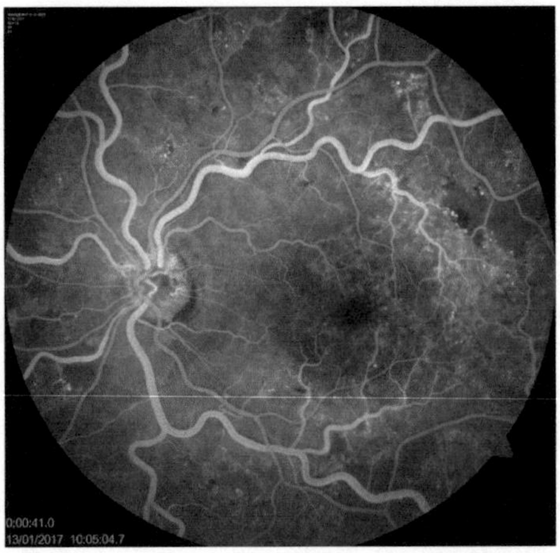

Figure 5. Fluorescein angiography of a patient with Behçet's disease revealing diffuse fluorescein leakage from retinal vessels and cystoid macular edema.

"Fern-like fluorescein leakage" due to inflammation at retinal capillaries is clearly demonstrated on the mid-phase FA, and it is a characteristic finding and the most frequent fluorescein angiographic appearance of BD (**Figure 6**). Fluorescein leakage from retinal capillaries is seen not only during the inflammatory period but also during the apparently quiescent periods between attacks. It may be the only sign of persistent inflammation in the posterior segment during clinically inactive periods. These findings have a high diagnostic value in BD [13, 19].

Determination of FA findings is important to evaluate the severity of the disease and the response to the treatment. All classifications were based on the late phase of angiogram. FA findings are classified based on the extent of the vascular leakage as focal and diffuse, according to macular involvement as incomplete perifoveal hyperfluorescence, mild 360° hyperfluorescence, moderate 360° hyperfluorescence (nearly 1 disc diameter across), and severe 360° hyperfluorescence (nearly 1.5 disc diameter across). Corresponding to optic disc hyperfluorescence in the late angiographic phases, the findings can be categorized as none (normal exiting of fluorescein and normal staining of the sclera rim), partial, diffuse without blurring of the disc margin, and diffuse with blurring of the disc margin [28].

Kim et al. investigated whether there is correlation between FA findings and visual acuity (VA) in Behçet patients with RV. Retinal vascular leakage, optic disc hyperfluorescence, and macular leakage were seen to be associated with a decreased VA [29].

Visualization of the peripheral retina by an ultrawide-field retinal imaging system may be useful to diagnose and monitor RV in Behçet patients and in the treatment of the disease. Conventional fundus cameras can capture only 30–60° of the fundus at a time and cannot image the entire retina simultaneously. The ultrawide-field imaging system provides 200° of photographic and angiographic views of the ocular fundus [30]. Improved visualization of the peripheral retina by ultrawide-field imaging has demonstrated that peripheral RV could be detected in 85% of eyes that did not have ophthalmoscopic evidence [31].

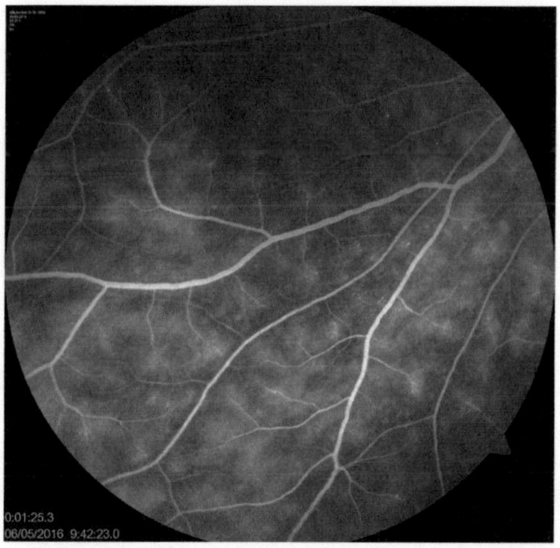

Figure 6. "Fern-like" fluorescein leakage from peripheral retinal vessels on fluorescein angiography.

Choroidal and retinal pigment epithelial changes are rarely seen in ocular BD. The BD patients with choroidal abnormalities could only be evaluated with ICGA and not with fundus examination or FA [32]. In these cases, ICGA may have an advantage over FA in showing lesions, choroidal vessel leakage, irregular filling of the choriocapillaris, and choroidal filling defects. ICGA was demonstrated with no clinically useful information on disease activity and monitoring the disease. ICGA is used to evaluate choroidal involvement in inflammation of the posterior segment [32, 33]. Since the choroidal infarcts are probably more common than they are usually estimated, simultaneous ICGA and FA would be useful for examining choroidal involvement in BD.

OCT provides both high-resolution cross-sectional imaging of the retina and quantitative measurement of the retinal thickness. For the detection and follow-up of macular edema in BD, OCT and FA are both necessary and complementary. The integrity of junctions between inner and outer segments of the photoreceptors (ISOS line) and the cone outer segment tip line (interdigitation zone) are correlated with visual function and prognosis in patients with uveitic macular edema, and these zones are best evaluated by OCT [34, 35].

Transient retinal infiltrates, which are commonly seen during exacerbations of Behçet's uveitis, are indicated as focal retinal thickening; increased hyper-reflectivity with blurring, especially of inner retinal layers; and optical shadowing by spectral-domain OCT. In Behçet's uveitis, retinal infiltrates rapidly resolve without any apparent retinochoroidal scarring. However, inner retinal atrophy is seen in the spectral-domain OCT sections [34].

Recently, the assessment of choroidal thickness has been possible by the enhanced depth imaging (EDI) mode of spectral-domain OCT in patients with Behçet's uveitis. Ishikawa et al. and Kim et al. reported that subfoveal choroidal thickness was significantly higher during an acute attack of Behçet's uveitis than in remission. Their choroid was found thicker than that of healthy control subjects not only during an attack of Behçet's uveitis but also during remission of the disease [36, 37].

Elevated erythrocyte sedimentation rate, positive C-reactive protein, and increased peripheral blood leukocytes, which are nonspecific factors indicative of immune system activation, may be abnormal during the acute phase of BD. The other acute phase reactants such as properdin factor-b and alpha-1-acid glycoprotein may also be elevated [16].

6. Management of ocular Behçet's disease

Behçet's uveitis has a remitting and relapsing course, and recurrent inflammatory attacks may result in irreversible damage and significant visual loss. It is one of the most difficult forms of uveitis to treat. The aim of the treatment should be to obtain a rapid resolution of inflammation, to prevent or at least reduce the frequency of attacks, and to avoid complications. There is no standard treatment protocol. The choice of therapy is based on the severity of the disease. Combination therapy is required in most of the patients. Early and aggressive treatment should be administered whenever following features are present: male sex, young age, characteristic geographical origin, complete BD (the presence of oral and genital ulcer, ocular and skin findings simultaneously or at different times), posterior segment and bilateral involvement, and central nervous system or vascular involvement [4]. The therapy in BD should be highly effective for preferably manifestations, should effect rapidly, have fewer side effects, and should be as cheap as possible.

6.1. Corticosteroid therapy

Local and systemic steroids especially during attacks are used very commonly. Corticosteroids help suppress the ocular inflammation rapidly but have potential side effects including glaucoma and cataract.

In the treatment of anterior uveitis, topical corticosteroid drops (prednisolone acetate, dexamethasone phosphate) should be used to suppress the inflammatory response. It can be discontinued upon vanishing the anterior chamber cells after nearly 6–8 weeks of application. Relapses and severe exacerbations may develop when dose is lowered. Therefore, stepwise tapering the corticosteroid dose is needed. Corticosteroid-induced ocular hypertension and cataract development are possible risks of the treatment. Topical nonsteroidal anti-inflammatory drugs such as indomethacin, diclofenac, and flurbiprophen could be added to topical corticosteroids to potentiate the corticosteroid activity. Topical mydriatic and cycloplegic agents should be added twice or three times a day (tropicamide 1%, cyclopentolate 1%, and phenylephrine 2.5 and 10%) in order to relieve photophobia, pain, and discomfort and prevent synechiae formation [38, 39].

Patients with severe anterior uveitis unresponsive to topical treatment may benefit from subtenon or subconjunctival injections of depot corticosteroids such as triamcinolone acetonide or methylprednisolone acetate every 2–4 weeks for 4–5 times. Depot steroids ensure long-lasting suppression of the inflammation. However side effects such as conjunctival hemorrhage or scarring, encapsulated cyst, ptosis, and accidental eye perforation may occur. Subconjunctival corticosteroid injection can be administered for treating hypopyon and severe anterior segment inflammation with fibrin clotting [38, 39].

When topical and local administration is not effective, a short course of oral corticosteroids (prednisolone, 1–2 mg/kg/day), colchicine, or methotrexate may be used in addition. High-dose systemic corticosteroids are used for the treatment of severe posterior uveitis and panuveitis attacks. Intravenous pulse methylprednisolone (1 g/day) is usually administered for 3 consecutive days to obtain a rapid anti-inflammatory effect. Then oral prednisone (1–1.5 mg/kg/day) is given in a single morning dose and slowly tapered to a maintenance dose of 7.5 mg/day or less after complete resolution of active inflammation. If exacerbation is encountered under the dose of 0.5 mg/kg/day, steroid may be stopped, and another immunosuppressant agent can be started. Long-term treatment with systemic corticosteroid should not be preferred. Elevation of intraocular pressure (IOP), cataract, cushingoid state, GI ulcers, osteoporosis, diabetes mellitus, and exacerbations of infections are some of the important side effects of systemic corticosteroid treatment [17, 38, 39].

6.2. Immunomodulatory therapy

Behçet patients with acute and severe posterior segment involvement may benefit from systemic corticosteroid treatment in early stages. The prolonged use of systemic corticosteroids must be avoided, because severe rebound attacks can occur during tapering the dose. Despite the fact that corticosteroids alone have failed to prevent vision loss in patients with BD, their immediate anti-inflammatory effect is useful while waiting for the immunosuppressant agents to effect fully. The corticosteroids should be tapered rapidly within weeks and immunosuppressant agents should start. A single long-term immunosuppressant agent is initially administered as monotherapy for at least 6–12 months. Conventional immunosuppressive agents that have been used for the treatment of BD uveitis with posterior segment involvement include antimetabolites (methotrexate, azathioprine, mycophenolate), calcineurin inhibitors (cyclosporine A, tacrolimus, sirolimus), and alkylating agents (chlorambucil, cyclophosphamide). If the disease does not respond to these drugs, the dose is increased or the drug is changed to another one. The combination of two cytotoxic immunosuppressants (methotrexate, azathioprine, chlorambucil, and cyclophosphamide) can be tried in patients with severe RV [17, 38].

In selected patients, low-dose corticosteroids, at the dose of equal or less than 10 mg/day, may be required chronically in combination with immunosuppressants for controlling uveitis. This combination is beneficial for reducing the adverse effects of either immunosuppressants or corticosteroids.

6.2.1. Azathioprine

Azathioprine is an antimetabolite drug that interferes with purine incorporation into DNA and affects rapidly proliferating cells such as activated lymphocytes [16]. Azathioprine can be administered alone or in combination with corticosteroids and other immunosuppressives at the dose of 2–2.5 mg/kg/day. Important side effects of Azathioprine are fever, reversible bone marrow suppression, hepatotoxicity, hyperuricemia, pancreatitis, and increasing risk of malignancies. Complete blood count (CBC) and liver function tests (LFT) should be performed every 2 weeks for the first month and then once every 3 months [17]. The patients who initially received azathioprine treatment especially within 2 years after disease onset have a better visual prognosis and less risk of new eye disease [40].

6.2.2. Methotrexate

Methotrexate is an antimetabolite drug that prevents the activation of folic acid, necessary for synthesis of DNA. Methotrexate is suggested at the dose of 7.5–20 mg/week perorally. Gastrointestinal upset, bone marrow suppression, hepatorenal toxicity, central nervous system toxicity, sterility, alopecia, and anorexia are potential side effects of methotrexate. CBC and LFT should be ordered every 2 weeks for the first month and then once a month [17].

6.2.3. Mycophenolate mofetil

Mycophenolate mofetil is an antimetabolite drug that blocks DNA synthesis by the inhibition of enzyme inosine monophosphate dehydrogenase. It does not inhibit the early production of cytokines of T-helper-cell clones (Th0 and Th2); it acts synergistically with other immunosuppressive agents [16]. Larkin and Lightman reported successfully treated Behçet patients by adding mycophenolate mofetil to their combination of steroid and cyclosporine [41].

6.2.4. *Cyclosporine A*

Cyclosporine A is a noncytotoxic immunomodulatory agent, which selectively and reversibly inhibits T-helper-lymphocyte-mediated immune responses. It binds to and inhibits calcineurin by forming cyclosporine-cyclophilin complex. Calcineurin catalyzes reactions necessary for early activation of T cells and production and expression of cytokines such as IL-2 [42]. Cyclosporine A has been shown to reduce frequency and severity of uveitis attacks and is administered at the dose of 3–5 mg/kg/day in two divided doses. It induces rapid suppression of intraocular inflammation. Cyclosporine A is safer than the cytotoxic agents in the management of posterior segment manifestations and inflammatory recurrences, and it is usually combined with systemic corticosteroids [43]. Cyclosporine A is shown to provide rapid improvement in VA and decrease in the frequency and severity of ocular attacks in ocular Behçet patients in three randomized controlled trials [44–46].

After corticosteroids are withdrawn, cyclosporine A is tapered down 10% of dose every month to the minimum effective dose to control the disease. But even at low doses, long-term treatment is limited to the development of side effects, including hypertension, nephrotoxicity, arrhythmia, headache, gum hyperplasia, hirsutism, female reproductive disorder, diabetes, hepatotoxicity, and myelosuppression. Rebound attacks may occur following discontinuation or even during tapering of the dose. Cyclosporine A is demonstrated to be associated with an increased risk of parenchymal neuro-Behçet's disease and is contraindicated in patients with neurological involvement [17, 38].

6.2.5. *Tacrolimus (FK-506)*

Tacrolimus suppresses CD4+ T lymphocytes similar to cyclosporine A. However, it has a better safety profile than cyclosporine. Favorable results in 75% of patients with refractory uveitis, who had been using corticosteroids, colchicine, cyclophosphamide, and cyclosporine, have been reported by the Japanese FK-506 Study Group on Refractory Uveitis [47]. However, the use of tacrolimus on the treatment of ocular BD is very limited.

6.2.6. *Chlorambucil*

Chlorambucil is a slow-acting alkylating agent. The usual dose of chlorambucil is 0.1 mg/kg/day. Immunosuppressive effect of chlorambucil appears in 1–3 months of therapy [16]. Chlorambucil has been reported to provide even a durable remission after its discontinuation, but its potential serious side effects including an increasing risk of malignancy and azoospermia in men have limited its use in ocular BD. It is suggested only as the last option before the biological agents are available [38].

6.2.7. *Cyclophosphamide*

Cyclophosphamide is a fast-acting alkylating agent. It can be administrated orally or intravenously. The recommended dose of cyclosporine is 1–2 mg/kg/day, which may be increased to 3–4 mg/kg/day for several weeks in selected, severe cases only. For long-term treatment, the dose must be adjusted according to the therapeutic response, renal function, and leukocyte count. The intravenous administration is indicated in cases like patients with occlusive RV where a fast onset of therapeutic effect is important to preserve VA. A bolus of 15–20 mg/kg is given every 3–4 weeks [48].

It has been reported that cyclophosphamide showed favorable results in controlling uveitis, preventing ocular attacks, and maintaining a good VA for a long time in patients with BD. There are also reports demonstrating that cyclophosphamide therapy is superior to steroids and cyclosporine in the management of ocular BD [43, 48, 49].

6.3. Biological agents

Severe RV secondary to BD is often treated with monoclonal antibody against TNF-α or IFN-α in some centers. Some authors prefer to use biological agents alone because of less risk of side effects and infection and less cost, but usually the authors add anti-TNF therapy to antimetabolites and then consider discontinuation of the antimetabolite therapy gradually in a period of 6–12 months, if complete control of ocular inflammation is achieved.

6.3.1. Antitumor necrosis factor agents

Several studies suggest a central pathogenic role of TNF-α in the pathogenesis of BD uveitis. TNF-α is produced by mononuclear cells in the peripheral blood as part of the inflammatory cascade in BD. Levels of TNF-α and soluble TNF receptors are elevated in serum and aqueous humor in patients with BD [50–52].

Currently, available anti-TNF-α agents include etanercept (a recombinant fusion protein, combining 2 human p75 TNF-α receptors linked to the Fc domain of human IgG1), infliximab (a mouse-human chimeric monoclonal IgG1 anti-TNF-α antibody), and adalimumab (a fully humanized monoclonal IgG1 anti-TNF-α antibody). Although it is useful in the management of many rheumatologic diseases, etanercept does not seem to be an effective treatment for ocular BD [16].

Refractory ocular involvement is the main indication for anti-TNF treatment in BD; the beneficial effects of these agents have been reported in extraocular manifestations such as gastrointestinal, vascular, and neurological manifestations of BD as well [53, 54].

6.3.1.1. Infliximab

Infliximab (Remicade, Bausch & Lomb, Rochester, New York, USA) is a chimeric monoclonal antibody directed against TNF-α. It neutralizes membrane-bound TNF-α and soluble TNF-α, suppresses the production of TNF-α by macrophages and lymphocytes, and induces T_{reg} cells that acquire suppressive function in the periphery. It is administered as intravenous infusions, at the dose of 5 mg/kg (3–10 mg/kg) at weeks 0, 2, and 6 and then every 8 weeks.

Infliximab is used in refractory sight-threatening cases. Regarding the safety profile, infliximab therapy is well tolerated with few adverse events including opportunistic infections, lupus-like reactions, multiple sclerosis, dyspnea, and hypotension and increased risk of malignancy.

Infliximab has been found to be efficient and well tolerated in ocular BD. Patients with two or more attacks of active posterior or panuveitis in a year and patients with chronic CME are likely to benefit biological agents. It is demonstrated that significant decrease in inflammation, improved VA, reduced ocular complications, and the number of relapses were observed in infliximab compared with corticosteroid and immunosuppressive therapy [55–57].

Summarizing recent reports evaluating the effect of repetitive infliximab therapy in BD, clinical responses to the therapy were achieved in 90, 89, 100, and 91% of patients with resistant mucocutaneous, ocular, gastrointestinal, and central nervous system involvement, respectively [58].

6.3.1.2. Adalimumab

Adalimumab (Humira, Abbvie Inc., North Chicago, IL, USA) is a fully recombinant human immunoglobulin G1 monoclonal antibody that specifically binds to membrane and soluble human TNF-α with high affinity and inhibits its binding to TNF receptors. Adalimumab is suggested to be administered at a dose of 40 mg/week, subcutaneously. In patients with sight-threatening Behçet's uveitis who were switched from infliximab to adalimumab, improvement in VA, decreasing in recurrences, and even complete resolution of inflammation have been demonstrated [59–61].

6.3.1.3. Golimumab

Another TNF-α inhibitor, golimumab, is a fully human monoclonal antibody with reduced immunogenicity. It has an advantage of longer half-life that allows monthly subcutaneous injections. Few data are available evaluating the efficacy of golimumab in BD uveitis [62].

6.3.2. Interferon-alpha

Interferon-alpha (IFN-α) is a natural cytokine produced by plasmacytoid dendritic cells. It induces T helper type 1 cells, T cytotoxic cells, and natural killer cells and increases the production of anti-IL-1 receptor antagonist. Interferons can influence both innate and adaptive immune responses [16, 38]. It is generally administered subcutaneously with a dose 3–6 million IU, most often three times weekly. IFN-α should not be used in pregnant patients. Immunosuppressive drugs should be stopped completely before the initiation of IFN-α. Systemic corticosteroids should be tapered to a dose of 10 mg prednisolone equivalent per day as soon as possible because of the antagonistic effect of corticosteroids [63, 64]. Adverse effects of IFN-α including flu-like reactions (90%), fever, mild leucopenia (30%), alopecia (10%), depression (8%), and thyroiditis are common. Gastrointestinal disturbances, increase of liver enzymes, transient paresthesia, and epilepsy may also be seen [64–66].

IFN-α is recommended for the treatment of severe eye involvement of BD by European League against Rheumatism (EULAR) in the light of several uncontrolled studies demonstrating a fast onset of action and high remission rates. The remission may persist after withdrawal of the agent. IFN-α has been included in the EULAR recommendation equal to TNF-α blockers [67]. It works fast enough to be used in the acute phase of BD with panuveitis and/or RV unresponsive to at least one immunosuppressive drug. A quick response within 2–4 weeks, complete or partial remission of uveitis, is achieved in almost all patients with BD [64, 68–70].

IFN-α has been shown to improve VA, resolve vitritis, and control RV and CME in most cases with BD [66, 68–70]. A reperfusion of occluded retinal vessels and complete regression of retinal neovascularization has been demonstrated with IFN-α. These effects may prevent the vision loss because occlusive vasculopathy develops despite the use of immunosuppressants [71, 72].

It is suggested that long-term remission seems to be associated with higher doses of IFN-α, but not with longer treatment durations. But IFN-α treatment with high initial doses, such as 3–6 million IU per day, may cause more side effects such as depression [64].

6.3.3. Interleukin-1 inhibition

IL-1β is a potent proinflammatory cytokine that is involved in the early response of the immune system in conditions of infection and tissue injury. In autoinflammatory disorders, IL-1 blockage results in a rapid and continuous reduction of disease manifestations. Serum levels of IL-1β and IL-1 receptor antagonist were found to be significantly higher in Behçet patients [38, 73, 74].

The three anti-IL-1 agents that have been used in BD are IL-1 receptor antagonist anakinra, anti-IL-1β monoclonal antibody canakinumab, and recombinant humanized anti-IL-1β gevokizumab. A retrospective multicenter study reported the efficacy and safety of anakinra and canakinumab in BD. Anakinra and canakinumab were well tolerated with no serious adverse effects except injection site reactions caused by anakinra. These agents should be interpreted with caution because of unavailability of controlled study [75].

IL-1 inhibition is a promising target in managing BD. The pathogenic, clinical, and therapeutic data supporting the use of IL-1 inhibitors in BD has been reviewed very recently. Anti-IL-1 therapy might also be a safer option than anti-TNF-α treatment because of lower risk of opportunistic infections such as tuberculosis [76, 77].

6.4. Intravitreal therapies

Intravitreal injections have advantage of avoiding systemic adverse events and disadvantages of decreased risk associated with intraocular administration and the absence of systemic benefits in patients with extraocular manifestations. When ocular inflammation is unilateral or asymmetric or when systemic administration is less desirable like during pregnancy, intravitreal injections may be preferable [39].

6.4.1. Intravitreal triamcinolone acetonide

Intravitreal triamcinolone acetonide (IVTA) has been administered in Behçet patients with CME, sight-threatening uveitis, or resistant posterior uveitis. Anatomical improvement and increase in VA have been demonstrated. Intravitreal treatment has been enabled tapering the dose of systemic medications. Triamcinolone acetonide is administered 4 mg (0.1 ml) intravitreally. Intravitreal triamcinolone is an effective, short-term therapeutic option. Repeated injections are usually needed. IVTA has no significant systemic side effects, but elevation of IOP and cataract progression is not rare. These side effects are limiting its efficacy and repeatability [78–82].

6.4.2. Intravitreal dexamethasone implant

Intravitreal dexamethasone implant (Ozurdex, Allergan Inc., Irvine, California, USA) has been shown to be effective in controlling intraocular inflammation and achieving reduction of central macular thickness in noninfectious intermediate and posterior uveitis in several studies. Therefore, the number of administration required in patients with uveitis is still controversial [83–85].

It was demonstrated that intravitreal dexamethasone implant has a side effect profile which include cataract formation with an incidence of 15% and IOP elevation with an incidence of 23% in patients with noninfectious uveitis [83].

6.4.3. Intravitreal fluocinolone acetonide implant

A long-term slow-release intravitreal fluocinolone acetonide implant (Retisert, Bausch & Lomb, Rochester, New York, USA) has been used in uveitis, and its efficacy and safety have been assessed by multicenter randomized clinical studies. Retisert is implanted surgically; it is placed through a pars plana incision and sutured to the sclera. It releases 0.59 mg of fluocinolone acetonide at a constant rate during 3 years [86, 87].

In a multicenter trial that compared fluocinolone acetonide implant with aggressive oral systemic therapy in patients with intermediate and posterior panuveitis, no significant difference between groups was found in VA, but the implant was found better and faster in controlling inflammation [88]. Another multicenter randomized study confirmed the superiority of the implant to control intraocular inflammation over standard systemic treatment in resistant noninfectious posterior uveitis.

6.4.4. Intravitreal antitumor necrosis factor

Intravitreal infliximab in the dose of 1–1.5 mg/0.05 ml and frequency of three times at 6-week intervals has been found to be effective and well tolerated. In the studies investigating the efficacy of intravitreal infliximab administration in patients with chronic noninfectious uveitis, improvement in vision, reduction in central foveal thickness, and reduction in inflammation have been demonstrated. Some cases have been reported such as vitreous opacifications and newly onset of severe panuveitis as adverse events after intravitreal infliximab. Infliximab has been suggested to be a promising agent for refractory eye disease in combination with other immunosuppressants. It is important to be cautious for reactivation of tuberculosis [89–94].

6.4.5. Intravitreal anti-VEGF agents

There are several studies that compared the use of intravitreal bevacizumab (IVB) with IVTA in the literature. IVTA was found superior to IVB in visual improvement and decreasing macular thickness in refractory uveitic CME [95, 96]. Conversely, Bae et al. concluded that IVB is a well-tolerated and effective supplementary therapy for persistent uveitic CME, especially in Behçet patients [97].

7. Prognosis and complications

Despite the use of steroids, immunomodulatory and biological agents, some patients may have poor final VA. Twenty-five percent to fifty percent of the patients have best corrected VA less than 20/200 after 5 years [98]. Aqueous protein and cells in anterior chamber, posterior synechiae formation, hypopyon, cataract formation, vitreous cells and exudates, posterior vitreous detachment, and CME may cause transient decrease in VA. Optic atrophy and resistant uveitic glaucoma may result in permanent visual loss at end-stage disease.

Attacks of RV, retinitis, retinal neovascularization, and vitritis lead to vitreous hemorrhage and retinal atrophy. In advance cases, fibrotic, attenuated retinal arterioles; narrowed and occluded "silver wired" vessels; alterations of retinal pigment epithelium; chorioretinal scars; and optic atrophy may be seen.

Inflammation and treatment modalities that are used in BD may cause complications. Complicated cataract and secondary glaucoma are usually associated with inflammation and steroid use. Repeated intraocular inflammation can lead to secondary glaucoma. Both open-angle and angle-closure glaucoma or even pupillary block may be seen. Retinal ischemia can cause neovascular glaucoma. Neovascular glaucoma appears in nearly 6% of patients with BD. Ciliary body involvement can cause a decrease in intraocular pressure, and finally phthisis bulbi may occur [15].

Vitreous hemorrhages are seen frequently in Behçet patients with severe retinal involvement. It can lead to organization with membrane formation, causing retinal holes and subsequent retinal detachment. Phthisis bulbi may finally occur. If the vitreous hemorrhage does not resolve spontaneously, it may be treated with pars plana vitrectomy.

Epiretinal membrane, membrane-shaped fibrosis especially in the macular region, is caused by posterior segment inflammation. Inflammation condensed over the macula and fibrous band between the posterior vitreous and retina result in macular hole formation. In the patients with epiretinal membrane, if the vision is seriously affected, the membrane may be removed surgically [16].

Recent advances in ophthalmic imaging methods have allowed to a better definition of visual prognosis in ocular BD. Identification of the high-risk group and the use of effective biologic agents as first line treatment will improve the prognosis in this potentially blinding disease.

Author details

Esra Sahli* and Ozlem Gurbuz-Koz

*Address all correspondence to: esracansizoglu@gmail.com

Ankara Numune Education and Research Hospital, Ankara, Turkey

References

[1] Ohno S, Namba K, Takemoto Y. Behçet's disease. In: Zierhut M, Pavesio C, Ohno S, Orefice F, Rao NA, editors. Intraocular Inflammation. 1st ed. Germany: Springer-Verlag Berlin Heidelberg; 2016. pp. 785-801. DOI: 10.1007/978-3-540-75387-2.ch.66.

[2] Yazıcı Y, Yurdakul S, Yazıcı H. Behçet's syndrome. Current Rheumatology Reports. 2010;**12**:429-435. DOI: 10.1007/s11926-010-0132-z

[3] Mishima S, Masuda K, Izawa Y, et al. Behçet's disease in Japan: Ophthalmological aspect. Transactions of the American Ophthalmological Society Journal. 1979;**77**:225-279

[4] Davatchi F, Shahram F, Akbarian M, et al. The prevalence of Behçet's disease in Iran. In: Nasution AR, Darmawan J, Isbagio H, editors. Proceedings of the 7th APLAR Congress of Rheumatology. Japan KK: Churchill Livingstone; 1992. pp. 95-98

[5] Palimeris G, Papakonstantinou P, Mantas M. The Adamantiades-Behçet's syndrome in Greece. In: Saari KM, editor. Uveitis Update. Amsterdam: Excerpta Medica; 1984. p. 321

[6] O'Duffy JD. Behçet's disease. In: Kelly WN, Harris ED, Ruddy S, Sledge CB, editors. Textbook of Rheumatology. Philadelphia: WB Saunders; 1985. pp. 1174-1178

[7] Takeno M, Kariyone A, Yamashita N, et al. Excessive function of peripheral blood neutrophils from patients with Behçet's disease and from HLA-B51 transgenic mice. Arthritis and Rheumatism. 1995;**38**:426-433

[8] International Study Group for Behçet's Disease. Criteria for diagnosis of Behcet's disease. Lancet. 1990; **335**:1078-1080

[9] Behçet's Disease Research Committee of Japan. Behçet's disease: Guide to diagnosis of Behçet's disease. Japanese Journal of Ophthalmology. 1974;**18**:291-294

[10] Lehner T, Barnes CM. Criteria for diagnosis and classification of Behçet's syndrome. In: Lehner T, Barnes CM, editors. Behçet's Syndrome. Clinical and Immunological Features. London: Academic Press. 1979:1-9

[11] Alpsoy E, Donmez L, Onder M, et al. Clinical features and natural course of Behcet's disease in 661 cases: A multicenter study. The British Journal of Dermatology. 2007;**157**:901-906. DOI: 10.1111/j.1365-2133.2007.08116.x

[12] Çakar Özdal MP, Yazici A, Tüfek M, Öztürk F. Epidemiology of uveitis in a referral hospital in Turkey. Turkish Journal of Medical Sciences. 2014;**44**:337-342

[13] Goto H, Mochizuki M, Yamaki K, Kotake S, Usui M, Ohno S. Epidemiological survey of intraocular inflammation in Japan. Japanese Journal of Ophthalmology. 2007;**51**:41-44. DOI: 10.1007/s10384-006-0383-4

[14] Tugal-Tutkun I, Onal S, Altan-Yaycioglu R, et al. Uveitis in Behcet disease: An analysis of 880 patients. American Journal of Ophthalmology. 2004;**138**:373-380. DOI: 10.1016/j.ajo.2004.03.022

[15] Kural-Seyahi E, Fresko İ, Seyahi N, et al. The long-term mortality and morbidity of Behçet's syndrome: A 2-decade outcome survey of 387 patients followed at a dedicated center. Medicine. 2003;**82**:60-76

[16] Zafirakis P, Foster CS. Adamantiades-Behçet's disease. In: Foster CS, Vitale A, editors. Diagnosis and Treatment of Uveitis. 2nd ed. New Delhi: Jaypee Brothers Medical Publishers Ltd; 2013. pp. 857-886

[17] Zierhut M, Stübiger N, Deuter C. Behçet's disease. In: Pleyer U, Mondino B, editors. Essentials in Ophthalmology: Uveitis and Immunological Disorders. 1st ed. Berlin: Springer-Verlag Berlin Heidelberg; 2005. pp. 173-200. DOI: 10.1007/3-540-26752-2.ch12

[18] Evereklioğlu C. Ocular Behcet disease: Current therapeutic approaches. Current Opinion in Ophthalmology. 2011;**22**:508-516. DOI: 10.1097/ICU.0b013e32834bbe91

[19] Namba K, Goto H, Kaburaki T, et al. A major review: Current aspects of ocular Behçet's disease in Japan. Ocular Immunology and Inflammation. 2015;**23**:1-23. DOI: 10.3109/09273948.2014.981547

[20] Yalcindag FN, Kiziltunc PB, Savku E. Evaluation of intraocular inflammation with laser flare photometry in Behçet uveitis. Ocular Immunology and Inflammation. 2017;**25**:41-45. DOI: 10.3109/09273948.2015.1108444

[21] Pantanelli SM, Khalifa YM. Retinal manifestations of autoimmune and inflammatory disease. International Ophthalmology Clinics. 2012;**52**:25-46. DOI: 10.1097/IIO.0b013e31823bbbe9

[22] Horiuchi T, Yoneya S, Numaga T. Vitreous involvement may be crucial in the prognosis of Behçet's disease. In: Blodi F, Brancato R, Cristini T, et al, editors. Acta XXV Concilium Ophthalmologicum. Rome: Kugler Ghedini;1986. pp. 2624-2631

[23] Rosenbaum JT, Sibley CH, Lin P. Retinal vasculitis. Current Opinion in Rheumatology. 2016;**28**:228-235. DOI: 10.1097/BOR.0000000000000271

[24] Stübiger N, Zierhut M, Kötter I. Ocular manifestations in Behçet's disease. In: Zierhut M, Ohno S, editors. Immunology of Behçet's Disease. Lisse, Netherlands: Swets & Zeitlinger; 2003. pp. 36-45

[25] Abu El-Asrar A, Almomen AM, Alamro S, Tabbara LK. Bilateral central retinal vein thrombosis in Behcet's disease. Clinical Rheumatology. 1996;**15**:511-513

[26] Lim JW, Kang SH. A case of Behçet's disease complicated by bilateral posterior ischemic optic neuropathy. International Ophthalmology. 2011;**31**:157-160. DOI: 10.1007/s10792-011-9415-2

[27] Atmaca LS. Fundus changes associated with Behçet's disease. Graefe's Archive for Clinical and Experimental Ophthalmology. 1989;**227**:340-344

[28] Tugal-Tutkun I, Herbort CP, Khairallah M, Mantovani A. Interobserver agreement in scoring of dual fluorescein and ICG inflammatory angiographic signs for the grading of

posterior segment inflammation. Ocular Immunology and Inflammation. 2010;**18**:385-389. DOI: 10.3109/09273948.2010.489730

[29] Kim M, Kwon HJ, Choi EY, et al. Correlation between fluorescein angiographic findings and visual acuity in Behçet retinal vasculitis. Yonsei Medical Journal. 2015;**56**:1087-1096. DOI: 10.3349/ymj.2015.56.4.1087

[30] Tugal-Tutkun I, Cakar Ozdal P, Oray M, Onal S. Review for diagnostics of the year: Multimodal imaging in Behçet uveitis. Ocular Immunology and Inflammation. 2017;**25**:7-19. DOI: 10.1080/09273948.2016.1205100

[31] Mesquida M, Llorenc V, Fontenla JR, et al. Use of ultra-wide-field retinal imaging in the management of active Behçet retinal vasculitis. Retina. 2014; **34**:2121-2127. DOI: 10.1097/IAE.0000000000000197

[32] Matsuo T, Sato Y, Shiraga F, et al. Choroidal abnormalities in Behcet disease observed by simultaneous indocyanine green and fluorescein angiography with scanning laser ophthalmoscopy. Ophthalmology. 1999;**106**:295-300. DOI: 10.1016/S0161-6420(99)90069-6

[33] Atmaca LS, Sonmez PA. Fluorescein and indocyanine green angiography findings in Behcet disease. The British Journal of Ophthalmology. 2003;**87**:1466-1468

[34] Onal S, Tugal-Tutkun I, Neri P, Herbort C. Optical coherence tomography imaging in uveitis. International Ophthalmology. 2014;**34**(2):401-435. DOI: 10.1007/s10792-013-9822-7

[35] Tortorella P, D'Ambrosio E, Iannetti L, et al. Correlation between visual acuity, inner segment/outer segment junction, and cone outer segment tips line integrity in uveitic macular edema. BioMed Research International. 2015;**2015**:853728. doi:10.1155/2015/853728

[36] Ishikawa S, Taguchi M, Muraoka T, et al. Changes in subfoveal choroidal thickness associated with uveitis activity in patients with Behçet's disease. The British Journal of Ophthalmology. 2014;**98**(11):1508-1513. DOI: 10.1136/bjophthalmol-2014-305333

[37] Kim M, Kim H, Kwon HJ, et al. Choroidal thickness in Behcet's uveitis: An enhanced depth imaging-optical coherence tomography and its association with angiographic changes. Investigative Ophthalmology & Visual Science. 2013;**54**(9):6033-6039. DOI: 10.1167/iovs.13-12231

[38] Zierhut M, Abu El-Asrar AM, Bodaghi B, Tugal-Tutkun I. Therapy of ocular Behçet disease. Ocular Immunology and Inflammation. 2014;**22**:64-76. DOI: 10.3109/09273948.2013.866257

[39] Fabiani C, Alio JL. Local (topical and intraocular) therapy for ocular Adamantiades-Behçet's disease. Current Opinion in Ophthalmology. 2015;**26**:546-552. DOI: 10.1097/ICU.0000000000000210

[40] Hamuryudan V, Ozyazgan Y, Hizli N, et al. Azathioprine in Behçet's syndrome: Effects on long-term prognosis. Arthritis and Rheumatism. 1997;**40**:769-774. DOI: 10.1002/1529-0131(199704)40:4<;769::AID-ART24>;3.0.CO;2-E

[41] Larkin G, Lightman S. Mycophenolate mofetil: A useful immunosuppressive in inflammatory eye diseases. Ophthalmology. 1999;**106**:370-374

[42] Siga NH, Dumont FJ. Cyclosporine, FK-506, and rapamycin: Pharmacologic probes of lymphocyte signal transduction. Annual Review of Immunology. 1992;**10**:519-560. DOI: 10.1146/annurev.iy.10.040192.002511

[43] Foster CS, Baer JC, Raizman MB. Therapeutic responses to systemic immunosuppressive chemotherapy agents in patients with Behçet's syndrome affecting the eyes. In: O'Duffy JD, Kokmen E, editors. Behçet's Disease: Basic and Clinical Aspects. New York: Marcel Dekker; 1991. pp. 581-588

[44] Ozyazgan Y, Yurdakul S, Yazici H, et al. Low dose cyclosporin A versus pulsed cyclophosphamide in Behçet's syndrome: A single masked trial. The British Journal of Ophthalmology. 1992;**76**:241-243

[45] Masuda K, Nakajima A, Urayama A, et al. Double-masked trial of cyclosporin versus colchicines and long-term open study of cyclosporin in Behçet's disease. Lancet. 1989;**1**:1093-1096

[46] BenEzra D, Cohen E, Chajek T, et al. Evaluation of conventional therapy versus cyclosporin A in Behçet's syndrome. Transplantation Proceedings. 1988;**20**:136-143

[47] Mochizuki M, Masuda K, Sakane T, et al. A multicenter clinical open trial of FK 506 in refractory uveitis, including Behçet's disease. Japanese FK 506 Study Group on refractory uveitis. Transplantation Proceedings. 1991;**23**:3343-3346

[48] Thurau SR, Wildner G. Immunomodulatory therapy. In: Pleyer U, Mondino B, editors. Essentials in Ophthalmology: Uveitis and Immunological Disorders. 1st ed. Berlin: Springer-Verlag Berlin Heidelberg; 2005. pp. 255-270. DOI:10.1007/3-540-26752-2.ch16

[49] Fain O, Du LTH, Wechsler B. Pulse cyclophosphamide in Behçet's disease. In: O'Duffy JD, Kokmen E, editors. Behçet's Disease: Basic and Clinical Aspects. New York: Marcel Dekker; 1991. pp. 569-573

[50] Misumi M, Hagiwara E, Takeno M, et al. Cytokine production profile in patients with Behçet's disease treated with infliximab. Cytokine. 2003;**24**:210-218

[51] Evereklioglu C, Er H, Turkoz Y, Cekmen M. Serum levels of TNF-alpha, sIL-2R, IL-6, and IL-8 are increased and associated with elevated lipid peroxidation in patients with Behçet's disease. Mediators of Inflammation. 2002;**11**:87-93. DOI: 10.1080/09629350220131935

[52] Santos Lacomba M, Marcos Martin C, et al. Aqueous humor and serum tumor necrosis factor-alpha in clinical uveitis. Ophthalmic Research. 2001;**33**:251-255. DOI: 55677

[53] Hatemi G, Seyahi E, Fresko I, et al. One year review 2016: Behçet's syndrome. Clinical and Experimental Rheumatology. 2016;**34**:10-22

[54] Fujikawa K, Aratake K, Kawakami A, et al. Successful treatment of refractory neuro-Behçet's disease with infliximab: A case report to show its efficacy by magnetic resonance

imaging, transcranial magnetic stimulation and cytokine profile. Annals of the Rheumatic Diseases. 2007;**66**:136-137. DOI: 10.1136/ard.2006.056804

[55] Accorinti M, Pirraglia MP, Paroli MP, et al. Infliximab treatment for ocular and extraocular manifestations of Behçet's disease. Japanese Journal of Ophthalmology. 2007;**51**:191-196. DOI: 10.1007/s10384-006-0425-y

[56] Tabbara KF, Al-Hemidan AI. Infliximab effects compared to conventional therapy in management of retinal vasculitis in Behçet disease. American Journal of Ophthalmology. 2008;**146**:845-850. DOI: 10.1016/j.ajo.2008.09.010

[57] Yamada Y, Sugita S, Tanaka H, et al. Comparison of infliximab versus ciclosporin during the initial 6-month treatment period in Behçet disease. The British Journal of Ophthalmology. 2010;**94**:284-288. DOI: 10.1136/bjo.2009.158840

[58] Arida A, Fragiadaki K, Giavri E, Sfikakis PP. Anti-TNF agents for Behçet's disease: Analysis of published data on 369 patients. Seminars in Arthritis and Rheumatism. 2011;**41**:61-70. DOI: 10.1016/j.semarthrit.2010.09.002

[59] Mushtaq B, Saeed T, Situnayake RD, Murray PL. Adalimumab for sight-threatening uveitis in Behçet's disease. Eye. 2007;**21**:824-825. DOI: 10.1038./sj.eye.6702352

[60] Bawazeer A, Raffa LH, Nizamuddin SH. Clinical experience with adalimumab in the treatment of ocular Behçet disease. Ocular Immunology and Inflammation. 2010;**18**:226-232. DOI: 10.3109/09273948.2010.483314

[61] Olivieri I, Leccese P, D'Angelo S, et al. Efficacy of adalimumab in patients with Behçet's disease unsuccessfully treated with infliximab. Clinical and Experimental Rheumatology. 2011;**29**:S54-S57. 75

[62] Santos Gomez M, Calvo Rio V, Blanco R, et al. The effect of biologic therapy different from infliximab or adalimumab in patients with refractory uveitis due to Behçet's disease: Results of a multicentre open-label study. Clinical and Experimental Rheumatology. 2016;**34**:34-40

[63] Deuter CME, Kötter I, Wallace GR, et al. Behçet's disease: Ocular effects and treatment. Progress in Retinal and Eye Research. 2008;**27**:111-136. DOI: 10.1016/j.preteyeres.2007.09.002

[64] Kötter I, Gü naydin I, Zierhut M, Stübiger N. The use of interferon a in Behçet disease: Review of the literature. Seminars in Arthritis and Rheumatism. 2004;**33**:320-355

[65] Deuter CM, Kötter I, Günaydin I, et al. Efficacy and tolerability of interferon alpha treatment in patients with chronic cystoid macular oedema due to non-infectious uveitis. The British Journal of Ophthalmology. 2009;**93**:906-913. DOI: 10.1136/bjo.2008.153874

[66] Bodaghi B, Gendron G, Wechsler B, et al. Efficacy of interferon alpha in the treatment of refractory and sight threatening uveitis: A retrospective monocentric study of 45 patients. The British Journal of Ophthalmology. 2007;**91**:335-339. DOI: 10.1136/bjo.2006.101550

[67] Hatemi G, Silman A, Bang D, et al. EULAR recommendations for the treatment of Behçet disease. Annals of the Rheumatic Diseases. 2008;**67**:1656-1662. DOI: 10.1136/ard.2007.080432

[68] Kötter I, Deuter C, Stübiger N, Zierhut M. Interferon-a (IFN-a) application versus tumor necrosis factor-a antagonism for ocular Behçet's disease: Focusing more on IFN. The Journal of Rheumatology. 2005;**32**:1633

[69] Kötter I, Zierhut M, Eckstein AK, et al. Human recombinant interferon alpha-2a for the treatment of Behçet's disease with sight threatening posterior or panuveitis. The British Journal of Ophthalmology. 2003;**87**:423-431

[70] Tugal-Tutkun I, Güney-Tefekli E, Urgancioglu M. Results of interferon-alfa therapy in patients with Behçet uveitis. Graefe's Archive for Clinical and Experimental Ophthalmology. 2006;**244**:1692-1695. DOI: 10.1007/s00417-006-0346-y

[71] Tugal-Tutkun I, Onal S, Altan-Yaycioglu R, Kir N, Urgancioglu M. Neovascularization of the optic disc in Behcet's disease. Japanese Journal of Ophthalmology. 2006;**50**(3):256-265. DOI: 10.1007/s10384-005-0307-8

[72] Gueudry J, Wechsler B, Terrada C, et al. Long-term efficacy and safety of low-dose interferon alpha2a therapy in severe uveitis associated with Behçet disease. American Journal of Ophthalmology. 2008;**146**:837-844. DOI: 10.1016/j.ajo.2008.08.038

[73] Yosipovitch G, Sholat B, Bshara J,Wysenbeek A, Weinberger A. Elevated serum interleukin 1 receptors and interleukin 1B in patients with Behçet's disease: Correlations with disease activity and severity. Israel Journal of Medical Sciences. 1995;**31**:345-348

[74] Düzgün N, Ayaslioglu E, Tutkak H, Aydintug OT. Cytokine inhibitors: Soluble tumor necrosis factor receptor 1 and interleukin-1 receptor antagonist in Behçet's disease. Rheumatology International. 2005;**25**:1-5. DOI: 10.1007/s00296-003-0400-6

[75] Emmi G, Talarico R, Lopalco G, et al. Efficacy and safety profile of anti-interleukin-1 treatment in Behçet's disease: A multicenter retrospective study. Clinical Rheumatology. 2016;**35**:1281-1286. DOI: 10.1007/s10067-015-3004-0

[76] Vitale A, Rigante D, Lopalco G, et al. Interleukin-1 inhibition in Behçet's disease. The Israel Medical Association Journal. 2016;**18**:171-176

[77] Dinarello CA. The many worlds of reducing interleukin-1. Arthritis and Rheumatism. 2005;**52**:1960-1967. DOI: 10.1002/art.21107

[78] Karacorlu M, Mudun B, Ozdemir H, et al. Intravitreal triamcinolone acetonide for the treatment of cystoid macular edema secondary to Behçet disease. American Journal of Ophthalmology. 2004;**138**:289-291

[79] Atmaca LS, Yalcindag NF, Ozdemir O. Intravitreal triamcinolone acetonide in the management of cystoid macular edema in Behçet's disease. Graefe's Archive for Clinical and Experimental Ophthalmology. 2007;**245**:451-456. DOI: 10.1007/s00417-006-0514-0

[80] Ohguro N, Yamanaka E, Otori Y, et al. Repeated intravitreal triamcinolone injections in Behçet disease that is resistant to conventional therapy: One year results. American Journal of Ophthalmology. 2006;**141**:218-220. DOI: 10.1016/j.ajo.2005.08.013

[81] Tuncer S, Yılmaz S, Urgancıoglu M, Tugal-Tutkun TI. Results of intravitreal triamcinolone acetonide (IVTA) injection for the treatment of panuveitis attacks in patients with Behçet disease. Journal of Ocular Pharmacology and Therapeutics. 2007;**23**:395-401. DOI: 10.1089/jop.2007.0015

[82] Park UC, Park JH, Yu HG. Long-term outcome of intravitreal triamcinolone acetonide injection for the treatment of uveitis attacks in Behçet disease. Ocular Immunology and Inflammation. 2014;**22**:27-33. DOI: 10.3109/09273948.2013.829109

[83] Lowder C, Belfort R Jr, Lightman S, et al. Dexamethasone intravitreal implant for noninfectious intermediate or posterior uveitis. Archives of Ophthalmology. 2011;**129**:545-553. DOI: 10.1001/archophthalmol.2010.339

[84] Khurana RN, Porco TC. Efficacy and safety of dexamethasone intravitreal implant for persistent uveitis cystoid macular edema. Retina. 2015;**35**:1640-1646. DOI: 10.1097/IAE.0000000000000515

[85] Zarranz-Ventura J, Carreno E, Johnston RL, et al. Multicenter study of intravitreal dexamethasone implant in noninfectious uveitis; indications, outcomes, and reinjection frequency. American Journal of Ophthalmology. 2014;**158**:1136-1145. DOI: 10.1016/j.ajo.2014.09.003

[86] Jaffe GJ, Martin D, Callanan D, et al. Fluocinolone acetonide implant (Retisert) for noninfectious posterior uveitis: Thirty-four week results of a multicenter randomized clinical study. Ophthalmology. 2006;**113**:1020-1027. DOI: 10.1016/j.ophtha.2006.02.021

[87] Sangwan VS, Pearson PA, Paul H, Comstock TL. Use of the fluocinolone acetonide intravitreal implant for the treatment of noninfectious posterior uveitis: 3-year results of a randomized clinical trial in a predominantly Asian population. Ophthalmology and Therapy. 2015;**4**:1-19. DOI: 10.1007/s40123-014-0027-6

[88] Kempen JH, Altaweel MM, Holbrook JT, et al. Randomized comparison of systemic anti-inflammatory therapy versus fluocinolone acetonide implant for intermediate, posterior, and panuveitis: The multicenter uveitis steroid treatment trial. Ophthalmology. 2011;**118**:1916-1926. DOI: 10.1016/j.ophtha.2011.07.027

[89] Giganti M, Beer PM, Lemanski N, et al. Adverse events after intravitreal infliximab (Remicade). Retina. 2010;**30**:71-80. DOI: 10.1097/IAE.0b013e3181bcef3b

[90] Pulido JS, Pulido JE, Michet CJ, Vile RG. More questions than answers: A call for a moratorium on the use of intravitreal infliximab outside of a well-designed trial. Retina. 2010;**30**:1-5. DOI: 10.1097/IAE.0b013e3181cde727

[91] Hamza MME, Macky TA, Sidky MK, et al. Intravitreal infliximab in refractory uveitis in Behcet's disease: A safety and efficacy clinical study. Retina. 2016;**36**:2408-2416. DOI: 10.1097/IAE.0000000000001109

[92] Farvardin M, Afarid M, Mehryar M, Hosseini H. Intravitreal infliximab for the treatment of sight-threatening chronic noninfectious uveitis. Retina. 2010;**30**:1530-1535. DOI: 10.1097/IAE.0b013e3181d3758a

[93] Farvardin M, Afarid M, Shahrzad S. Long-term effects of intravitreal infliximab for treatment of sight-threatening chronic noninfectious uveitis. Journal of Ocular Pharmacology and Therapeutics. 2012;**28**:628-631. DOI: 10.1089/jop.2011.0199

[94] Markomichelakis N, Delicha E, Masselos S, et al. Intravitreal infliximab for sight-threatening relapsing uveitis in Behçet disease: A pilot study in 15 patients. American Journal of Ophthalmology. 2012;**154**:534-541. DOI: 10.1016/j.ajo.2012.03.035

[95] Lasave AF, Zeballos DG, El-Haig WM, et al. Short-term results of a single intravitreal bevacizumab (avastin) injection versus a single intravitreal triamcinolone acetonide (kenacort) injection for the treatment of refractory noninfectious uveitic cystoid macular edema. Ocular Immunology and Inflammation. 2009;**17**:423-430. DOI: 10.3109/09273940903221610

[96] Soheilian M, Rabbanikhah Z, Ramezani A, et al. Intravitreal bevacizumab versus triamcinolone acetonide for refractory uveitic cystoid macular edema: A randomized pilot study. Journal of Ocular Pharmacology and Therapeutics. 2010;**26**:199-206. DOI: 10.1089/jop.2009.0093

[97] Bae JH, Lee CS, Lee SC. Efficacy and safety of intravitreal bevacizumab compared with intravitreal and posterior sub-tenon triamcinolone acetonide for treatment of uveitic cystoid macular edema. Retina. 2011;**31**:111-118. DOI: 10.1097/IAE.0b013e3181e378af

[98] Kacmaz RO, Kempen JH, Newcomb C, et al. Ocular inflammation in Behcet disease: Incidence of ocular complications and of loss of visual acuity. American Journal of Ophthalmology. 2008;**146**:828-836. DOI: 10.1016/j.ajo.2008.06.019

Chapter 8

Joint Involvement and Synovial Histopathology in BD

Yuki Nanke and Shigeru Kotake

Additional information is available at the end of the chapter

http://dx.doi.org/10.5772/68078

Abstract

Behcet's disease (BD) is a polysymptomatic and recurrent systemic vasculitis with a chronic course and unknown cause. Joint involvement in BD is common. Arthritis and arthralgia in BD are known to be the most common rheumatologic findings. Arthropathy in BD is monoarthritis or asymmetrical oligoarthritis affecting larger joints, and it is usually acute or recurrent with a self-limiting course. Bone deformity and destruction are rare. Autoantibodies are typically negative, and the presence of anti-CCP antibodies at high titers favors a diagnosis of rheumatoid arthritis (RA). Although joint involvement is clinically well recognized, few histologic studies have been reported. In this chapter, we focused on the synovitis and synovial histopathology in BD.

Keywords: Behcet's disease, arthritis, joint, synovia, synovitis

1. Introduction

Behcet's disease (BD) is a polysymptomatic and recurrent systemic vasculitis with a chronic course and unknown cause [1]. Joint involvement in BD is very common. Arthropathy in BD is monoarthritis or asymmetrical oligoarthritis, and it is usually acute or recurrent [2, 3]. In addition, arthritis associated with BD is usually self-limiting and non-deforming; bone erosive change of joints is extremely rare [4]. It typically affects larger joints (knees, ankles, wrists, and elbows). Unusual findings include arthritis with deformities and/or destruction. The synovial histopathology shows a wide range of features, including lining cell hyperplasia, angiogenesis, granulation tissue, and lymphoid follicle formation. Usually, autoantibodies are typically negative, and the presence of anti-CCP antibodies at high titers favors a diagnosis of RA. First-line treatment includes non-steroidal anti-inflammatory drugs, or corticosteroids for severe cases, whereas colchicine has shown some efficacy for the treatment of recurrent and refractory arthritis. Although joint involvement is clinically well recognized, few histologic studies have been reported. We review joint involvement in BD patients with both typical and atypical findings. In this chapter, we focused on the synovitis and synovial histopathology in BD. In addition, we introduce rare cases, and we have encountered with synovial findings.

1.1. Typical joint involvement

Joint manifestations are very common, being present in 40–75% of BD patients. According to a retrospective review of 340 cases, joint involvement is the initial manifestation of BD in 18.2% [5]. The knees, ankles, wrists, and elbows are frequently affected, while the involvement of small joints in the hands and feet is less common. Most cases demonstrate monoarthritis or oligoarthritis and usually run an acute or recurrent course [2]. Polyartritis and the chronic form are rare. In addition, arthritis associated with BD is usually benign, self-limiting, and non-deforming. Bone erosive change of the joints is extremely rare [4]. Joint deformities and destruction have been reported in only a few cases [6].

According to another retrospective review of 176 cases [7], rheumatic manifestations were noted in 45%. Articular manifestations were the initial disease manifestation in 16.5%. Inflammatory arthralgia was observed in 81% mainly in the large lower limb joints. Arthritis was less common: oligoarthritis, 7.5%; monoarthritis, 6.5%; and polyarthritis, 5%. The disease course was acute in most patients. Axial involvement was noted: spinal pain in 2.9%, isolated sacroiliitis in 7.5%, and definite ankylosing spondylitis in 5%.

Frikha et al. [8] reviewed the medical records of 553 BD patients. Rheumatologic manifestations were observed in 71.1%, being second after cutaneo-mucosal involvement. Rheumatologic manifestations in BD are defined as inflammatory arthralgia, peripheral arthritis, intermittent hydrarthrosis, popliteal cysts, and spondylarthropathy (low back pain with sacroiliitis). Definite arthritis was noted in 50%. The most frequent manifestation is a non-erosive and non-deforming monoarthritis or asymmetrical oligoarthritis, commonly subacute and self-limiting, typically affecting the larger joints.

1.2. Hand involvement

In a recent randomized study in Turkey, clinical hand involvement was investigated in 57 BD patients [9], and the prevalence of hand involvement in BD was found to be relatively high. Thus, terminal phalangeal pulp resorption was observed in 29.8%, which might be induced by the vasculitic process due to repeated digital infarcts. Rheumatoid-like hand findings were noted in 28.1%, dorsal interosseous atrophy was observed in 20.1%, and erythema of the digitis was identified in 20%. Twenty-four patients (42.1%) showed scintigraphic abnormalities.

1.3. Atypical joint involvement: erosive changes

Erosive changes due to joint involvement by BD are also infrequent. Thus, Vernon-Roberts et al. [6] reported that two of six patients with BD showed radiologically erosive changes in the hip and manubriosternal joints. Armas et al. [10] reported radiologically well-defined "punched-out" erosive arthropathy in the head of the first metacarpophalangeal (MCP) joints. Düzgün and Ateş [11] reviewed erosive arthropathy in BD patients with references to 11 papers. Erosive changes were reported in axial joints (sacroiliac) and peripheral joints such as intertarsal and MTP (metatarsophalangeal) joints of the foot, intercarpal and MCP joints of the hand, knee, wrist, and hip joints [2, 4–6, 10–13]. Enthesis was also noted in calcaneal joints. More recently, Aydin et al. [14] reported an unusual case of BD with extensive erosive arthropathy radiologically mimicking psoriatic arthritis. In their case, erosive changes at the styloid process of the left ulnar bone were notable. Yurdaku et al. reported five out of 47 BD patients who had radiologically erosive lesions in a prospective study [2]. We also reported [15] a female patient with BD who demonstrated arthritis in the sternocostal joint showing erosive changes, which rarely occur in BD [16]. Taken together, erosive change can be found in various joints, although it is an atypical change in BD.

1.4. Atypical joint involvement: destructive arthritis

In the review of 553 BD patients by Frikha et al., as mentioned above, only eight patients (1.4% overall, 2% of patients with rheumatic involvement) had destructive arthritis (defined by radiological changes: erosions and/or geodes and/or global narrowing of the joint space and/or ankylosis) [8]. The involved joints included knee joints, sternoclavicular joints, the wrist, foot, and tarsal scaphoid, whereas the spine or sacroiliac joint was not affected. On the other hand, sacroiliitis and enthesitis have been reported in BD, although their prevalence is low [17, 18].

1.5. Synovial histology

It has been reported that approximately 40–50% of patients with BD have synovitis [2, 19], although there have been a limited number of reports on the synovial histology in BD [2, 6, 20]. Yuradakul et al. reported the findings of synovial biopsy in 12 patients, revealing superficial ulceration, paucity of plasma cells, and, in five instances, lymphoid follicle formation [2]. Vernon-Roberts et al. indicated that only superficial zones of the synovial tissue were affected. In seven of eight specimens, the superficial zones were replaced by densely inflamed granulation tissue composed of lymphocytes mixed with macrophages, vascular elements, fibroblasts, and neutrophils [6]. Gibson et al. [20] noted that synovial changes in BD are similar to those observed in early RA, and demonstrated hypertrophy and hyperplasia of synovial lining cells, hypervascularity, subsynovial accumulation of inflammatory cells, and replacement of superficial zones of the synovial membrane by densely inflamed granulation tissue. However, immunofluorescent studies indicated that the consistent deposition of IgG might be characteristic of BD [20]. Moll et al. [21] described the macroscopic features of early untreated knee synovitis in BD and psoriatic arthritis (PsA). They reported the presence of extensive fibrinoid membranes and large areas of erythematous synovitis without villi or a distinctive vascular pattern in early and untreated BD. Cañete et al. [22] noted that polymorph nuclear neutrophils and lymphocytes were indicators of cytotoxic molecules in early untreated synovitis in BD. Thus, the histopathological characteristics of synovial tissue in BD may be diverse.

1.6. Presentation of synovial histology in our cases

We previously reported the synovial histology and destructive joint manifestations in three BD patients who underwent orthopedic surgery [23]. *They all had morning stiffness.* The joints affected in these cases were the ankle, wrist, elbow, and knee. Case 1 *presented bleeding from ulcers of the small intestine* and complained of polyarthritis (both ankles, wrists, and PIP joints) and severe recurrent pain in the left ankle and intermittent claudication. *The patient was diagnosed as having BD (incomplete type) was with oral prednisolone (15 mg/day).* Radiographs of the left ankle revealed a sclerotic joint space and osteoporotic change, for which arthrodesis was performed. Histological studies of synovial tissues revealed non-specific chronic synovitis and the infiltration of lymphoid cells around the vascular cells with fibrinoid changes. There was no sign of vasculitis.

Case 2 underwent Darrach's procedure for the right wrist joint. Histological findings showed neither the formation of lymphoid follicle formation nor infiltration of plasma cells, although some neutrophils and lymphocytes were detected. She had the chronic form of polyarthritis of the right wrist and elbow, left knee, both ankles, and PIP joints and received synovectomy. *She had been treated with NSAIDs for arthritis.* Radiographs revealed joint space narrowing in the right elbow and left knee. Synovial tissue from the elbow showed hyperplasia of the synovial lining cells and the infiltration of plasma cells, with the formation of numerous lymphoid follicles. Synovial tissue from the knee showed hyperplasia of the synovial lining cells, and the perivascular infiltration of lymphoid cells.

Case 3 had chronic arthritis *on left knee, both wrists and PIP joints,* and radiography revealed bone atrophy and ankylosis of the left knee, erosive changes of the PIP joints, and destructive changes of the wrists, mimicking rheumatoid arthritis. Synovectomy was then performed, and histopathological findings showed hyperplasia of the lining cells, the deposition of fibrin, infiltration of inflammatory cells, and marked vascularity. These features cannot be differentiated from those of rheumatoid arthritis.

1.7. Synovial immunopathology in BD

Cañete et al. [22] investigated the differences in synovial immunopathology between early active and untreated BD and PsA. There was marked $CD15^{+}$neutrophilic inflammation in the intimal lining layer in BD synovitis. This increased number of polymorphonuclear neutrophils (PMNs) has been reported not only in the synovium but also in the skin and central nervous system. As for lymphocytes, $CD3^{+}$T cells, but neither $CD20^{+}$ B cells nor $CD138^{+}$ plasma cells, were increased in BD [22]. Specific T-cell subsets are associated with sterile neutrophil-rich inflammation as observed in BD synovitis, and this may explain the simultaneous increase of both T cells and PMN [24]. The analysis of the T-cell population in SF showed that there was no clear shift in the CD4/CD8 ratio or Th1/Th2/Th17 profile. The synovial fluid levels of perforin, an effector molecule of cytotoxic cells, showed a significant increase in BD [22]. This suggests the relevance of cytotoxicity in BD synovitis [25, 26]. Suh et al. [27] reported that antigen-driven clonal B-cell proliferation occurs in the synovium in BD. They identified immunoglobulin transcripts clonally expanded in the synovium in BD.

http://dx.doi.org/10.5772/68078

1.8. Humoral protective factors in synovial fluid or blood

As with BD, the pathogenesis of arthritis and protective mechanisms against erosive changes needs to be elucidated. The plasminogen activation system can contribute to the pathogenesis of destructive joint disease. Ertenli et al. [28] demonstrated that *synovial fluid* (SF) in BD is inflammatory in nature. They reported increased SF IL-1β levels in BD patients. In SF, levels of IL-1β, IL-1ra, and TGF-β were higher in BD than *osteoarthritis* (OA) [28]. Thus, they speculated that IL1ra and TGF-β might serve as protective factors against cartilage destruction. Pay et al. [29] also reported that BD and RA patients had higher synovial IL-1β than OA patients. MMP-3 and proinflammatory cytokines except IL-1β were expressed in small quantities in BD synovitis; this may explain the non-erosive character of BD arthritis. Thus, IL-β may be involved in the pathogenesis of BD synovitis. In addition, relatively lower levels of IL-18 in the SF of BD patients might be the cause of less marked inflammation in BD arthritis. Recently, Karasneh et al. [30] reported that IL-1 gene cluster polymorphisms, including the *IL-1B* gene, are associated with an increased risk of BD. Therefore, the detection of increased synovial IL-1β levels in BD patients could be determined genetically by functional polymorphism, leading to differential gene regulation and expression.

Ozturk et al. [31] reported that systemic bloodstream and local SF plasminogen activator inhibitor-1 (PAI-1) antigen levels and PAI-1 activities were higher in BD patients than RA patients and healthy controls. PAI-1 may promote hypofibrinolysis of BD vasculopathy and also plays a protective role against arthritis in BD patients. They speculated that elevated PAI-1 antigen and activities in the synovial fluid of BD patients contribute to the unique nonerosive character of BD.

1.9. Proinflammatory factors in synovial fluid or blood

Aktas Cetin et al. [32] reported that in peripheral blood mononuclear cells (PBMCs), CD4, CD25, HLA-DR expression and intracellular IL-12, and TNF-αlevels of CD3+ T cells were increased in BD compared with HC. Compared with AS patients, CD25, HLA-DR surface expression, and intracellular IFN-γ and TNF-αlevels in T cells were elevated in BD. Th1 polarization occurred in both the peripheral blood and SF of BD patients with arthritis. Duygulu et al. [33] demonstrated that the levels of both serum and erythrocyte nitric oxide (NO), the most abundant free radial in the body, were elevated in BD patients and associated with disease activity. In addition, synovial NO levels were positively correlated with serum levels. Turan et al. [34] analyzed the production of soluble TNF receptors, sTNFR1 and sTNFR2, in BD patients. STNFR2 plasma concentrations are closely linked with active BD and especially with arthritis. The expression of TNFR molecules in mast cells of mucocutaneous lesions indicates the fundamental role of the TNF/TNFR pathway in BD.

Erdem et al. [35] demonstrated that the expression of CXC chemokines, including IL-8, GRO-a, and ENA-78, was lower in the SF of patients with BD than in those with RA. All CXC chemokines and VEGF were induced by IL-18, which are involved in angiogenesis and the development of pannus. Thus, the lower levels of these chemokines in the SF of BD patients may explain the lack of pannus formation or erosion in BD arthritis.

Ertenli et al. [28] reported higher levels of synovial IL-8 in BD than OA patients. They suggested that elevated synovial IL-8 might play a pivotal role in the process of neutrophil migration in BD synovitis and reflect a nonspecific inflammatory process. Erdem et al. [35] speculated that synovial IL-8 levels increased via the attraction of more neutrophils to SF, and this, in addition to its angiogenic properties, might be responsible for the development of acute synovitis.

1.10. Metabolomic evaluation of BD in synovial fluid: potential biomarkers

Ahn et al. [36] investigated possible metabolic patterns and potential biomarkers of BD with arthritis on metabolic profiling of SF from BD patients with arthritis and seronegative arthritis (SNA). They identified 123 metabolites. Compared with SNA, BD patients with arthritis exhibited relatively high levels of glutamate, valine, citramalate, leucine, methionine sulfoxide, glycerate, phosphate, lysine, isoleucine, urea, and citrulline. Finally, they identified two markers, elevated methionine sulfoxide and citrulline, associated with increased oxidative stress, providing a potential link to BD-associated neutrophil hyperactivity. Gultamate, citramalate, and valine were selected as putative biomarkers for BD with arthritis.

1.11. Anti-cyclic citrullinated peptide (Anti-CCP) antibodies and BD

Anti-CCP antibodies are a more reliable diagnostic marker for RA and closely associated with the prognosis in RA patients [37]. Recently, a significant correlation was reported between anti-CCP antibodies and joint symptoms in patients with familial Mediterranean fever [38]. In a study of 189 Korean BD patients, only seven patients (3.7%) were positive for anti-CCP antibodies, five of which (71.4%) had polyarticular joint involvement, and the other two (28.6%) had oligoarticular involvement. Among the seven patients, one patient with an anti-CCP antibody titer of over 100 U/mL fulfilled the diagnostic criteria for both BD and RA. Of course, all BD patients without articular involvement were negative on an anti-CCP antibody test [39]. Since it has been demonstrated that anti-CCP antibodies are elevated prior to the development of RA, we need to be careful when diagnosing BD patients who show arthritis in the presence of positive anti-CCP antibodies.

1.12. Sonographic study

Ultrasound (US) evaluation is useful for the detection of joint involvement. Synovial proliferation, joint effusion, and bone surface erosions are detectable, and even asymptomatic joint involvement showed US alterations [40]. Ceccarelli et al. performed knee United States in 30 BD patients and found that 60% of patients showed knee involvement based on United States. They detected synovial proliferation in 14%, joint effusion in 46%, and bone surface erosions in 10% of patients. They also pointed out that subjects with a higher US score showed a positive correlation with disease activities such as acneiform skin lesions. Gok et al. performed high-frequency United States and power Doppler ultrasonography (PDUS) examination of knee joints [41]. By ultrasonography, synovial hypertrophy scores were lower in patients with BD than in those with RA and spondyloarthropahy. However, no difference was found between BD, RA, and spondyloarthropahy patients based on PD signal scores using PDUS. Gok et al. also investigated ultrasonographic findings and synovial angiogenesis modulators.

Cumulative effusion scores were positively correlated with angiopoietin-1, angiostatin, and basic fibroblast growth factor (bFGF), while they were negatively correlated with thrombospondin-1 levels. Synovial hypertrophy scores were positively correlated with angiostatin and bFGF levels and negatively correlated with thrombospondin-1. No correlation was found between PD scores and modulators of angiogenesis.

1.13. Magnetic resonance imaging study and Tc-99m-MDP bone scintigraphy

Magnetic resonance imaging has been reported to be sensitive for detecting early arthritis of BD. Choi et al. showed syovial thickening and effusion based on a high signal intensity on T2-weighted images of two BD patients with arthropathy [42].

Sugawara et al. reported radiography and magnetic resonance imaging of hand and wrist arthritis in four BD patients [43]. They concluded that characteristics on imaging of arthritis in BD patients vary and may be similar to those of psoriatic arthritis patients. Erosion in the distal interphalangeal joint was seen, but the type of erosion was of the gull-wing type, being different from RA variants.

Joint scanning with 99m Tc is a more valuable tool for the prediction of hand joint inflammation than radiography [44]. Bone scintigraphy is also more sensitive for the earlier diagnosis of joint involvement, especially in sacroileal joints [45].

2. Conclusion

In summary, arthritis and arthralgia are common in BD patients, and joint manifestations of BD patients are diverse: sometimes mimicking rheumatoid arthritis, PsA, and spodyloarthritides radiologically. In addition, the histopathological characteristics of synovial tissue in BD may be various.

Thus, despite the rarity of destructive arthropathies, this unusual form should be known and considered in the differential diagnosis of other rheumatic diseases.

Abbreviation

BD	Behcet's disease

Author details

Yuki Nanke* and Shigeru Kotake

*Address all correspondence to: ynn@ior.twmu.ac.jp

Institute of Rheumatology, Tokyo Women's Medical University, Shinjuku-ku, Tokyo, Japan

References

[1] Nanke Y, Kotake S, Ogasawara K, Shimakawa M, Takasawa S, Ujihara H, et al. Raised plasma adrenomedullin level in Behcet's disease patients. Mod Rheumatol 2003; 13: 139–142.

[2] Yurdakul S, Yazici H, Tüzün Y, Pazarli H, Yalçin B, Altaç M, et al. The arthritis of Behcet's disease: a prospective study. Ann Rheum Dis 1983; 42: 505–515.

[3] Calguneri M, Kiraz S, Ertenli I, Erman M, KaraasalanYCelik I. Characteristics of peripheral arthritis in Behcet's disease. N Z Med J 1997; 10: 80–81.

[4] Ben-Dov I, Zimmerman J. Deforming arthritis of the hands in Behcet's disease. J Rheumatol 1982; 9: 617–618.

[5] Benamour S, Zeroual B, Alaoui FZ. Joint manifestations in Behcet's disease, a review of 340 cases. Rev Rheum 1998; 65: 299–307.

[6] Vernon-Roberts B, Barnes CG, Revell PA. Synovial pathology in Behcet's syndrome. Ann Rheum Dis 1978; 37: 139–145.

[7] AitBadi MA, Zyani M, Kaddouri S, Niamane R, Hda A, Algayres JP. Skeletal manifestations in Behcet's disease. A report of 79 cases. Rev Med Interne 2008; 4: 277–82. doi: 10.1016/j.revmed.2007.09.031. Epub October 22, 2007.

[8] Frikha F, Marzouk S, Kaddour N, Frigui M, Bahloul Z. Destructive arthritis in Behcet's disease: a report of eight cases and literature review. Int J Rheuma Dis 2009; 12: 250–255. doi: 10.1111/j.1756-185X.2009.01419.x

[9] Yurtkuran M, Yurtkuran M, Alp A, Sivrioglu K, Dilek K, Tamgaç F, et al. Hand involvement in Behcet's disease. Joint Bone Spine 2006; 73: 679–683.

[10] Armas JB, Davies J, Davis M, Lovell C, McHugh N. Atypical Behcet's disease with peripheral erosive arthropathy and pyoderma gangrenosum. Clinical Exp Rheum 1992; 10: 177–180.

[11] Düzgün N, Ateş A. Erosive arthritis in a patient with Behcet's disease. RheumatolInt 2003; 23: 265–267.

[12] Kötter I, Dürk H, Eckstein A, Zierhut M, Fierlbeck G, Saal JG. Erosive arthritis and posterior uveitis in Behcet's disease: treatment with interferon alpha and interferon gamma Clinical Exp Rheum 1996; 14: 313–315.

[13] Jawad AS, Goodwill CJ. Behcet's disease with erosive arthritis. Ann Rheum Dis 1986; 45: 961–962.

[14] Aydin G, Keleş I, Atalar E, Orkun S. Extensive erosive arthropathy in a patient with Behcet's disease: case report. Clin Rheumatol 2005; 24: 645–647.

[15] Nanke Y, Kobashigawa T, Yago T, Ichikawa N, Yamanaka H, Kotake S. Bone erosion of the sternocostal joint in a patients with Bechet's disease. Jpn J ClinImmnol 2009; 32: 186–188.

[16] Crozier F, Arlaud J, Tourniaire P, Bodiou Y, Christides C, Paris M, et al. Manubrio-sternal arthritis and Behcet's disease: report of 3 cases. J Radiol 2003; 84: 1978–1981.

[17] Chang HK, Lee DH, Jung SM, Choi SJ, Kim JU, Choi YJ, et al. The comparison between Behcet's disease and spondyloarthritides: does Behcet's disease belong to the spondyloarthropathy complex? J Korean Med Sci 2002; 17: 524–529.

[18] Chamberlain MA, Robertson RJ. A controlled study of sacroiliitis in Behcet's disease. British J Rheumatol 1993; 32: 693–698.

[19] Sakane T, Takeno M, Suzuki N, Inaba G. Behcet's disease. N Eng J Med 1999; 21: 1284–1291.

[20] Gibson T, Laurent R, Highton J, Wilton M, Dyson M, Millis R. Synovial histopathology of Behcet's syndrome. Ann Rheum Dis 1981; 40: 376–381.

[21] Moll C, Bogas M, Gómez-Puerta JA, Celis R, Vázquez I, Rodríguez F, et al. Macroscopic features of knee synovitis in early untreated Behcet's disease and psoriatic arthritis. Clinical Rheumatol 2009; 28: 1053–1057. doi: 10.1007/s10067-009-1205-0

[22] Cañete JD, Celis R, Noordenbos T, Moll C, Gómez-Puerta JA, Pizcueta P, et al. Distinct synovial immunopathology in Behcet's disease and psoriatic arthritis. Arthritis Res Therapy 2009; 11: R17. doi: 10.1186/ar2608

[23] Nanke Y, Kotake S, Momohara S, Tateishi M, Yamanaka H, Kamatani N. Synovial histology in three Behcet's disease patients with orthopedic surgery. Clinical Exp Rheum 2002; 20(4 Suppl 26): S35–S39.

[24] Keller M, Spanou Z, Schaeri P, Britschagi M, Yawalkar N, Seitz M et al. T cell-regulated neutrophilic inflammation in autoimflammatory disease. J Immunol2005; 175: 7678–7686.

[25] Yasuoka H, Okazaki Y, Kawakai Y, Hirakata M, Inoko H, Ikeda Y et al. Autoreactive CD8+ cytotoxic T lymphocytes to major histocompatibility complex class I chain-related gene A in patients with Behcet's disease. Arthritis Rheum 2004; 50: 3658–3662.

[26] Ahn JK, Chun H, Lee DS, Yu YS, Yu HG. CD8bright CD51+T cells are cytotoxic effectors in patients with active behcet's uveitis. J Immunol 2005; 175: 6133–6142.

[27] Suh OH, Park YB, Song J, Lee CH, Lee SK. Oligoclonal B lymphocyte expansion in the synovium of a patient with Behcet's disease. Arthritis Rheum 2001; 44(7): 1707–1712.

[28] Ertenli I, Kiraz S, Calguneri M, Celik I, Erman M, Haznedaroglu IC et al. Synovial fluid cytokine levels in Behcet's disease. Clin Exp Rheumatol 2001; 19: S37–S41.

[29] Pay S, Erdem H, Pekel A, Simsek I, Musabak U, Sengul A et al. synovial proinflammatory cytokines and their correlation with matrix metalloproteinase-3 expression in Behcet's disease. Does interleukin-1 beta play a major role in Behcet's synovitis? Rheumatol Int 2006; 26(7): 608–613.

[30] Karasneh J, Hajeer AH, Barrett J, Ollier WER, Thornhill M, Gul A. Association of specific interleukin 1 gene cluster polymorphisms with increase susceptibility for Behcet's disease. Rheumatology 2003; 42: 860–864. doi: 10.1093/rheumatology/keg232R

[31] Ozturk MA, Ertenli I, Kiraz S, Haznedaroglu IC, Celik I, Kirazh S et al. Plasminogen activator inhibitor-1 as a link between pathological fibrinolysis and arthritis of Behcet's disease. Rheumatol Int 2004; 24: 98–102.

[32] Aktas Cetin E, Kucuksezer UC, Bilgic S, Cagaatay Y, Gul A, Deniz G. Behcet's disese: immunological relevance with arithritis of ankylosing spondylitis. Rheumatol Int 2013; 33(3) :733–741. doi: 10.1007/s00296-012-2446-9

[33] Duygulu F, Evereklioglu C, Calis M, Borlu M, Cekmen M, Ascioglu O. Synovial nitric oxide concetrations are increased and correlated with serum levels in patients with active Behcet'sdisese: a pilot study. Clin Rheumatol 2005; 24(4): 324–330.

[34] Turan B, Pfister K, Diener PA, Hell M, Moller B, Boyvat A et al. Soluble tumor necrosis factor receptors stNFR1 and sTNFR2 are produced at site of inflammation and are markers of arthritis activity in Behcet's disease. Scand J Rheumatol 2008; 37(2): 135–141. doi: 10.1080/03009740701747137

[35] Erdem H, Pay S, Serdar M, Simsek I, Dinc A, Musabak U et al. Different ELR(+) angiogenic CXC chemokine profiles in synovial fluid of patients with Behcet's disease, familial Mediterranean fever, rheumatoid arthritis, and osteoarthritis. Rheumatol Int 2005; 26(2): 162–167.

[36] Ahn JK, Kim S, Kim J, Hwang J, Kim KH, Cha HS. A comparative metabolomic evaluation of Behcet's disease with arthritis and seronegative arthritis using synovial fluid. PLoS One 2015; 10(8): e0135856. doi: 10.1371/journal.pone.0135856

[37] Koca SS, Akbulut H, Dag S, Artas H, Isik A. Anti-cyclic citrullinated peptide antibodies in rheumatoid arthritis and Behcet's disease. Tohoku J Exp Med 2007; 213: 297–304.

[38] Uyanik A, Albayrak F, Uyanik MH, Dursun H, keles M, Cetinkaya R et al. Antibodies directed to cyclic citrullinated peptide in familial Mediterranean fever. Rheumatol Int 2010; 30: 467–470. doi: 10.1007/s00296-009-0993-5

[39] Cho SB, Lee JH, Ahn KJ, Bae BG, Kim T, Park YB, et al. Anti-cycle citrullinated peptide antibodies and joint involvement in Behcet's disease. Yonsei Med J 2012; 53: 759–764. doi: 10.3349/ymj.**2012**.53.4.759

[40] Ceccarelli F, Priori R, Iagnocco A, Coari G, Accorinti M, PivettiPezzi P, et al. Knee joint synovitis in Behcet's disease: a sonographic study. ClinExpRheumatol 2007; 45: S76–S79.

[41] Gok M, Erdem H, Gogus F, Yilmaz S, Karadag O, Simsek I et al. Relationship of ultrasonographic findings with synovial angiogenesis modulators in different forms of knee arthritides. Rheumatol Int 2013; 33: 879–885. doi: 10.1007/s00296-012-2452-y

[42] Choi JA, Kim JE, Koh SH, Chung HW, Kang HS. Arthropathy in Behcet's disease: MR imaging findings in two cases. Radiology 2003; 226(2): 387–389.

[43] Sugawara S, Ehara S, Hitachi S, Sugimoto S. Hand and wrist arthritis of Behcet disease: imaging features. Acta Radiologica 2010;51(2):183–6. doi: 10.3109/02841850903401349

[44] Backhaus M, Kamradt T, Sandrock D, Loreck D, Fritz J, Wolf KJ, et al. Arthritis of the finger joints: a comprehensive approach comparing conventional radiography, scintigraphy, ultrasound, and contrast-enhanced magnetic resonance imaging. Arthritis Rheum 1999; 42: 1232–1245.

[45] Sahin M, Yildiz M, Tunc SE, Cerci S, Suslu H, Cure E, et al. The usefulness of Tc-99m-MDP bone scintigraphy in detection of articular involvement of Behcet's disease. Ann Nucl Med 2006; 10: 649–653.

Chapter 9

Vascular Manifestations of Behçet's Disease

Orhan Saim Demirtürk, Hüseyin Ali Tünel and

Utku Alemdaroğlu

Additional information is available at the end of the chapter

http://dx.doi.org/10.5772/intechopen.68765

Abstract

Behçet's disease (BD), a very morphologically diverse systemic disease, may involve the vascular system. The venous system is the most frequently attacked vessel system. The arterial system, when involved, increases the severity and morbidity of Behçet's disease. Cardiac involvement, although rare, can be very subtle and in itself increases the mortality. Vasculitis is the hallmark pathology resulting in occlusion, aneurysms, or both. Vascular involvement may be very challenging in all phases of treatment beginning from diagnosis till recovery and remission.

Keywords: vascular involvement, vasculitis, arterial occlusion, venous thrombosis, arterial aneurysm

1. General cardiovascular involvement and findings associated with Behçet's disease (BD)

Behçet's disease (BD) is the only systemic vasculitis involving both arteries and veins in any sizes [1]. The most frequent vascular involvement is of the venous system. Both genders in their 20s and 30s can be affected. Prevalences differ.

BD has a decidedly increased mortality when the disease is seen in young male patients, while it is not as severe in female and aged patients. In most patients the severity of BD abates with the transition of time. The largest cause of mortality in BD is large-vessel vascular disease, especially hemorrhage because of pulmonary artery aneurysms (PAAs), which are almost always seen in men.

Etiology and pathophysiology of BD are still obscure and as of today unilluminated [2].

BD is a vasculitis which can involve all arteries and veins irrespective of diameter. The entire venous system from subcutaneous superficial veins to the vena cava and all deep lower extremity veins are under risk of thrombosis. The location of these thromboses determines the clinical picture. Cardiac involvement is one of the prognostically devastating manifestations of Behçet's disease (BD). Cardiac involvement is relatively uncommon [3]. The heart and great vessels are not primary targets of BD, but although not well recognized, arterial or cardiac involvement is life-threatening with associated strong prognostic implications in BD.

Therefore, physicians caring for BD patients should work closely with cardiologists, cardiovascular surgeons, and endovascular interventionists to increase awareness of these silent and potentially fatal vascular complications and form multidisciplinary groups to more successfully manage BD and its cardiovascular complications in the future.

2. Venous involvement and treatment modalities in Behçet's disease

2.1. Introduction

Vascular and neurological involvements make up the largest causes of mortality in BD. Men are more frequently affected than women. The entire venous system from subcutaneous superficial veins to the vena cava and all deep lower extremity veins are under risk of thrombosis. The clinical characteristics differ with regard to both clinical course and treatment in comparison to venous diseases due to other etiologies, and unfortunately, as of 2017, there is no set of algorithm for treatment.

As the world integrates and becomes a global village, our colleagues in both the traditional Silk Road countries and in countries receiving immigrants from these countries should have a practical knowledge and remember the particulars of the venous manifestations of this disease in order to differentially diagnose BD among a variety of venous diseases.

We will give clinicians information about the etiopathogenesis and clinical course of the venous manifestations of BD in light of literature and discuss related treatment options in this chapter.

2.2. Epidemiology

Although the incidence of BD does not differ according to sex, vascular involvement, the factor which determines the prognosis of the disease, is more frequently seen in men. Female to male ratio is 1 to 9 and does not change according to whether the thrombosis is venous or arterial. Vascular disease usually commences in the fourth decade within the first 5 years of the manifestation of other symptoms of BD. Although vascular involvement is seen in 15–38% of BD patients, this ratio was found 35% after 20 years of BD in a long-term prognostic study [4].

Even though the 1990 ISG criteria does not have vascular involvement as a prerequisite for diagnosis, this stems not from the fact that vascular involvement is insignificant, but because it does

http://dx.doi.org/10.5772/intechopen.68765

not carry significance in the differential diagnosis of BD. This matter was finally resolved when the International Criteria for Behçet's Disease (ICBD) was revised in 2014 [5]. In all discussions of criteria for diagnosis of BD, venous involvement is again put on the discussion table [6].

Ten percent of patients applied to clinics with a vascular incident before being diagnosed with BD and twenty percent of them applied after BD diagnosis were made having other coincidental symptoms of BD. A new incidence of vascular involvement in the next 5 years increases by 38% after the first vascular event [7].

Venous disease comprises the largest part within the aforementioned vascular incidences. Nearly 882 BD patients had vascular incidents in a cohort of 1272 patients applying to the clinic in an investigation conducted between 1977 and 2006. Almost 67 vascular BD patients verified by retrospective radiological methods in 6 different centers in Ankara, Turkey, were studied, and in 63 patients, a venous lesion was found in 200 locations. Both arterial and venous lesions were detected in 8 of these patients [8].

2.3. Pathogenesis

The fact that BD, although seen now almost everywhere throughout the world after migrations and distribution of refugees after civil wars, is originally seen along the so-called Silk Road, makes one think that the probable factors having a role in the pathogenesis of BD and genetic tendencies like having HLA-B5(51) have also spread along the same geography.

Although genetic factors were emphasized mostly in older studies, the detection of less disease incidence in Turkish people residing in Germany in comparison to the Turkish resident population in Anatolia and Eastern Thrace (consisting of the territory of modern Turkey) and more disease than Germans living in Germany revealed that both genetic and environmental factors were individually or jointly decisive in the development of BD [9]. Clinical disease symptoms and mortality appear to vary by geography as well as ethnic group.

In the Far East, BD usually coexists with inflammatory gastrointestinal diseases, whereas this is rare in Anatolia and Eastern Thrace. While the relationship between pathergy test positivity and HLA-51 is strong in Mediterranean countries and Japan, it is not the case in North America and patients in the USA [10].

BD, whose underlying pathology is vasculitis, is encountered in patients with familial Mediterranean fever (FMF) more frequently than the normal population. The reason for this may be the gene mutation related to the HLA region involved in BD (A9 allele of MICA [class I–related chain A (MICA) antigens]) which concurrently plays a role in the FMF pathogenesis. In a gene research conducted in the Jewish population, 54 BD patients were investigated. In 24 of these patients, one or two mutations were encountered in the MEFV gene playing a key role in FMF. Also, reported in this study is that this mutation does not only lead to BD but concurrently is related to more venous occlusive course in BD [11].

According to a survey conducted by Kural-Seyahi et al., the beginning of ocular disease and its greatest destruction usually occurred within the first early years after the initial attack. This finding led to the suggestion that the "disease burden" of BD is generally confined to the early years of the course of the disease and as the authors expressed, the disease "burns out" in time. Nonetheless, the important distinction comes from the fact that central nervous system involvement and vascular disease are exceptions to this rule. Vascular BD and central nervous BD have their beginnings later (5–10 years after onset of BD). The mortality numbers showed a less severe course in almost all disease involvement in female patients. No female patients had arterial aneurysms in the abovementioned survey [12].

No Behçet-specific factor initiating thrombosis or increasing the tendency for thrombosis could be found in studies directed at pathogenesis. BD differs from classical autoimmune diseases because of the absence of female dominance, classical pathognomonic antibodies, and being unrelated to syndromes like Sjogren's syndrome. Factors like factor V mutation, which increase the general tendency for thrombosis, may be responsible for the initial and recurrent thromboses [11]. Antithrombotic factors like protein C, S, and antithrombin III were not found deficient when all Behçet patients were examined. In the light of all these studies, it is now thought that in BD venous thrombosis develops as a result of an inflammation on the vein wall. There is a vessel wall damage and nonspecific inflammation especially in the vein adventitia [13].

T1 helper cell immune response is predominant in this inflammation, and CD4+ lymphocytes are dominant in the lesions [14]. Coagulation begins with tissue factor activation, and thrombocytes, by adhering to the present fibrin, grow ascendingly and fill the lumen.

The presence of anticardiolipin antibodies (aCL), similarly, cannot explain the increased risk of thrombosis in BD [15]. Biochemical marker negativity is not limited to anticardiolipin antibodies. RF (rheumatoid factor), ANA (antinuclear antibody), and ANCAs (antineutrophil cytoplasmic antibodies) are also negative.

Patients with BD do not have decreased protein C, protein S levels or antithrombin III activity, presence of activated protein C resistance, circulating LAC (Lupus anticoagulant) , or elevated levels of IgM aCL (anticardiolipin antibodies). A significant number of patients have elevated levels of IgG aCL, but they are not associated with venous or arterial thrombosis. No correlation was found between any variable and other clinical manifestations of the disease [15, 16].

The reason for observing so few thromboembolic events in a disease where a great number of venous thromboses are seen is the fact that thrombi have been found to be spread in an ascending and smearing fashion strongly attached to the inflammation on the vessel wall in unpublished autopsy series [17]. Histopathological specimens taken from the thromboses on the venous wall at different phases during thrombosis are needed in illuminating this specific subject.

2.4. Superficial vein thrombosis (SVT)

Superficial vein thrombosis (SVT) is a sign that can be as frequently encountered as DVT (deep vein thrombosis) with a commonly acute beginning which may be accompanied by symptoms of thrombophlebitis (an increase of skin temperature along a superficial vein, erythema, and pain).

It presents with symptoms like extensive body pain, chills, and tremors. There is no registered data about fever which may accompany SVT. Because the inflammation may reveal itself as nodular lesions in the vein rather than thrombophlebitis in some patients, BD may be impossible to differentiate from erythema nodosum. Vein wall thickening and intraluminal thrombus are detected upon superficial Doppler ultrasonography.

Superficial vein thrombosis (SVT) may be simultaneously seen in BD patients with previous DVT or concomitantly with DVT [18]. SVT is more frequently observed in the presence of venous insufficiency background and appears like diffuse erythematous indurated plaques in the dermal-epidermal tissue. SVT leaves a pigmented trace or thinned but hardened vein after recovery.

2.5. Deep vein thrombosis

DVT is the initial and most frequently appearing vascular incident in BD (two-thirds of the cases). Even though it can be seen anywhere along the venous system, it is most commonly observed in the femoral and popliteal veins. There are no criteria differentiating DVT in BD from classical DVT. There is no clear data concerning the frequency or time about the development of venous insufficiency in Behçet patients with DVT. Edema due to venous insufficiency, pigmentation, and venous claudication can be observed in patients who have been followed for a long time [19]. While some studies declare the rate of postthrombotic syndrome (PTS) incidence as 20–50% in patients who have been affected by proximal DVT (DVT in iliac, common femoral veins), this rate is given as 5–10% in severe PTS patients with venous ulcers [20]. It is important to differentiate between venous insufficiency and vasculitis in patients who present with venous ulcer. Venous claudication which directly affects daily quality of life occurs in one-third of the patients [19].

Roumen-Klappe et al. in their 2009 work demonstrated that elevated IL-6, C-reactive protein (CRP), and intercellular adhesion molecule 1 (ICAM-1) levels after DVT development are directly related to PTS [21]. The increase in ICAM-1 level is also directly proportional to the severity of PTS.

Although Behçet patients who have DVT are under risk of PTS, the clinical course differs to a large extent from that in classical DVT with regard to the frequency of pulmonary thromboembolus (PTE) development. This leads to a great difference in DVT treatment protocols in BD. The chance of recanalization of the affected veins is low. Clinical relief comes more from collateral development which is copious in the venous system. DVT also can be ameliorated using thromboaspiration as an adjunct to conventional low-molecular-weight heparin treatment which is usually advised for a duration of 6 months. It has been reported that endovascular treatment with US-guided percutaneous aspiration thrombectomy can be considered as a safe and effective way to remove thrombus from the deep veins in pregnant women with acute and subacute iliofemoral deep vein thrombosis [22]. The effectiveness of this method is also corroborated in studies reporting about endovascular treatment of postpartum deep vein thrombosis [23, 24].

2.6. Vena cava thrombosis (VCT)

Vena cava thrombosis (VCT) is the second most commonly encountered venous incident after DVT. It is seen in approximately 15% of the patients, and the superior vena cava (SVC) is more commonly involved than the inferior vena cava (IVC).

Occlusion of the SVC causes the classical superior vena cava syndrome. Edema and erythema of the upper extremities and nonpulsatile congestion of the jugular veins are seen. Rarely, increased intracranial pressure and papilledema are also observed. Venous collaterals with caudal flow may be encountered upon physical examination. Pleural effusion is seen when the bronchial and pleural venous return is disrupted, and chylothorax is seen when the thoracic duct does not function properly. Contrast-enhanced computed tomography (CT) portraying the absence of venous flow is diagnostic.

IVC thrombosis shows symptoms similar to DVT. Computed tomography is again the diagnostic tool of choice. IVC thrombosis causes serious complications in the long run if intra-abdominal organs, especially the liver, are affected.

2.6.1. Budd-Chiari syndrome (BCS)

In Turkey BD is responsible for 40% of Budd-Chiari syndrome (BCS) cases [25]. The best known common characteristics of BCS cases that have been reported are the close relationship of BCS with vena cava thrombosis. Hepatic vein thrombosis coexists with IVC thrombosis in 80% or more patients with BCS [12].

Hepatic vein thrombosis should come to mind when a patient with the diagnoses of DVT or IVC thrombosis has or develops accompanying abdominal pain, ascites, and splenomegaly. High albumin gradient ascites, elevation of transaminase levels, and alkaline phosphatase may be seen in laboratory tests. In the long term, prognosis is determined by thrombosed vessels. While the prognosis is favorable in patients with solitary occurrence of the hepatic vein, the prognosis worsens when the portal vein or IVC is attacked, hitherto, the largest patient series reveals that two-thirds of 493 patients with Budd-Chiari syndrome have been lost by the end of the first year [25].

2.7. Cerebral venous thrombosis (CVT)

Cerebral venous thrombosis (CVT) as venous involvement in BD is a relatively rare vascular incident. 2.5% of Behçet patients are affected by CVT. It appears mostly in male patients over the age of 30. In a study conducted in 3908 patients, the rate of incidence was found 0.31%. This rate may differ between clinics because headache is encountered frequently in BD and diagnosis of CVT is difficult to make. The clinical course and prognosis are different from parenchymal neurological involvement [26].

CVT is the most frequent cause of intracranial hypertension [27]. Hyperhomocysteinemia as an independent factor has been held responsible for CVT [28]. In a meta-analysis it has been reported that hyperhomocysteinemia may be considered to be associated with thrombosis in BD [30]. 4.77% of CVT patients have already entered the subacute or chronic phase when diagnosis is established. The superior sagittal sinus (64%) or the transverse sinus is the most frequently involved locations. The sigmoid sinus follows in the frequency of involvement [29].

Differential diagnosis of CVTs encountered in BD can be made from other CVTs seen in different diseases or coagulation defects because of their characteristic male dominance, scarcity of neurological signs, and unusual venous infarcts [30]. CVT should be suspected in a young male patient consulting the emergency department with headache, especially if the headache is recent and papilledema is present upon examination. Seen less is lateral rectus muscle weakness due to an increase in intracranial pressure resulting in diplopia and vomiting.

Cranial magnetic resonance imaging (MRI) and MR venography are the diagnostic golden standards. In two-thirds of the patients, the cerebrospinal fluid pressure is increased, and if no parenchymal disease accompanies CVT, the cerebrospinal fluid is normal.

Optic atrophy and resultant loss in vision are the main sequelae subsequent to long-standing papilledema in the long-term course of CVT in BD. Ventriculoperitoneal shunt may be needed in patients with elevated cerebrospinal fluid pressure. Prognosis is fair even though generally no anticoagulation is given. Early and differential diagnosis amiliorate the prognosis [31].

2.8. Treatment in venous involvement

DVT has the largest share in venous involvement. Its treatment is open to discussion. Especially for individually practicing vascular surgeons and other primary care physicians, the greater part of the treatment consists of anticoagulation. However, anticoagulation is not recommended for venous incidents in BD because the course of venous thrombosis is different in comparison to classical venous thromboses [32]. As evident from these conflicting reports, the discussion about coagulation defects is not settled yet.

It was reported in 2015 that procoagulant factors like coagulation factor V G1691A (factor V Leiden mutation) and prothrombin G20210A polymorphisms exist in BD. This led to the suggestion that these factors may be additional risk factors for thrombosis in certain people [33].

It has been reported that factor V Leiden mutation was more frequent in Turkish, but not in Italian, Spanish, and Israeli patients [34–37]. Prothrombin gene mutation was not reported to be relevant in several studies, but a meta-analysis by Ricart et al. demonstrated an interrelationship between the presence of prothrombin G20210A mutation and thrombosis in BD after excluding Turkish patients [37].

Lenk et al. reported that deficiencies of protein C, protein S, and antithrombin have not been linked to thrombosis in BD patients [15]. It has been reported that high levels of lipoprotein found in BD patients may be involved in the development of thrombosis by weakening fibrinolysis [25]. Moreover, high plasma levels of thrombin-activatable fibrinolysis inhibitor, which could lead to a substantial decrement of the clot lysis process, were documented in BD patients [38].

Although not clearly established as yet, there is conflicting data concerning the preventive potential immunosuppressive therapy on vascular diseases and complications [39]. Immunosuppressive drug therapy alone or in combination with steroids is advised during early stages of BD before the development of irreversible damage to the arterial wall [39]. Colchicine, which is a commonly used and very effective drug for mucocutaneous lesions, is not effective on vascular or ocular lesions. Colchicine may decrease nodular lesions in women, but it is not clear what percentage of these lesions is superficial thrombophlebitis.

Treatment in SVT is usually symptomatic. Nonsteroidal anti-inflammatory drugs and topical cold applications will ameliorate the local symptoms. 20–40 mg of prednisolone may be added to the treatment for patients with severe clinical course. Two weeks of steroids with mild doses may be added to the symptomatic treatment of patients with DVT.

It should be born in mind that a Behçet patient with prior history of a vascular incident is under risk for a second recurrent event. All Behçet patients who have DVT are given 2.5 mg/kg/day of azathioprine. This should be continued until the fifth decade (mid-1940s) when BD activity usually decreases. Azathioprine may prevent superficial thrombophlebitis [40].

Postthrombotic syndrome (PTS) is the most serious complication in the long term. Treatment of PTS is treated classically as in PTS due to other conditions. Compression stockings, bandages, and venoactive agents can prevent venous ulcer formation, and ulcer stockings are indicated when needed.

In SVC thrombosis corticosteroids and diuretics are effective if headache and diffuse edema are present. Although prognosis is fair in the long run, azathioprine should be added to the treatment.

Endovenous interventions (IVC filter placement and thrombectomy) should be avoided in BD because they may result in pathergy like symptoms and also because PTE practically does not occur. When treatment is planned for IVC thrombosis, BCS, which is the most mortal complication of venous involvement in BD, should always be born in mind. For portal hypertension diuretics and sodium restriction and for hepatic vein thrombosis, high doses of corticosteriods and monthly pulse doses of cyclophosphamides should be considered especially if de novo thrombosis has developed in the IVC or if the anatomical level of the thrombus is near the hepatic veins. Anti-TNF treatment has been tried in some patient groups but was not successful. Azathioprine used in combination with interferon causes serious leukopenia.

Symptoms improve, and the clinical course ameliorates with corticosteroids and azathioprine in CVT. If treatment is begun early, the prognosis is fairly good. Ventriculoperitoneal shunts may be needed for stubborn diseases with increased intracranial pressure and papilledema.

3. Arterial involvement and treatment modalities in Behçet's disease

3.1. Introduction

Behçet's disease (BD) is a vasculitis which can involve all arteries and veins irrespective of diameter. Changes in endothelial function due to this involvement cause different grades of clinically observable organ lesions [41]. Vascular involvement, especially arterial involvement, is one of the major causes of morbidity and mortality [42].

BD has a high incidence along the ancient "Silk Road" stretching from the Far East to the Mediterranean. The prevalence in Turkey is 80–370/100,000, while it is only 0.12–7.5/100,000 in the United States of America and Europe [43, 44]. But recently it can be seen anywhere in the world due to immigration.

Studies performed in Turkey, Iran, Japan, and Europe report that the prevalence of vascular involvement in Behçet's disease in their respective countries is 17, 9, 9, and 10–37% [45].

Vascular involvement rarely occurs as the initial clinical appearance of BD. It was reported that in a cohort of BD patients more than 94% exibited oral and genital ulceration at the first visit, while only 20.6% displayed vascular involvement in their very first clinical examination [44].

Since the first report in Japan by Mishima et al. in 1961, written in 1973, vascular involvement in BD has been reported to be about 2–46% and seen four to five times more in men in endemic regions [46]. In a retrospective study consisting of 882 BD patients with vascular involvement, the rate of vascular recurrence 2 years after the initial episode was found to be 23% and 38% after 5 years. Only male gender was found as a potential risk factor among potential predictive factors in the same study. Arterial attack is less frequent in comparison to venous involvement. Worldwide prevalence of arterial involvement is around 1.5–3% [47]. Patients with arterial involvements tend to have multiple lesions and usually have accompanying deep vein thrombosis. Aneurysm is usually more commonly reported than occlusion [47].

Regarding the site of occurrence, there have been some geographic variations in cohorts studied so far [47, 48]. Reports from Turkey and Korea described the femoral artery and the abdominal aorta as the most common locations of aneurysm formation [49, 50]. However, a report from a Chinese registry showed the lower extremity and the abdominal aorta as the most frequently attacked sites and the femoral artery as a rarely attacked location [47]. This is a typical example of geographical difference in frequency and locations of vascular lesions.

3.2. Pathogenesis

Autoinflammatory diseases have been described as diseases characterized by increased immune response mediated by the immune system cell and molecules with a significant degree of genetic predisposition and dominant congenital characteristics. BD also falls in this group because of various clinical and inflammatory characteristics [48].

3.2.1. Genetic predisposition: HLA-B51

BD is not a Mendelian disease. However, it has an important genetic component due to its familial characteristics [48]. HLA-B51 is the strongest identified factor for genetic predisposition. The presence of this association has been proven in various ethnic groups [50].

HLA-B51 may contribute to the pathogenesis of BD by both adaptive (presentation of some pathogenic peptides to CD8 T cells) and congenital mechanisms (activation with natural killer cells and by activating intracellular inflammatory pathways) affecting the immune system [48].

The evidence obtained in the recent research established the correlation between HLA-B51 and the clinical severity of BD [51].

3.2.2. Abnormally increased inflammatory response

Increased inflammatory response against nonspecific stimuli is a known feature of BD. This particular feature forms the basis of the pathergy test which is widely used for diagnosis [6].

The distinctly marked congenital immune response in BD patients is an enhanced expression of cytokines such as IL-1, IL-6, IL-8, and tumor necrosis factor (TNF) [52]. IL-1 levels released by monocytyes, an action induced by lipopolysaccharides, can also be high in BD patients [51]. Similarly, activated neutrophils are frequently observed in pathological specimens, and BD is generally classified among neutrophilic dermatoses [53]. Systemic vasculitis and occlusive perivasculitis and thrombosis are observed [53]. The hallmark histopathologic pattern of neutrophilic vasculitides is denoted as leukocytoclastic vasculitis, which is characterized by angiocentric segmental inflammation, endothelial cell swelling, and fibrinoid necrosis of blood vessel walls (postcapillary venules). Alavi et al. reported that the cellular infiltrate around and within dermal blood vessel walls is composed mainly of neutrophils. Direct immunofluorescence demonstrates deposition of complement C3, immunoglobulin IgM, IgA, and/or IgG in a granular pattern within the vessel walls. Circulating immune complex deposition increases adhesiveness between inflammatory cells and the endothelium and neutrophil-mediated damage to postcapillary venules. Therefore, many factors play a role in the pathogenesis of BD. Vascular damage triggered by inflammation increases the risk of thrombosis [41]. Increased plasma levels of nitric oxide (NO) and its metabolites seen in BD patients demonstrate also the presence of an endothelial dysfunction [54].

The presence of hypercoagulability also has been broadly demonstrated in BD patients. The findings supporting this observation are a decrease in physiological fibrinolysis together with high thrombin levels, low activated protein C concentrations, increase in thrombocyte activation, and the presence of lower tissue plasminogen activator levels [44, 55, 56].

The pathogenesis of aneurysms in BD is also another interesting pathological discussion. The pathogenesis of aneurysms in BD has not been clearly revealed. However, it is presumed to be caused by obliterative endarteritis of vasa vasorum concomitant with intense inflammation primarily involving the media and adventitia. Infiltration of inflammatory cells, as reported by Al-Basheer et al., causes destruction of the media and fibrous thickening of the intima and adventitia. The weakened arterial wall leads to the distension of the vessel wall which at the end causes development of a true aneurysm or perforation of the vessel wall which in turn leads to the development of a false aneurysm or arterial dissection [57].

Although the underlying causative factor is not yet well understood, BD can affect the mucocutaneous tissues, eyes, blood vessels, both arteries and vein, brain, nervous system, and gastrointestinal system with recurrent attacks. Ultimately, BD, as initially described by Hulusi Behçet, is a multifactorial disease in which many triggering factors like infections and viruses may play a role [58].

3.3. Clinical findings

Like in other vasculitides, in BD, fever, weakness, and an increase in acute-phase reactants (CRP, Erythrocyte sedimentation rate [ESR]) are the systemic findings in the acute stage of the disease [59]. The following findings can be monitored in the acute inflammatory phase and the following recovery—fibrosis phase:

1. In the vessel lumen: irregularities, narrowing, and occlusion
2. In the vessel wall: necrosis, aneurysm, rupture, and fibrosis
3. In the tissues distal to the lesion: ischemia, necrosis, and dysfunction [59]

Arterial lesions are associated with the inflammation of the adventitia and media consisting of the aseptic infiltration of tissues with neutrophils and mononuclear cells. Initially, active arteritis develops in the affected arteries. This inflammation is followed by medial destruction and fibrosis. Arterial involvements include aneurysm, stenosis, and occlusions [60]. Perforation, the most frequently seen lesion in the arterial wall, develops probably as a result of endothelial dysfunction, necrosis of elastic and smooth muscle cells. This in turn paves the way for sinister pseudoaneurysm formation or an ominous rupture.

The most frequently affected artery is the abdominal aorta. This is followed in frequency by the pulmonary, femoral, subclavian, and common carotid arteries [46]. Although rare, we may encounter visceral artery involvement such as in jejunal arteries as reported by Wu et al. [61].

3.3.1. *Aneurysms*

Aneurysms are encountered more frequently than arterial occlusions [47]. Aneurysms are frequent in Behçet patients whose course is severe and complicated by uveitis or deep vein thrombosis and cause high mortality rates [62]. It approximately takes 7 years for aneurysm development after the onset of BD [12].

Although aneurysms can occur in almost all arteries, the abdominal aorta is the most frequently involved artery. Rupture is the most commonly seen complication of aneurysms and the most frequently encountered cause of vascular death [63]. Multiple aneurysms are also relatively common in comparison to the normal population [47].

3.3.2. *Systemic arterial aneurysms*

Aneurysms in BD differ from degenerative aneurysms in many ways. They diverge from degenerative aneurysms because they are observed in young patients, suprarenal location is more frequent in aneurysms detected in Behçet patients, and the shape of these aneurysms is more often saccular rather than fusiform. Often multiple aneurysms coexist, and patient symptoms more frequently appear under emergency conditions [47]. Aneurysms are the most complex vascular lesions encountered in BD. They are among the most challenging pathologies for vascular surgeons because of technical difficulties they present and their association with high recurrence rates [64]. It is a unique fact that BD is the only vasculitis known to lead to pulmonary artery aneurysms [57]. Also, it is a unique fact for BD that there is no correlation between the diameter of an aneurysm and the risk of rupture [65].

Pseudoaneurysms develop as a result of frequent rupture of saccular aneurysms. Defects are usually located on the posterior walls of arteries. There is a thick fibrous tissue containing reactional lymph nodes in the retroperitoneum in abdominal aortic aneurysms. It may be surgically difficult to expose the aorta because of this reason.

Peripheral artery aneurysms may present as painful swellings. Following the aorta and the pulmonary arteries, the carotid, femoral, popliteal, and subclavian arteries are the most frequently affected sites. Apart from these usual locations, all visceral arteries may be attacked [64, 66, 67]. Involvement of cerebral and renal arteries is rare. Abdominal aortic aneurysms are often discovered in the chronic stage, with vague symptoms like back pain or abdominal discomfort [51].

3.3.3. Pulmonary artery aneurysms

BD may attack any pulmonary artery in the pulmonary arterial tree regardless of diameter causing aneurysm or occlusion in a similar fashion akin to what it does in the arterial system [60]. Pulmonary artery aneurysms (PAAs) usually involve large- or medium-sized arteries. Hemoptysis is the most frequent and generally the initial symptom [68]. Fatal hemorrhages can occur when aneurysmatic arteries rupture into the bronchi [68, 69]. PAAs tend to occur more in men and appear in younger patients in comparison to arterial involvement in other areas. PAA can be multiple and bilateral. These patients generally also have DVT, caval or intracardiac thrombi, and systemic arterial aneurysms [45, 70, 71].

The inflammatory process in PAA occurs in the vasa vasorum of the artery. Consequent ischemia occuring in the artery wall causes weakening in the vessel wall and causes rupture [55]. It is rather rare to have concomitant true and false PAA side by side. These lesions frequently erode bronchi and cause massive and potentially mortal hemoptyses [72].

3.3.4. Occlusive lesions

Arterial lesions are usually solitary, but they may sometimes be multiple. They are generally accompanied by venous thromboses [73]. Arterial lesions may be asymptomatic depending on the sufficiency of the collateral circulation or may present with ischemic symptoms. Thrombi may develop within the aneurysmal sac, and very rarely distal embolization may occur leading to threatening limb ischemia [74]. The femoral artery is frequently affected. But an extremity artery or coronary and splenic or visceral arteries like the mesenteric artery can be occluded [60].

3.4. Diagnosis

The revised International Criteria for Behçet's Disease (ICBD) published in 2014 is the latest diagnosis/classification criteria. The diagnosis is made clinically. Although the classical triad includes urogenital ulcer, chronic ocular inflammation (uveitis), and mucocutaneous lesions, BD is a multisystemic disease [74]. The new criteria include oral aphthosis, genital aphthosis, ocular lesions, neurological manifestations, skin lesions, vascular manifestations, and positive pathergy test. Oral aphthosis, genital aphthosis, and ocular lesions each get two points, whereas skin lesions, vascular manifestations, neurological manifestations, and positive pathergy test each get one point. A patient scoring four points or above is classified/diagnosed as BD [5].

As reported by Wu et al., various symptoms in BD do not necessarily manifest themselves at the same time. Sarica-Kuçukoğlu report that in 6.8% of their cases, vascular involvement preceded or occurred during the diagnosis of BD, and 33.7% of the patients developed vascular disease within 5 years of diagnosis [75].

Early diagnosis of BD in young males with aneurysms is critical to avoid any ruptured aneurysms. Early diagnosis may be based on radiographic imaging such as ultrasound angiography, CT, and magnetic resonance angiography. CT has become the procedure of choice in evaluating patients with aneurysm. Selective angiography has proven useful for both the diagnosis and treatment of intestinal bleeding.

Patients with diagnosis of BD must be investigated with regard to multiple silent aneurysms; close follow-up should be conducted and must especially be reinvestigated after major activation phases of BD [74].

Noninvasive methods such as Doppler ultrasonography, CT, MRI, or PET/CT should be preferred in evaluation and follow-up of arterial lesions. Arterial punctures made in classical angiography may cause pseudoaneurysm development, a process similar to the reaction produced by the pathergy test in the skin [76, 77].

3.5. Treatment modalities

The treatment strategy for a peripheral artery aneurysm associated with BD is determined by the anatomical location and clinical presentation, including rupture or impending rupture and the active or remission stage of disease.

The presence of arterial involvement changes the course of BD dramatically and is associated with bad prognosis [74]. Surgery or endovascular treatment used without immunosuppressive medical therapy increases the risk of development of complications and pseudoaneurysm after the operation or intervention [61]. Because of this important fact, endovascular or surgical treatment must be combined with medical therapy.

3.5.1. Medical treatment

Steroids are the mainstay of treatment. They may be used systemically or topically. It is critically important to begin cyclophosphamide or prednisolone with aggressive immunosuppressive therapy in a combined fashion for the inhibition of progression of vascular lesions and causes good prognosis [78]. Medical therapy should be the first choice for the treatment of asymptomatic occlusive or stenotic lesions [60].

Anticoagulant, fibrinolytic, or antiplatelet agent use increases the risk of aneurysm rupture. Serious hemorrhages can lead to death. There is no proof supporting the use of anticoagulants in the treatment of arterial lesions. Anticoagulant use is not advised [61]. Nevertheless, the use of anticoagulants or antiaggregants in combination with immunosuppressive and anti-inflammatory agents in order to prevent graft occlusions in the postoperative period may be useful [60].

3.5.2. *Surgical treatment*

Surgical treatment is indicated generally for the treatment of systemic arterial aneurysms because of increased risk of rupture. Since the risk of rupture of arterial aneurysms in BD is not directly proportional to their diameter, they should be treated even if they are less than 5 cm in the abdominal aorta [47, 74]. Nevertheless, arterial repair under emergency conditions can be complicated because of recurrent disease, graft occlusion, or development of anastomotic pseudoaneurysm [57, 79]. Due to these difficulties, strenghthening of the anastomotic sites with prosthetic material thus decreases the dead space, and omental wrapping for fistula prevention can be protective [47, 62].

Because the inflammatory process in BD may involve the autologuous venous material, sythetic material (Dacron or polytetrafluoroethylene [PTFE]) should be used instead of the saphenous vein for graft material. Anastomoses should be performed at healthy-looking zones [60].

Reconstruction should always be performed in a disease-free–looking segment of the artery. To avoid suture line problems of development of pseudoaneurysms, the suture lines can be reinforced with plagets made of Teflon, and the graft can be wrapped with omentum. The choice of graft material is significant in decreasing long-term complications. Vasculitis may be present in the veins of the patient, and because of this factor, the use of autologous grafts should be avoided, and synthetic grafts should be preferred. The graft of choice in the abdominal area should be Dacron, whereas it should be polytetrafluoroethylene (PTFE) in the extremities [74].

Especially if collateral circulation is deemed adequate, ligation of the aneurysmatic artery is an alternative surgical treatment in distal aneurysms like popliteal artery aneurysm and for unstable patients with ruptured aneurysms [80, 81].

Mortality of emergency surgery for ruptured pulmonary artery aneurysms is very high. Therefore, it is advisable to avoid surgery as much as possible if there is no life-threatening hemorrhage [82].

Recurrent false aneurysms at anastomotic sites may result in as high as 30–50% of cases. Therefore, anastomoses should be done in macroscopically disease-free segments [83].

3.5.3. *Endovascular treatment*

Endovascular methods are increasingly widely used treatment modalities for patients with BD. Endovascular treatment became popular because of being less invasive. They are more preferred in BD because in BD the length of aneurysmatic segments is shorter, and these aneurysms are in relatively younger group of patients in comparison to the older patients with atherosclerotic aneurysms [65].

The endovascular approach is an alternative for treating arterial lesions. According to a report by Kim et al., which stresses the importance of induction of remission of active disease by preoperative immunosuppression, successful results have been achieved with an acceptable complication rate [65]. Endovascular treatment looks like a safe and less invasive modality for arterial pathologies linked with BD. In cases in which ligation cannot be performed because of the risk of peripheral ischemia, the endovascular approach may be a treatment option for arterial involvement associated with BD.

Surgical and endovascular surgery, whichever is suitable for the patient, must be combined with preoperative, perioperative, and postoperative medical therapy in order to increse the chance of success.

3.6. Prognosis

The presence of BD increases morbidity and mortality significantly. This is even higher in patients with vascular involvement. The highest morbidity and mortality rates in BD are seen in patients who have pulmonary artery aneurysm. One-year survival is 50% in these patients [84].

The most important reason of mortality is aneurysm rupture. One- and five-year mortalities are 1.2 and 3.3 %, respectively [42]. Mortality rates, which are higher between ages 15 and 34, decrease after age 35 [42].

In a multivariate analysis conducted by Sadooun et al., male gender, arterial involvement, and multiple disease exacerbations were found independent factors of mortality [85].

3.7. Future and recommendations

Predicting which patients will have cardiovascular complications is the major concern of recent investigations. Early diagnosis of vascular involvement is helpful for planning effective management and improving the prognosis. Long-term follow-up is also essential in patients with BD because of the relapsing nature of the disease [86]. The cornerstone in the treatment of Behçet patients is the avoidance of surgical intervention during the active stage of the disease. But this is not possible in many cases [87]. Kasirajan suggests that all patients after the age of 55 with aneurysms involving large- and medium-sized vessels should have an ESR and a CRP evaluation [76].

The infrequent nature of aneurysms in patients with BD precludes a large prospective study evaluating open surgery versus endovascular technique. Nevertheless, the data at the present time compels one to take the endovascular route if feasible. An increased awareness of BD and its vascular complications is essential.

Management for arterial involvements associated with BD requires perioperative and postoperative comprehensive medical therapy to control the inflammation [88]. Consensus regarding the graft of choice for arterial vasculature in BD is debatable. For example, successful treatment of celiac artery aneurysm with extra-anatomical aorta-common hepatic artery bypass using e-PTFE graft has been reported by Maeda et al. [89]. Koksoy et al. declared that the choice of graft material did not affect the outcomes [90].

After surgical management, a high incidence of anastomotic dehiscence is one of the major problems in the treatment of vasculo-BD (VBD) [65]. There is no universally accepted method for assessing disease activity in these patients, and no standard immunosuppressive protocol exists for pre-/postendograft treatment. Nevertheless, the results of a small pilot study supported the usefulness of immunosuppressive treatment combined with endovascular pseudoaneurysm repair (exclusion) in BD when the immunosuppressive agent kept the serum ESR level within the normal range [90].

There are no data or evidence of benefit from anticoagulant, antiplatelet, or antifibrinolytic agents in the management of DVT or for the use of anticoagulation for arterial lesions of BD.

The thrombus in BD adheres to the vessel wall and does not result in emboli, so pulmonary embolism is rare. Another reason to avoid these agents is the possibility of a coexisting pulmonary arterial aneurysm, which might result in fatal bleeding.

In the EULAR (European League Against Rheumatism) recommendation, immunosuppressive agents, such as corticosteroids, azathioprine, and cyclophosphamide, are suggested to reduce this inflammation because the primary pathology leading to DVT in BD is inflammation of the vessel wall [90]. Several case reports showed the efficacy of antitumor necrosis factor-alpha (TNF-α) agents for BD patients with complications of vascular involvement, such as PAA, aortitis, and deep vein thrombosis. But only a limited number of studies about these agents have been published [91–94]. In contrast, several studies have raised caution regarding the possibility of development of thrombophlebitis as a side effect of infliximab in BD patients [95, 96]. Further research is needed to clarify the efficacy and safety of anti-TNF-α agents in the treatment of vascular involvement in BD.

4. Cardiac involvement and treatment modalities in Behçet's disease

4.1. Introduction

Cardiac involvement is one of the prognostically devastating manifestations of Behçet's disease (BD). Cardiac involvement is relatively uncommon [97]. The heart and great vessels are not primary targets of BD, but although not well recognized, arterial or cardiac involvement are life-threatening with associated strong prognostic implications in BD [3]. Cardiac involvement is one of the most severe complications in patients with BD despite its sporadic occurrence, being greatly correlated with mortality [98]. The incidence and nature of cardiac involvement in Behçet's disease are not yet clearly documented [99].

Cardiac involvement includes pericarditis, coronary artery aneurysms, or stenoses independent of atherosclerosis because of BD per se. Spontaneous coronary artery dissection, myocarditis, cardiomyopathy, congestive cardiac failure, valvular diseases due to endomyocardial fibrosis called Behçet's valvulitis, intracardiac thrombosis (ICT), sinus of Valsalva aneurysms, ventricular aneurysms, aneurysms of the ascending aorta or branches of the aorta such as the carotid arteries, and aneurysms of the thoracic aorta are the other phenomena associated with BD that will be discussed in this section.

BD may attack the myoendothelial damaging valves leading to conduction disturbances. Endomyocardial fibrosis or valve dysfunction usually in the form of insufficiencies rather than stenoses occur. Coronary arteritis may induce thrombi within ventricles, most commonly the right ventricle [100]. Several cardiac manifestations may occur in the same patient [2].

4.2. Epidemiology

BD is common in countries along the ancient Silk Road (from the Far East to the Mediterranean region). The highest prevalence is in Turkey 40–370/100,000 [2]. In the Eastern Mediterranean and the Middle East, middle-aged men suffer a more aggressive course especially when the vascular system is affected. But nowadays, due to immigrations, BD is seen in almost everywhere throughout the world [101].

4.3. Pathogenesis

Over the past few years, pathophysiology of cardiovascular disease has been substantially revised, and new facts have been discovered. Mechanisms of atherothrombogenesis have been associated with inflammation and immune disorders [2]. In the recent past, many authors began to classify BD as an autoinflammatory disease rather than an autoimmune disease [3].

The pathogenic mechanism underlying thrombotic propensity in patients with BD is not however yet completely understood. It is believed that endothelial cell ischemia or disruption leads to enhancement of platelet aggregation. It is important to consider BD as a prototypic example of thrombotic diseases associated with T-cell–mediated neutrophilic inflammation. In various studies it was shown that TNF-α-103 C allele and polymorphism in IL-21, IL-10, and IL-8 genes are related to the pathogenesis if BD [1]. In addition, similar to the other disorders with increased risk of thrombosis formation, there is endothelial cell injury and a hypercoagulable state in BD. Furthermore, selectins, a group of adhesion molecules consisting of P- and E-selectins mediating leukocyte adhesion to platelets and endothelium, have a role in thrombogenesis. Increased E- and P-selectin levels were reported in BD in some studies [102].

Prothrombin gene mutation was identified in some BD patients. Increased plasma homocysteine levels are also a risk factor for thrombosis in BD. It was shown that mean plasma homocysteine levels in BD patients were substantially higher in comparison to that in healthy subjects, which led to the suggestion that another conceivable pathogenic mechanism of thrombosis in BD may be related to the presence of antiphospholipid antibodies, which have been reported in 18% of cases in a study [103].

The vessel wall attracts cytokinergic and neutrophilic reactions causing damage by excessive production of superoxide anion radicals and lysosomal enzymes leading to vascular wall destruction with aneurysm formation [3]. Endothelial dysfunction, release of von Willebrand factor, activation of platelets, enhanced thrombin and fibrin generation coupled with antithrombin deficiency, and impaired fibrinolysis lead to increased thrombocoagulation associated with perivasculitis [104, 105]. In a case series, histological samples of right-sided intracardiac masses secondary to BD were studied which demonstrated dense inflammatory infiltration, neovascularization, endocardial fibrin deposition, and fibrosis [106].

The pathogenesis of valvular regurgitation in BD was suggested as resulting from dilatation of the aortic or mitral annulus caused by a typical inflammation [107]. Diffuse aortitis leads to proximal aortic dilatation and aortic regurgitation requiring aortic valve replacement. Histopathology of the aorta reveals features similar to those observed in other systemic diseases with aortic involvement, destruction of the valve tissue itself, diffuse aortitis of the ascending aorta, and aneurysm of the sinus of Valsalva. Several specific echocardiographic discoveries have been made like redundant aortic valve cusps with prolapse, vegetation-like masses, and echolucencies in Behçet's valvulitis [108].

There is uncertainty about whether the coronary lesions are caused by atherosclerosis or vasculitis in these patients. Many studies investigated the possibility of increased atherosclerosis in BD. Most findings refute this hypothesis. Atherosclerosis by itself does not seem to be enhanced by BD [109].

Three additional mechanisms have been proposed for development of coronary artery disease (CAD) in BD in the past decade:

1. Subclinical atherosclerosis
2. Silent ischemia
3. Spontaneous coronary artery dissection

A Spanish group reported about spontaneous coronary artery dissection of the LAD in a Behçet patient. They proposed that spontaneous coronary artery dissection could possibly be a cause of coronary ischemia in BD [110]. A recent meta-analysis pointed to the fact that subclinical atherosclerosis, not clinically apparent atherosclerosis, is increased in BD as depicted by impaired flow-mediated dilatation and increased intima-media thickness but whether this translates into coronary artery disease in time is controversial [111].

4.4. Clinical findings

Estimated incidence of cardiac involvement is reported 1–5% in a case series. Mortality is rather high (around 20%). Cardiac involvement in BD could be asymptomatic [112]. Cardiac involvement, when occurs, coexists with mucocutaneous manifestations.

Pericarditis is the most common cardiac complication in BD. Acute pericarditis, tamponade, and constrictive pericarditis have been reported. Myocarditis, cardiomyopathy causing diastolic and systolic dysfunction, valvular pathology coronary thromboses, coronary aneurysms, coronary rupture, predominantly right-sided intracardiac thrombus, aneurysm of the aorta, and its branches including the arch of aorta are other important cardiac complications of BD [112]. Several cardiac manifestations may occur in one patient [2]. This manifests itself such as ICT accompanied by peripheral arterial or venous involvement. Pulmonary, venous, and arterial involvements are more common in patients with ICT than in patients without ICT. Recurrent ICT formation, especially right ventricular or atrial thrombosis due to BD, is therefore another important problem.

ICT was noted in 1.9% of 626 BD patients in a 2016 study. ICT typically involves the ventricles rather than the atria and usually the right ventricle. The ICT is usually multiple, hyperechoic, and homogenous with well-demarcated margins and mostly immobile with a broad-based attachment to the ventricle or atrium [108].

Coronary artery disease (CAD) is rare in BD. It is more common in males younger than 40 years of age. CAD can lead to clinical manifestations such as stable or unstable angina which usually leads to myocardial infarction (MI). Sometimes silent ischemia occurs which may later cause problems. Aneurysms readily occur in coronary arteries, sometimes multiple and accompanied by stenoses. Coronary lesions tend to be proximal and easily cause MI leading to development of ventricular aneurysm formation or cardiomyopathy [113]. Aneurysm formation and occlusion of coronary arteries are the most common etiologies for CAD in BD.

Coronary aneurysms are more frequent than stenoses and can present as acute coronary syndrome and MI but sometimes are symptomatic [112]. In young adults with myocardial infarction, BD should be considered as a nonatherosclerotic cause of CAD. Silent myocardial infarction and subclinical disease may also be present in cardiac involvement of BD [114]. Therefore, understanding the etiology of acute myocardial infarction in BD is important for determination of treatment strategy.

Although coronary arteritis may cause MI (myocardial infarction), in some of the patients with MI, the coronary arteries are normal. Severe cases of BD look more prone to AMI (acute myocardial infarction), and it was also demonstrated that occlusion of coronary arteries usually developed because of thrombus formation in CAD (coronary artery disease) leading to AMI.

Intracardiac thrombus that often precedes other manifestations of BD has been reported. These thrombi are found mainly in the right ventricle and are often associated with pulmonary artery aneurysm. Endomyocardial fibrosis plays a role in the intracardiac thrombus development in some patients. Due to high specificity of the right heart thrombus in BD, in any patient with this finding, diagnosis of BD should be considered. Intracardiac thrombus is the major differential diagnosis when a young patient presents with an intracardiac mass. It is especially common in young adult BD patients from the Middle East or the Mediterranean basin.

The right and left ventricular function may also be subtly impaired in patients with BD. There is a relationship between the duration of BD and cardiac involvement. As the duration of BD lengthens, the development of left ventricular diastolic dysfunction increases [115, 116].

Interatrial septal aneurysm, atrial septal defect, mitral valve prolapse, and mitral failure are also seen, albeit rarely [113]. It was reported that valvular prolapse including mitral valve prolapse can be related to vasculitis and tissue derangement [112].

Most of the aneurysms of the sinus of Valsalva observed in BD have been seen in the right coronary sinus, which may protrude into the right atrium or ventricle [112]. Most unfortunately this pathology is discovered after rupture. A few cases of the sinus of Valsalva aneurysm, which usually developed in the active phase of BD, have been reported. Heart failure may occur because of the ruptured aneurysm necessitating urgent surgical intervention [112].

Conduction abnormalities that could directly be ascribed to BD and those that could not be ascribed directly to BD were reported in the past [112].

Aortic valve involvement occurs late in the course of the disease as in the case of arterial lesions. They usually occur 3.2–7.9 years after diagnosis [107]. Aortitis by itself or seen with valvulitis in BD is very rare and frequently causes clinically important aortic regurgitation leading eventually to hemodynamic decompensation for which surgical treatment is generally needed. Surgical treatment is demanding because of the presence of inflamed, fragile aortic tissue. The most dangerous complications seen postoperatively are prosthetic valve detachment, bypass graft occlusion, and pseudoaneurysm development leading to more morbid and sometimes mortal second operations. A high rate of prosthetic valve detachment rate of 40% and a low rate of 5-year freedom from reoperation (64%) in patients with BD were reported [117]. In a study, the reoperation rate was 7.4% per patient-year, and the mortality rate was 3.7% per patient-year [118].

Radiographic evidence of ascending aortic dilatation has been reported in 48% of BD patients in a series [99]. Other cross-sectional studies have reported various prevalences of thoracic aortic aneurysm: 5% in a Turkish cohort and 5.4% in a French cohort of BD patients in similar-sized BD cohorts [119, 120]. In a longitudinal study, eight patients diagnosed with thoracic aortic aneurysm were followed up for a median of 7.6 years. During this follow-up period, three deaths occurred, and the cause of death was recorded as due to thoracic aortic aneurysm [120]. However, despite many advances over recent years in imaging techniques for thoracic aortic aneurysm, international recommendations, such as those currently provided by the European League Against Rheumatism (EULAR), do not provide any guidance about screening and monitoring thoracic aortic aneurysm [121]. Aortic root inflammation can cause mural thickening, dilatation, valvulitis, and aortic valve insufficiency in a variety of infectious and noninfectious aortitides. Specific echocardiographic findings have been described as redundant aortic valve cusps with prolapse, vegetation-like masses, and echolucencies with Behçet's valvulitis [122].

As early as 1997, Morelli et al. reported mitral valve prolapse which was observed in 50% and proximal aorta dilatation in 30% of their patients. There was a significant difference in the rate of these abnormalities in comparison to their control group. The positivity rate of antinuclear and anticardiolipin autoantibodies was found to be very low (7%), with no difference between the study and control groups. HLA-B51 was detected in 82.7% of the patients in comparison to 21.7% in the control group ($p < 0.00001$). As a result, this study showed a high rate of cardiac abnormalities in patients with BD [123].

4.5. Diagnosis

Because BD lacks proper, clear-cut pathognomonic clinical and especially laboratory findings, the diagnosis may be difficult to reach. Also, it is important to bear in mind the fact that autoinflammatory diseases such as BD are heterogeneous diseases showing heterogeneous symptoms and clinical courses. Diagnosis is, therefore, clinically made [101]. Cardiac BD affects males more than females and is prone to delayed diagnosis because some patients do not have typical clinical manifestations at cardiac onset [124].

Cardiac valve involvement is a rare entity in BD, but when it occurs, it presents as a critical problem that necessitates urgent and correct diagnosis and treatment. Echocardiography is very useful for the necessary timely diagnosis. Diagnosis of FDG-PET scans may have a clinical value as a workup study for patients with BD who have cardiovascular presentations [125].

The right and left ventricular function is impaired in patients with BD. Novel methods such as tissue Doppler echocardiography (TDE) or Doppler-derived myocardial performance index (MPI) allow more objective estimation of cardiac functions [126].

4.6. Treatment

Treatment of BD is still unfortunately based on the low level of evidence (experts' opinion) [127]. Treatment of Behçet's disease is symptomatic and empirical but remains unsatisfactory because of variable, heterogeneous manifestations with uncertain etiology and pathogenesis. In addition, clinical disease manifestations and mortality appear to vary by ethnic group [128].

4.6.1. Medical treatment

Corticosteroids, cyclophosphamide, methotrexate, azathioprine, cyclosporine, and colchicine provide remissions of variable remissions in most patients. Experience with the use of anti-TNF agents in BD has advanced in recent years. Colchicine is shown to be effective in cases of pericarditis.

Corticosteroids plus immunosuppressants reduce the thrombus formation and improve aortic regurgitation and heart failure in cardiac BD, whereas surgery alone does not lead to complete resolution of thrombus [129].

In cases of ICT, the current therapy is built according to the severity of the disease and the location of the lesion. Since BD usually has an ever-changing fiery and silent-phase variations, it is generally difficult to monitor the effectivity of treatment. Like in other serious vasculitides, the mainstay of treatment in BD is immunosuppressive therapy.

Standard anticoagulation with heparin or oral anticoagulants is not recommended in all BD cases. However, anticoagulation with immunosuppression is the recommended treatment in BD cases with ICT. Aneurysms may reduce in size or may even disappear with medical treatment (combination of cyclophosphamide and methylprednisolone) [127].

It was reported that recurrent right atrial thrombus due to BD is commonly observed despite continued anticoagulation therapy. It is important to know that thrombus disappears after the initiation of immunosuppressive therapy [129]. Medical treatment with immunosuppressants may be the first choice for patients with BD who have ICT [111]. To avoid a progression to thrombus or cardiac dysfunction in recurrent cases, the early identification of cardiac involvement of BD using echocardiography and/or cardiac magnetic resonance imaging is of great importance. Combined immunosuppressive therapy with prednisolone and cyclophosphamide are usually needed to treat recurrent thrombosis due to BD [111, 129].

4.6.2. Surgical and endovascular treatment

There is surprisingly limited evidence of quality in planning a consistent treatment strategy for cardiovascular involvement of BS, especially in the potential role for surgery [130].

In patients with BD, aortitis or other cardiovascular complications should be evaluated carefully in those with chest discomfort. Steroid administration is important, especially preoperatively, which not only decreases inflammatory reactions but also reduces the postoperative steroid dosage and diminishes the associated side effects.

Coronary arterial disease is generally treated with either conservative or invasive procedures and by surgery when indicated. Less invasive therapies are the first choice because many perioperative complications may await the patient. Graft failure due to thrombosis and development of aneurysms at anastomotic sites are such complications. Moreover, complications such as disseminated venous thrombosis leading to pleural effusion, Budd-Chiari syndrome, and central nervous system involvement following coronary artery bypass grafting (CABG) surgery treated with anticoagulant and anti-inflammatory therapy have been reported [131].

In the course of CABG, the use of arterial grafts and avoidance of aortic manipulation, in order to decrease the risk of pseudoaneurysmal formation, are strongly recommended [132]. The use of free arterial grafts is advised because of the risk of possible left subclavian arterial occlusion after CABG which may cause a devastating MI [133].

Behçet's disease involves all types of vessels, but coronary arterial involvement is extremely rare. The patients are generally young, and they are frequently treated medically. CABG is performed with care on these patients, and off-pump techniques are generally preferred. Surgical treatment of Behçet patients is itself challenging because the tissues are fragile and the coronary arteries are inflamed [132]. Therefore, some surgeons prefer not to perform CABG because the tissues are fragile, the grafts are affected by inflammation, and hypercoagulopathy may be a problem perioperatively [134]. Others recommend percutaneous interventions (PCI) or minimally invasive procedures such as off-pump no-touch aorta techniques [135].

Major problems after CABG surgery are also bleeding and anastomotic pseudoaneurysm. Minimal manipulation of the tissues, meticulous hemostasis, and concomitant use of corticosteroids and immunosuppressants are important to circumvent these devastating complications [131, 132, 134].

Hematoma and/or pseudoaneurysm, especially of the femoral artery after coronary angiography, may be encountered. Multiple punctures must be avoided, and catheters should be removed as early as the patient's condition allows to prevent such complications [134].

Advances in noninvasive imaging modalities such as CT coronary angiography increased our noninvasive capability of evaluating coronary artery disease. When control imaging like angiography is needed, this ever-developing cost-effective method should be utilized [136].

There are no comprehensive studies on the long-term patency of the grafts used for coronary bypass because the grafts may be affected by the disease. Therefore, patients must be informed about possible reoperations and reinterventions.

Surgery alone in treating ICT leads to recurrences. ICT has risk of recurrence [129]. Combined immunosuppressive therapy with steroids (prednisolone) and cyclophosphamide is needed to treat ICT and prevent recurrences. Immunosuppressive therapy reduces ICT relapse [137]. EULAR does not recommend anticoagulants in the treatment of thrombosis [121]. Unfortunately, as of now, there are no controlled studies or evidence of benefit from experience with anticoagulants, antiplatelet, or antifibrinolytics in vascular BD [129].

Rates of prosthetic valve detachment in BD of the aortic valve are significantly higher than in other valvular diseases such as rheumatic valve disease. Performing prosthetic aortic valve replacements for a Behçet-related valvulopathy carries an increased risk of dehiscence if no preoperative immunosuppression is administered; on the other hand, total aortic root replacement may allow more durable results.

The surgical implications and management of Behçet's aortitis with associated severe aortic insufficiency remain a serious challenge, because the aortic tissue involved not only is inflamed but also may be irrevocably fragile. The postoperative period may be affected by complications that may be both costly and life-threatening. Reoccurrence and reoperation rates in BS are high contributing to higher morbidity and mortality. Modified surgical techniques like valved conduit procedures and perioperative and postoperative continuous immunosuppression are advised.

There is a high recurrence rate of complications in PAA stemming from inadequate medical therapy and the inherent disadvantages of surgical treatment. This fact makes PAA candidates for endovascular management. Successful treatment of PAA with endovascular embolization using n-butyl cyanoacrylate (NBCA) has been reported [138–140].

Percutaneous NBCA embolization of PAAs is also reported as a safe and effective front-line treatment in BD patients presenting with life-threatening massive hemoptysis [139].

Emergency surgery after the diagnosis of PAA has a high potential of complications like perivascular leaks, graft thrombosis, and anastomotic leaks due to the very nature of PAA. Anastomotic leaks causing recurrence of hemoptysis have also been reported. Surgical treatment may have the disadvantage of the potential need for repeated thoracotomy because of recurrence of aneurysm. Postoperative healing has been shown to be compromised because of long-term corticosteroid usage. The risk of infection is high. PAAs commonly occur bilaterally. Increased pulmonary artery pressure after lobectomy on one hemithorax may cause increased size of other PAAs with eventual rupture and mortality. Due to these setbacks and the possible high mortality rate associated with surgical treatment, endovascular treatment looks like a reliable alternative instead of surgery when life-threatening hemoptysis and a narrow window of opportunity to save patients' lives are present [139]. PAA patients treated by embolization with or without immunosuppressive therapy were reported to have a better prognosis than patients who underwent surgery with or without immunosuppressive therapy [139].

Delaying surgery in cases with active-phase inflammation and initiating immunosuppressive therapy before and after surgery is recommended when the patients' lives are not immediately threatened. Moreover, because of high reoperation and mortality rates, long-term follow-up is mandatory after surgery.

4.7. Prognosis

BD significantly increases mortality especially in young male patients, while it is less severe among females and the aged with regard to cardiac and vascular involvement. In many patients, the disease tends to abate with the passage of time. The main cause of mortality is large-vessel disease, especially bleeding PAA, almost exclusively among male patients [84]. BD is a chronic inflammatory disease which shows exacerbations and remissions. Especially, young male patients have severe prognoses. With advancing age remission periods lengthen and the severity of exacerbations decrease. A five-year survival rate of BD was 95.8% without cardiac complications. But this rate drops to 83.6% if cardiac BD is present [113]. Annual BD mortality varies between 2 and 4% [3]. Prognosis of coronary artery involvement is poor. MI accounted for 25% of deaths in a cohort published in 2012 [113].

Poor prognostic factors in BD include vascular and cardiac involvement per se, male gender, and early age of onset. Involvement of the aortic valve is also a bad prognostic factor with a given 44% mortality rate in a study [141].

Follow-up is also problematic. In a study conducted in Korea about long-term mortality after treatment for aortic involvement revealed 47% mortality of which none occurred at the operating room but all in the postoperative period. Also, in this study event-free survival at 13 years in patients who were administered immunosuppressive therapies versus no immunosuppression was 34% to zero (0%), respectively, underlining the importance of continuation of immunosuppressive therapy perioperatively. It was also reported that aortic root replacement in comparison to solitary aortic valve replacement had much better prognosis, namely, 39% versus 4%, respectively [142].

4.8. Suggestions and future

In young male patients with intracavitary thrombus, BD must come to mind as a probable diagnosis.

Arterial, venous, and pulmonary involvements are generally more frequently seen in BD patients in whom ICT occurs in comparison to the general BD population As DVT has been documented in almost half of the BD patients with ICT, we recommend that all BD patients with ICT should be examined for venous disease using duplex ultrasonography. Because pulmonary involvement (PAA and PTE) and ICT are oftentimes encountered concomitantly, we suggest that pulmonary involvement should be investigated by thoracic CT in all BD patients with ICT.

In patients with BD who are in the active inflammatory stage of the disease, periodic echocardiography examination for early detection of an aneurysm or valvular involvement should be made even if there are no symptoms. We recommend for all BD patients a systematic echocardiographic examination not only when clinically indicated but also routinely once every year [130].

The prevalence of SMI is high in patients with BD. Therefore, myocardial perfusion scintigraphy should be recommended for patients with duration of BD greater than 10 years.

Physicians caring for BD patients, internists, rheumatologists, and dermatologists should work closely with cardiologists and cardiovascular surgeons to increase awareness of these silent and potentially fatal vascular complications and form multidisciplinary groups to address this problem not only for individual cases as they arise but also in order to generate the future evidence bases to more successfully manage BD and its cardiovascular complications in the future.

5. Behçet's disease and vascular involvement in the pediatric age group

BD occasionally involves children before the age of 16 in 4–26% of BD cases [143]. Large-vessel vasculitis is the leading cause of vascular mortality seen in the pediatric age group. In children with vascular involvement, male patients are predominantly affected with a ratio of 6 to 1.

BD manifests itself differently in children. Ocular disease is usually absent, and establishment of diagnosis is usually late. The diagnosis of BD is difficult to establish in itself, and because of the insidious onset in children it is more subtle and challenging [144]. Because of this difficulty, several new pediatric BD classifications were proposed [145].

In a study conducted in children, vascular involvement was observed in 25% of the children affected by BD, and all of them had venous thrombi [146]. Half of these were cerebral thrombi and the other half was peripheral thrombi. These rates were also found in similar percentages in another study conducted in children [147]. The main locations of thrombosis were the cerebral sinuses in 11 patients (52.4%) and lower limbs in 9 patients (40.9%)

Although very rare, Budd-Chiari syndrome and rupture of pulmonary artery aneurysms have all been reported in children [144].

In a comprehensive study comprising four countries, the mortality rate in pediatric BD (3%) was generally related to large-vessel involvement [148]. In this study, 18 episodes of venous thrombosis were observed in 10 (15%) patients: 7 boys and 3 girls. They occurred six times in the lower extremities (both legs in two cases). It was reported that one patient experienced eight episodes of IVC thrombosis and died eventually of multiple deep vein thromboses. Arterial involvement including arterial aneurysms (four) and arterial thrombosis (five) occurred in six patients (four boys, two girls). Pulmonary arteries were the most frequently attacked (three), causing life-threatening hemoptyses. Geographic differences among patients with vascular complications were reported as not statistically significant [148].

In a study conducted on vascular BD patients in the pediatric age group, out of seven patients two had superficial vein thrombosis, two patients exhibited atrial or ventricular thrombosis, and one showed arterial involvement with PAA. Two of the patients had thrombosis of the venous sinuses in the central nervous system. The average apperance of vascular involvement was reported 4 months after the diagnosis of BD. All of these patients were administered with colchicine and steroids. The ones with thrombosis in the venous system received additional azathioprine, whereas those with pulmonary arterial or cardiac involvement initially received cyclophosphamide and then were changed to azathioprine for 6 more months. All patients other than the PAA patient were administered with a course of anticoagulation treatment as well. These patients were then followed up for at least 18 months and were free of vascular relapses as of reporting [149].

The abovementioned study had some recommendations for both physicians and families. They suggested that pediatricians should follow and monitor their patients with BD for arterial and venous vascular disease. All families should be informed about the possible characteristics and appearances of peripheral venous involvement, signs of sinus thrombi, and be warned and informed about chest pain. When pertinent symptoms arise, urgent medical care and diagnostic techniques should be used. They reported that effective management and the judicious use of immunosuppressives are successful in disease control and recommended avoidance of biological agents [149].

6. Behçet's disease and vascular involvement in pregnancy

6.1. Introduction

Because BD occurs more prevalently during fertile years and is multisystemic in its involvements, disease activity in pregnancy and its obstetric and neonatal outcomes deserve special attention.

BD is often diagnosed in women in the childbearing age [150]. The rate of de novo occurrence of BD in pregnancy is rare [151]. BD presents itself with similar symptoms observed in nonpregnant patients. Patients with BD do not have a higher rate of vascular complications during pregnancy. Similarly, the obstetric complication rate is not increased.

6.2. Clinical course

Symptoms are inclined to improve in pregnancy, and most patients have a symptom-free pregnancy. Remission of disease activity is seen in a minority of pregnant BD patients [152]. Because of this reason, vascular complications are very rare in pregnant patients with BD.

Regression of disease activity during pregnancy is attributed to the inhibition of T cell, macrophage, and natural killer cell activity [153]. Interleukin 10 (IL-10) levels have been found elevated during pregnancy, but those levels were decreased at the end of pregnancy. The anti-inflammatory properties of IL-10 may have reduced the occurrence of BD exacerbations during the obstetric period, but decreased levels of IL-10 may explain some of the symptoms occurring in the postpartum period [154]. Estrogen also has anti-inflammatory actions like suppression of IL12 production and suppression of antigen-presenting capacity and stimulation of anti-inflammatory IL-10 production [155].

6.2.1. The neonatal outcome

The neonatal outcome is debatable. In a study presented in 2014, a series of 298 pregnancies of which 94 had BD were compared with 95 healthy controls, and it was reported that BD patients delivered smaller babies and miscarriages were more numerous in the BD group that could be attributed to vasculitis of the placenta [156]. However, in a study conducted in Turkey, among 342 deliveries 41 deliveries occurred in patients with BD. The rates of stillbirth, preeclampsia, preterm delivery, and intrauterine growth retardation did not differ in pregnant patients with BD. Perinatal mortality, neonatal intensive care unit admissions, and low birth weight incidences were similar to those without BD [152].

6.2.2. *Vascular complications*

The overall incidence of vascular complications in pregnant patients with BD was 5%, which was significantly higher than the normal pregnant patients [152]. Various types of thrombotic attacks have been reported during pregnancy and in the postpartum period. The postpartum period may be complicated by thromboses refractory to anticoagulation.

It was reported that complications during pregnancy in Behçet patients who had prior vascular involvement were higher in comparison to the normal population [154]. The annual rate of BD flare was threefold lower during pregnancy. The rate of obstetric complications was 16% and was increased in BD patients with a history of venous thrombosis [154]. In a study the presence of venous involvement increased the odds of obstetric complications by sevenfold [157]. All of such patients in a French cohort who had venous BD exacerbations had experienced prior DVT, and two had associated cerebral venous thrombosis [154].

The risk of fetal loss in BD is, however, lower than the risk of fetal loss observed in antiphospholipid syndrome [158].

Most BD flares during pregnancy are mucocutaneous or ocular in character [159]. Vascular involvement usually includes the venous system similar to the nonpregnant population. Heart failure due to tricuspid regurgitation and related right ventricular dysfunction resulting from ventricular endomyocardial fibrosis has been reported [151]. BD exacerbation developed in 29.7% of the pregnancies in a series [154]. This rate ranges from 8% to 60% in the literature [150, 160]. In the above-mentioned series, the main symptoms during BD activity were oral ulceration (58.3% [range 50–66.7%]) and genital ulceration (44.4% [range 25–55.6%]), followed by skin lesions (25% [range 8.3–33.3%]) and ocular inflammation (5.6% [0–25%]) [150, 160].

Vascular manifestations were reported in two series: one patient experienced Budd-Chiari syndrome, and one patient had DVT [150, 157]. Apart from these series, some case reports have been published and described exceptionally severe disease exacerbations such as DVT with nephrotic syndrome, SVC thrombosis, dural sinus thrombosis, or intracardiac thrombosis [161–164].

6.3. Treatment

Surgical thrombectomy has been used for DVT [12]. Thrombolytic therapy is effective for DVT and intracardiac thrombus and may be safer and more effective than surgery [164]. Thrombolysis and stent placement are viable options in SVC thrombosis [165].

Medical treatments, especially acetylsalicylic acid and low-molecular heparin, are safe in pregnancy and are widely used. The use of colchicine is reported to reduce the risk of severe BD exacerbations, because the proportion of disease exacerbations was twofold lower in BD patients treated with colchicine [154]. Because colchicine crosses the human placenta, the safety of colchicine treatment in pregnant BD patients is an important point. Although colchicine has antimitotic effects, the safety of this drug during pregnancy was recently assessed in a prospective comparative cohort study in which 238 colchicine-exposed pregnancies were followed up [166]. No increase in teratogenicity or congenital abnormalities was observed. Therefore, colchicine treatment is safe in pregnant women with BD and could even reduce the risk of disease exacerbations. Other medications such as azathioprine, glucocorticoids, and biological agents like infliximab can also be used during pregnancy, apparently without an increased risk of complications [167].

7. Conclusion

Since the first description by Hulusi Behçet in 1937, BD has been one of the most thoroughly researched diseases. But the enigma continues. The mechanisms of vascular involvement are still very obscure. Cardiac Behçet, since continuous perioperative immunosuppression administration became the rule, and thrombolysis became available, began to have fair results after intervention or surgery. Moreover, in the last two decades, vascular manifestation of BD has at least begun to be amenable to vascular and endovascular surgery increasing hopes for better quality of life for BD patients.

Author details

Orhan Saim Demirtürk*, Hüseyin Ali Tünel and Utku Alemdaroğlu

*Address all correspondence to: osdemirturk@yahoo.com

Department of Cardiovascular Surgery, Başkent University, Adana Dr. Turgut Noyan Medical Center, Adana,, Turkey

References

[1] Owlia MB, Mostafavi Pour Manshadi SM, Naderi N. Cardiac manifestations of rheumatological conditions: A narrative review. ISRN Rheumatology. 2012;**2012**:463620. DOI: 10.5402/2012/463620

[2] Cocco G, Gasparyan AY. Behçet's disease: An insight from a cardiologist's point of view. Open Cardiovascular Medicine Journal. 2010 Feb 23;**4**:63–70. DOI: 10.2174/1874192401004020063

[3] Demirelli S, Degirmenci H, Inci S, Arisoy A. Cardiac manifestations in Behcet's disease. Intractable & Rare Diseases Research. 2015 May;**4**(2):70–75. DOI: 10.5582/irdr.2015.01007. Review

[4] Azizlerli G, Köse AA, Sarica R, Gül A, Tutkun IT, Kulaç M, Tunç R, Urgancioğlu M, Dişçi R. Prevalence of Behçet's disease in Istanbul, Turkey. International Journal of Dermatology. 2003 Oct;**42**(10):803–806

[5] The International Criteria for Behçet's Disease (ICBD): A collaborative study of 27 countries on the sensitivity and specificity of the new criteria. International Team for the Revision of the International Criteria for Behçet's Disease (ITR-ICBD). Journal of the European Academy of Dermatology and Venereology. 2014 Mar;**28**(3):338–347. DOI: 10.1111/jdv.12107. Epub 2013 Feb 26

[6] International Study Group for Behçet's Disease. Criteria for diagnosis of Behçet's disease. International Study Group for Behçet's Disease. Lancet. 1990;**335**(8697):1078–1080. DOI: 10.1016/0140-6736(90)92643-V

[7] Yurdakul S, Günaydin I, Tüzün Y, Tankurt N, Pazarli H, Ozyazgan Y, Yazici H. The prevalence of Behçet's syndrome in a rural area in northern Turkey. Journal of Rheumatology. 1988;**15**(5):820–822

[8] Cakir N, Dervis E, Benian O, Pamuk ON, Sonmezates N, Rahimoglu R, Tuna S, Cetin T, Sarikaya Y. Prevalence of Behçet's disease in rural western Turkey: A preliminary report. Clinical and Experimental Rheumatology. 2004 Jul-Aug;**22**(4 Suppl 34):S53-S55

[9] Yurdakul S, Yazıcı Y. Epidemiology of Behçet's syndrome and regional differences in disease expression. In: Yazıcı Y, Yazıcı H, editors. Behçet's Syndrome. 1st ed. New York: Springer; 2010. pp. 35–52

[10] Shimizu T, Ehrlich GE, Inaba G, Hayashi K. Behçet disease (Behçet syndrome). Seminars in Arthritis and Rheumatism. 1979 May;**8**(4):223–260

[11] Rabinovich E, Shinar Y, Leiba M, Ehrenfeld M, Langevitz P, Livneh A. Common FMF alleles may predispose to development of Behcet's disease with increased risk for venous thrombosis. Scandinavian Journal of Rheumatology. 2007 Jan-Feb;**36**(1):48–52

[12] Kural-Seyahi E, Fresko I, Seyahi N, Ozyazgan Y, Mat C, Hamuryudan V, Yurdakul S, Yazici H. Medicine (Baltimore). 2003 Jan;**82**(1):60–76

[13] Gül A, Ozbek U, Oztürk C, Inanç M, Koniçe M, Ozçelik T. Coagulation factor V gene mutation increases the risk of venous thrombosis in behçet's disease. British Journal of Rheumatology. 1996 Nov;**35**(11):1178–1180

[14] Yurdakul S, Tüzüner N, Yurdakul I, Hamuryudan V, Yazici H. Gastrointestinal involvement in Behçet's syndrome: A controlled study. Annals of the Rheumatic Diseases. 1996;**55**(3):208–210

[15] Lenk N, Ozet G, Alli N, Coban O, Erbasi S. Protein C and protein S activities in Behcet's disease as risk factors of thrombosis. International Journal of Dermatology. 1998;**37**:124–125

[16] La Regina M, Gasparyan AY, Orlandini F, Prisco D. Behcet's disease as a model of venous thrombosis. Open Cardiovascular Medicine Journal. 2010;**4**:71–77

[17] Taşçılar K, Melikoğlu M. Venous involvement in Behçet's syndrome. Turkiye Klinikleri Journal of Cardiovascular Surgery Special Topics. 2011;**3**(29):11–17

[18] Nalçaci M, Pekçelen Y. Antithrombin III, protein C and protein S plasma levels in patients with Behçet's disease. Journal of International Medical Research. 1998 Aug-Sep;**26**(4):206–208

[19] Mader R, Ziv M, Adawi M, Mader R, Lavi I. Thrombophilic factors and their relation to thromboembolic and other clinical manifestations in Behçet's disease. Journal of Rheumatology. 1999 Nov;**26**(11):2404–2408

[20] Kahn SR. How I treat postthrombotic syndrome. Blood. 2009 Nov 19;**114**(21):4624–4631. DOI: 10.1182/blood-2009-07-199174. Review

[21] Roumen-Klappe EM, Janssen MC, Van Rossum J, Holewijn S, Van Bokhoven MM, Kaasjager K, Wollersheim H, Den Heijer M. Inflammation in deep vein thrombosis and the development of post-thrombotic syndrome: A prospective study. Journal of Thrombosis and Haemostasis. 2009 Apr;**7**(4):582–587. DOI: 10.1111/j.1538-7836.2009.03286.x

[22] Gedikoglu M, Oguzkurt L. Endovascular treatment of iliofemoral deep vein thrombosis in pregnancy using US-guided percutaneous aspiration thrombectomy. Diagnostic and Interventional Radiology. 2017 Jan-Feb;**23**(1):71–76. DOI: 10.5152/dir.2016.16199

[23] Demirtürk OS, Oğuzkurt L, Coşkun I, Gülcan Ö. Endovascular treatment and the long-term results of postpartum deep vein thrombosis in 18 patients. Diagnostic and Interventional Radiology. 2012 Nov-Dec;**18**(6):587–593. DOI: 10.4261/1305-3825.DIR.5808-12.1. Epub 2012 Sep 27

[24] Srinivas BC, Patra S, Nagesh CM, Reddy B, Manjunath CN. Catheter-directed thrombolysis in management of postpartum lower limb deep venous thrombosis—A case series. Indian Heart Journal. 2015 Dec;**67** Suppl 3:S67-S70. DOI: 10.1016/j.ihj.2015.08.002. Epub 2016 Jan 15

[25] Bayraktar Y, Balkanci F, Bayraktar M, Calguneri M. Budd-Chiari syndrome: A common complication of Behçet's disease. American Journal of Gastroenterology. 1997 May;**92**(5):858–862

[26] Tokay S, Direskeneli H,Yurdakul S,Akoglu T. Anticardiolipin antibodies in Behçet's disease: A reassessment. Rheumatology (Oxford). 2001 Feb;**40**(2):192–195

[27] Leiba M, Seligsohn U, Sidi Y, Harats D, Sela BA, Griffin JH, Livneh A, Rosenberg N, Gelernter I, Gur H, Ehrenfeld M. Thrombophilic factors are not the leading cause of thrombosis in Behcet's disease. Annals of the Rheumatic Diseases. 2004;**63**:1445–1449

[28] Er H, Evereklioglu C, Cumurcu T, Türköz Y, Ozerol E, Sahin K, Doganay S. Serum homocysteine level is increased and correlated with endothelin-1 and nitric oxide in Behçet's disease. British Journal of Ophthalmology. 2002 Jun;**86**(6):653–657

[29] Aguiar de Sousa D, Mestre T, Ferro JM. Cerebral venous thrombosis in Behçet's disease: A systematic review. Journal of Neurology. 2011 May;**258**(5):719–727. DOI: 10.1007/s00415-010-5885-9. Epub 2011 Jan 6

[30] Yesilot N, Bahar S, Yilmazer S, Mutlu M, Kurtuncu M, Tuncay R, Coban O, Akman-Demir G. Cerebral venous thrombosis in Behçet's disease compared to those associated

with other etiologies. Journal of Neurology. 2009 Jul;**256**(7):1134–1142. DOI: 10.1007/s00415-009-5088-4

[31] Wechsler B, Vidailhet M, Piette JC, Bousser MG, Dell Isola B, Blétry O, Godeau P. Cerebral venous thrombosis in Behçet's disease: Clinical study and long-term follow-up of 25 cases. Neurology. 1992 Mar;**42**(3 Pt 1):614–618

[32] Ahn JK, Lee YS, Jeon CH, Kho EM, Cha HS. Treatment of venous thrombosis associated with Behcet's disease: Immunosuppressive therapy alone versus immunosuppressive therapy plus anticoagulation. Clinical Rheumatology. 2008;**27**:201–205

[33] Emmi G, Silvestri E, Squatrito D, Amedei A, Niccolai E, D'Elios MM, Della Bella C, Grassi A, Becatti M, Fiorillo C, Emmi L, Vaglio A, Prisco D. Thrombosis in vasculitis: From pathogenesis to treatment. Thrombosis Journal. 2015 Apr 16;**13**:15. DOI: 10.1186/s12959-015-0047-z

[34] Gul A, Ozbek U, Ozturk C, Inanc M, Konice M, Ozcelik T. Coagulation factor V gene mutation increases the risk of venous thrombosis in Behcet's disease. British Journal of Rheumatology. 1996;**35**:1178–1180

[35] Ates A, Duzgun N, Ulu A, Tiryaki AO, Akar N. Factor V gene (1691A and 4070G) and prothrombin gene 20210A mutations in patients with Behcet's disease. Pathophysiology of Haemostasis and Thrombosis. 2003;**33**:157–163

[36] Silingardi M, Salvarani C, Boiardi L, Accardo P, Iorio A, Olivieri I, Cantini F, Salvi F, La Corte R, Triolo G, Ciccia F, Ghirarduzzi A, Filippini D, Paolazzi G, Iori I. Factor V Leiden and prothrombin gene G20210A mutations in Italian patients with Behcet's disease and deep vein thrombosis. Arthritis and Rheumatism. 2004;**51**:177–183

[37] Ricart JM, Vaya A, Todoli J, Calvo J, Villa P, Estelles A, Espana F, Santaolaria M, Corella D, Aznar J. Thrombophilic risk factors and homocysteine levels in Behcet's disease in eastern Spain and their association with thrombotic events. Thrombosis and Haemostasis. 2006;**95**:618–624

[38] Evereklioglu C. Current concepts in the etiology and treatment of Behcet disease. Survey of Ophthalmology. 2005;**50**:297–350

[39] Tunaci M, Ozkorkmaz B, Tunaci A, Gül A, Engin G, Acunaş B. CT findings of pulmonary artery aneurysms during treatment for Behçet's disease. AJR Am J Roentgenol 1999;**172**(3): 729–33

[40] Yazici H, Pazarli H, Barnes CG, Tüzün Y, Ozyazgan Y, Silman A, Serdaroğlu S, Oğuz V, Yurdakul S, Lovatt GE, Yazici B, Soman Si, Müftüoğlu A. A controlled trial of azathioprine in Behçet's syndrome. New England Journal of Medicine. 1990 Feb 1;**322**(5):281–285

[41] Mazzoccoli G, Matarangolo A, Rubino R, Inglese M, De Cata A. Behçet syndrome: From pathogenesis to novel therapies. Clinical and Experimental Medicine. 2016 Feb;**16**(1):1–12. DOI: 10.1007/s10238-014-0328-z

[42] Saadoun D, Wechsler B. Behçet's disease. Orphanet Journal of Rare Diseases. 2012 Apr 12;**7**:20. DOI: 10.1186/1750-1172-7-20. Review

[43] O'Neill TW, Rigby AS, Silman AJ, Barnes C. Validation of the International Study Group criteria for Behcet's disease. British Journal of Rheumatology. 1994;**33**(2):115–117

[44] Calamia KT, Wilson FC, Icen M, Crowson CS, Gabriel SE, Kremers HM. Epidemiology and clinical characteristics of Behçet's disease in the US: A population-based study. Arthritis and Rheumatism. 2009;**61**(5):600-604. DOI: 10.1002/art.24423

[45] Uzun O, Akpolat T, Erkan L. Pulmonary vasculitis in behcet disease: A cumulative analysis. Chest. 2005;**127**(6):2243–2253. DOI: 10.1378/chest.127.6.2243

[46] Park JH, Han MC, Bettmann MA. Arterial manifestations of Behcet disease. American Journal of Roentgenology. 1984;**143**(4):821–825. DOI: 10.2214/ajr.143.4.821

[47] Kwon TW, Park SJ, Kim HK, Yoon HK, Kim GE, Yu B. Surgical treatment result of abdominal aortic aneurysm in Behçet's disease. European Journal of Vascular and Endovascular Surgery. 2008 Feb;**35**(2):173–180. DOI: 10.1016/j.ejvs.2007.08.013. Epub 2007 Oct 26

[48] Gül A. Pathogenesis of Behçet's disease: Autoinflammatory features and beyond. Seminars in Immunopathology. 2015 Jul;**37**(4):413–418. DOI: 10.1007/s00281-015-0502-8. Epub 2015 Jun 12

[49] Melikoglu M, Kural-Seyahi E, Tascilar K, Yazici H. The unique features of vasculitis in Behçet's syndrome. Clinical Reviews in Allergy and Immunology. 2008;**35**(1-2):40–46. DOI: 10.1007/s12016-007-8064-8

[50] Maldini C, Lavalley MP, Cheminant M, de Menthon M, Mahr A. Relationships of HLA-B51 or B5 genotype with Behcet's disease clinical characteristics: Systematic review and meta-analyses of observational studies. Rheumatology (Oxford). 2012;**51**(5):887–900. DOI: 10.1093/rheumatology/ker428

[51] Gül A, Uyar FA, Inanc M, Ocal L, Tugal-Tutkun I, Aral O, Koniçe M, Saruhan-Direskeneli G. Lack of association of HLA-B*51 with a severe disease course in Behçet's disease. Rheumatology (Oxford). 2001 Jun;**40**(6):668–672

[52] Gul A. Behcet's disease: An update on the pathogenesis. Clinical and Experimental Rheumatology. 2001;**19**(s24):S6-s12

[53] Alavi A, Sajic D, Cerci FB, Ghazarian D, Rosenbach M, Jorizzo J. Neutrophilic dermatoses: An update. American Journal of Clinical Dermatology. 2014;**15**(5):413–423. DOI: 10.1007/s40257-014-0092-6

[54] Evereklioglu C, Turkoz Y, Er H, Inaloz HS, Ozbek E, Cekmen M. Increased nitric oxide production in patients with Behçet's disease: Is it a new activity marker? Journal of the American Academy of Dermatology. 2002;**46**(1):50–54

[55] Akar S, Ozcan MA, Ateş H, et al. Circulated activated platelets and increased platelet reactivity in patients with Behçet's disease. Clinical and Applied Thrombosis/Hemostasis. 2006;**12**(4):451–457. DOI: 10.1177/1076029606293430

[56] Yurdakul S, Hekim N, Soysal T, et al. Fibrinolytic activity and d-dimer levels in Behçet's syndrome. Clinical and Experimental Rheumatology. 2005;**23**(4 Suppl 38):S53-S58

[57] Al-Basheer M, Hadadin F. Aneurysm formation type of vasculo-Behcet's disease. Heart, Lung and Circulation. 2007 Dec ;**16**(6):407–409. DOI: 10.1016/j.hlc.2007.04.010. Epub 2007 Jun 18

[58] Behçet H, Matteson EL On relapsing, aphthous ulcers of the mouth, eye and genitalia caused by a virus. 1937. Clinical and Experimental Rheumatology. 2010 Jul-Aug;**28**(4 Suppl 60):S2-S5. Epub 2010 Sep 23

[59] Dinç A. Vascular involvement and its treatment in Behçet's disease. Turkiye Klinikleri Journal of Dermatology Special Topics. 2011;**4**(4):66–72. [Original article in Turkish -Behçet Hastalığında Vasküler Tutulum ve Tedavisi. Türkiye Klin Dermatoloji Özel Derg. 2011;4(4):66–72.]

[60] Calamia KT, Schirmer M, Melikoglu M. Major vessel involvement in Behçet disease. Current Opinion in Rheumatology. 2005;**17**(1):1–8. DOI: 10.1097/01.bor.0000145520.76348.dd

[61] Wu XY, Wei JP, Zhao XY, Wang Y, Wu HH, Shi T, Liu T, Liu G. Spontaneous intra-abdominal hemorrhage due to rupture of jejunal artery aneurysm in behcet disease: Case report and literature review. Medicine (Baltimore). 2015 Nov;**94**(45):e1979. DOI: 10.1097/MD.0000000000001979

[62] Tüzün DH, Arslan DC. Aneurysms in Behçet's syndrome and their treatment Turkiye Klinikleri Journal of Cardiovascular Surgery Special Topics. 2011;**3**(2):23–26. [Original article in TurkishTürkiye Klin Kalp Damar Cerrahisi Özel Derg. 2011;3(2):23–26.]

[63] Tüzün H, Beşirli K, Sayin A, et al. Management of aneurysms in Behçet's syndrome: An analysis of 24 patients. Surgery. 1997;**121**(2):150–156

[64] Sasaki S, Yasuda K, Takigami K, Shiiya N, Matsui Y, Sakuma M. Surgical experiences with peripheral arterial aneurysms due to vasculo-Behçet's disease. The Journal of Cardiovascular Surgery. 1998;**39**(2):147–150

[65] Kim WH, Choi D, Kim JS, Ko YC, Jang Y, Shim WH. Effectiveness and safety of endovascular aneurysm treatment in patients with vasculo-Behçet disease. Journal of Endovascular Therapy. 2009 Oct;**16**(5):631–636. DOI: 10.1583/09-2812.1

[66] Ohshima T, Miyachi S, Hattori K-I, et al. A case of giant common carotid artery aneurysm associated with vascular Behçet disease: Successfully treated with a covered stent. Surgical Neurology. 2008 Mar;**69**(3):297–301. DOI: 10.1016/j.surneu.2006.12.063. Review

[67] Liu Q, Ye W, Liu C, Li Y, Zeng R, Ni L. Vascular outcomes of vascular intervention and use of perioperative medications for nonpulmonary aneurysms in Behçet disease. Surgery. 2016 May;**159**(5):1422–1429. DOI: 10.1016/j.surg.2015.11.022. Epub 2016 Jan 5

[68] Hamuryudan DV. Pulmonary arterial involvement in Behçet's disease Turkiye Klinikleri Journal of Cardiovascular Surgery Special Topics. 2011;**3**(2):18–22. [Original article in

Turkish Hamuryudan DV Behçet Hastalığında Pulmoner Arter Tutulumu. Türkiye Klin Kalp Damar Cerrahisi Özel Derg. 2011;3(2):18–22]

[69] Kaieda S, Zaizen Y, Nomura Y, Okabe K, Honda S, Kage M, Ida H, Hoshino T, Fukuda T. An autopsy case of refractory vasculo-Behçet's disease. Modern Rheumatology. 2015 Mar;**25**(2):307–311. DOI: 10.3109/14397595.2013.874755. Epub 2014 Feb 18

[70] Hamuryudan V, Er T, Seyahi E, et al. Pulmonary artery aneurysms in Behçetsyndrome. American Journal of Medicine. 2004;**117**(11):867–870. DOI: 10.1016/j.amjmed.2004.05.027

[71] Vivante A, Bujanover Y, Jacobson J, Padeh S, Berkun Y. Intracardiac thrombus and pulmonary aneurysms in an adolescent with Behçet disease. Rheumatology International. 2009;**29**(5):575–577. DOI:10.1007/s00296-008-0730-5

[72] Hamuryudan V, Oz B, Tüzün H, Yazici H. The menacing pulmonary artery aneurysms of Behçet's syndrome. Clinical and Experimental Rheumatology. 2004 Jul-Aug;**22**(4 Suppl 34):S1-S3

[73] Jayachandran NV, Rajasekhar L, Chandrasekhara PKS, Kanchinadham S, Narsimulu G. Multiple peripheral arterial and aortic aneurysms in Behcet's syndrome: A case report. Clinical Rheumatology. 2008;**27**(2):265–267. DOI: 10.1007/s10067-007-0713-z

[74] Iscan ZH, Vural KM, Bayazit M. Compelling nature of arterial manifestations in Behcet disease. Journal of Vascular Surgery. 2005 Jan;**41**(1):53–58. DOI: 10.1016/j.jvs.2004.09.018

[75] Sarica-Kucukoglu R, Akdag-Kose A, KayabalI M, et al. Vascular involvement in Behcet's disease: A retrospective analysis of 2319 cases. International Journal of Dermatology. 2006;**45**:919–921

[76] Kasirajan K. Commentary: Endovascular aneurysm treatment in patients with vasculo-Behçet disease. Journal of Endovascular Therapy. 2009;**16**(5):637. DOI: 10.1583/09-2812C.1

[77] Denecke T, Staeck O, Amthauer H, Hänninen EL. PET/CT visualises inflammatory activity of pulmonary artery aneurysms in Behçet disease. European Journal of Nuclear Medicine and Molecular Imaging. 2007;**34**(6):970. DOI: 10.1007/s00259-007-0429-y

[78] Li S, Chen A-J, Huang K, Li H. Successful treatment of vasculo-Behcet's disease presenting as recurrent pseudoaneurysms: The importance of medical treatment. Dermatology and Therapy. 2013;**3**(1):107–112. DOI: 10.1007/s13555-013-0024-z

[79] Mercan S, Sarigül A, Koramaz I, Demirtürk O, Böke E. Pseudoaneurysm formation in surgically treated Behçet's syndrome—A case report. Angiology. 2000;**51**(4):349–353; discussion 354. http://www.ncbi.nlm.nih.gov/pubmed/10779007

[80] Kim H-K, Choi HH, Huh S. Ruptured iliac artery stump aneurysm combined with aortic pseudoaneurysm in a patient with Behçet's disease. Annals of Vascular Surgery. 2010;**24**(2):255.e5–255.e8. DOI: 10.1016/j.avsg.2009.07.012

[81] Goz M, Cakir O, Eren MN. Huge popliteal arterial aneurysms in Behçet's syndrome: Is ligation an alternative treatment? Vascular. 2007 Jan-Feb;**15**(1):46–48

[82] Aroussi AA, Redai M, Ouardi F El, Mehadji B-E, Casablanca M. Bilateral pulmonary artery aneurysm in Behçet syndrome: Report of two operative cases. Journal of Thoracic and Cardiovascular Surgery. 2005 May;**129**(5):1170–1171. DOI: 10.1016/j.jtcvs.2004.08.038

[83] Nitecki SS, Ofer A, Karram T, Schwartz H, Engel A, Hoffman A. Abdominal aortic aneurysm in Behçet's disease: New treatment options for an old and challenging problem. The Israel Medical Association Journal. 2004 Mar;**6**(3):152–155

[84] Yazici H, Esen F. Mortality in Behçet's syndrome. Clinical and Experimental Rheumatology. 2008;**26**(5 Suppl 51):S138-S140

[85] Saadoun D, Wechsler B, Desseaux K, et al. Mortality in Behçet's disease. Arthritis and Rheumatism. 2010;**62**(9):2806–2812. DOI: 10.1002/art.27568

[86] Kutay V, Yakut C, Ekim H. Rupture of the abdominal aorta in a 13-year-old girl secondary to Behçet disease: A case report. Journal of Vascular Surgery. 2004;**39**:901–902

[87] Kalko Y, Basaran M, Aydin U, Kafa U, Basaranoglu G, Yasar T. The surgical treatment of arterial aneurysms in Behçet disease: A report of 16 patients. Journal of Vascular Surgery. 2005 Oct;**42**(4):673–677

[88] Sato T, Matsumoto H, Kimura N, Okamura H, Adachi K, Yuri K, Yamaguchi A, Yamada S, Adachi H. Urgent surgical management of deep femoral artery aneurysm in a patient with pre-vasculo-behcet status. Annals of Vascular Diseases. 2015;**8**(2):116–119. DOI: 10.3400/avd.cr.15-00017. Epub 2015 May 26

[89] Maeda H, Umezawa H, Goshima M, Hattori T, Nakamura T, Negishi N, Oinuma T, Sugitani M, Nemoto N. An impending rupture of a celiac artery aneurysm in a patient with Behçet's disease—Extra-anatomic aorto-common hepatic artery bypass: Report of a case. Surgery Today. 2008;**38**(2):163–165. DOI: 10.1007/s00595-007-3584-7

[90] Koksoy C, Gyedu A, Alacayir I, Bengisun U, Uncu H, Anadol E. Surgical treatment of peripheral aneurysms in patients with Behcet's disease. European Journal of Vascular and Endovascular Surgery. 2011 Oct;**42**(4):525–530. DOI: 10.1016/j.ejvs.2011.05.010

[91] Lee SW , Lee SY , Kim KN , Jung JK , Chung WT . Adalimumab treatment for life threatening pulmonary artery aneurysm in Behcet disease: A case report . Clinical Rheumatology. 2010;**29**:91–93

[92] Yoshida S, Takeuchi T , Yoshikawa A , Ozaki T , Fujiki Y , Hata K, et al . Good response to infliximab in a patient with deep vein thrombosis associated with Behcet disease . Modern Rheumatology. 2012;**22**:791–795

[93] Baki K , Villiger PM , Jenni D , Meyer T , Beer JH . Behcet's disease with life-threatening haemoptoe and pulmonary aneurysms: Complete remission after infliximab treatment. Annals of the Rheumatic Diseases. 2006;**65**:1531–1532

[94] Rokutanda R, Okada M, Yamaguchi K, Nozaki T, Deshpande GA, Kishimoto M. Infliximab for Behcet disease with aortic involvement: Two novel case reports without concurrent use of immunosuppressive agents or corticosteroids. Modern Rheumatology. 2013;**23**:412–413

[95] Seyahi E, Hamuryudan V, Hatemi G , Melikoglu M, Celik S, Fresko I, et al. Infliximab in the treatment of hepatic vein thrombosis (Budd-Chiari syndrome) in three patients with Behcet's syndrome. Rheumatology. 2007;**46**:1213–1214

[96] Puli SR, Benage DD. Retinal vein thrombosis after infliximab (Remicade) treatment for Crohn's disease. Am J Gastroenterol 2003;98(4):939-40.

[97] Zehir R, Karabay CY, Aykan AÇ, Özkan M. The role of two-dimensional speckle-tracking echocardiography in a patient with Behçet's disease. Anadolu Kardiyoloji Dergisi. 2013 Feb;**13**(1):74–76. DOI: 10.5152/akd.2013.012. Epub 2012 Nov 15

[98] Veilleux SP, O'Connor K, Couture C, Pagé S, Voisine P, Poirier P, Dubois M, Sénéchal M. What the cardiologist should know about cardiac involvement in Behçet disease. Canadian Journal of Cardiology. 2015 Dec;**31**(12):1485–1488. DOI: 10.1016/j.cjca.2015.04.030. Epub 2015 May 9

[99] Gürgün C, Ercan E, Ceyhan C, Yavuzgil O, Zoghi M, Aksu K, Cinar CS, Türkoglu C. Cardiovascular involvement in Behçet's disease. Japanese Heart Journal. 2002 Jul;**43**(4):389–398

[100] Dogan SM, Birdane A, Korkmaz C, Ata N, Timuralp B. Right ventricular thrombus with Behçet's syndrome: Successful treatment with warfarin and immunosuppressive agents. Texas Heart Institute Journal. 2007;**34**(3):360–362

[101] Davatchi F, Shahram F, Chams-Davatchi C, Shams H, Nadji A, Akhlaghi M, Faezi T, Ghodsi Z, Faridar A, Ashofteh F, Sadeghi Abdollahi B. Behcet's disease: From East to West. Clinical Rheumatology. 2010 Aug;**29**(8):823–833. DOI: 10.1007/s10067-010-1430-6. Review

[102] Haznedaroglu IC, Ozcebe OI, Dündar SV. Behçet's disease. New England Journal of Medicine. 2000 Feb 24;**342**(8):588; author reply 588–9

[103] Aksu T, Tufekcioglu O. Intracardiac thrombus in Behçet's disease: Four new cases and a comprehensive literature review. Rheumatology International. 2015 Jul;**35**(7):1269–1279. DOI: 10.1007/s00296-014-3174-0. Review

[104] Koşar A, Oztürk M, Haznedaroğlu IC, Karaaslan Y. Hemostatic parameters in Behçet's disease: A reappraisal. Rheumatology International. 2002 May;**22**(1):9–15

[105] Kiraz S, Ertenli I, Oztürk MA, Haznedaroğlu IC, Celik I, Calgüneri M. Pathological haemostasis and "prothrombotic state" in Behçet's disease. Thrombosis Research. 2002 Jan 15;**105**(2):125–133. Review

[106] Wang H, Guo X, Tian Z, Liu Y, Wang Q, Li M, Zeng X, Fang Q. Intracardiac thrombus in patients with Behcet's disease: Clinical correlates, imaging features, and outcome: A retrospective, single-center experience. Clinical Rheumatology. 2016 Oct;**35**(10):2501–2507. DOI: 10.1007/s10067-015-3161-1. Epub 2016 Jan 11

[107] Lee I, Park S, Hwang I, Kim MJ, Nah SS, Yoo B, Song JK. Cardiac Behçet disease presenting as aortic valvulitis/aortitis or right heart inflammatory mass: A clinicopathologic

study of 12 cases. American Journal of Surgical Pathology. 2008 Mar;**32**(3):390–398. DOI: 10.1097/PAS.0b013e31814b23da

[108] Tai YT, Fong PC, Ng WF, Fu KH, Chow WH, Lau CP, Wong WS. Diffuse aortitis complicating Behçet's disease leading to severe aortic regurgitation. Cardiology. 1991;**79**(2):156–160

[109] Ugurlu S, Seyahi E, Yazici H. Prevalence of angina, myocardial infarction and intermittent claudication assessed by Rose Questionnaire among patients with Behcet's syndrome. Rheumatology (Oxford). 2008 Apr;**47**(4):472–475. DOI: 10.1093/rheumatology/kem385

[110] Díez-Delhoyo F, Sanz-Ruiz R, Casado-Plasencia A, Rivera-Juárez A, Gutiérrez-Ibañes E, Sarnago-Cebada F, Vázquez-Álvarez ME, Clavero-Olmos M, Elízaga J, Fernández-Avilés F. Not just thrombi occlude coronary arteries in Behçet's disease: A case of spontaneous coronary artery dissection. International Journal of Cardiology. 2016 Jul 1;**214**:317–319. DOI: 10.1016/j.ijcard.2016.03.208

[111] Merashli M, Ster IC, Ames PR. Subclinical atherosclerosis in Behcet's disease: A systematic review and meta-analysis. Seminars in Arthritis and Rheumatism. 2016 Feb;**45**(4):502–510. DOI: 10.1016/j.semarthrit.2015.06.018. Epub 2015 Jul 4

[112] Owlia MB, Mehrpoor G. Behcet's disease: New concepts in cardiovascular ınvolvements and future direction for treatment. ISRN Pharmacology. 2012;**2012**:760484. DOI: 10.5402/2012/760484

[113] Geri G, Wechsler B, Thi Huong duL, IsnardR, PietteJC, AmouraZ, Resche-RigonM, CacoubP, SaadounD. Spectrum of cardiac lesions in Behçet disease: A series of 52 patients and review of the literature. Medicine (Baltimore). 2012 Jan;**91**(1):25–34. DOI: 10.1097/MD.0b013e3182428f49. Review

[114] Türkölmez Ş, Gökçora N, Alkan M, Gürer MA. Evaluation of myocardial perfusion in patients with Behçet's disease. Annals of Nuclear Medicine. 2005;**19**(3):201–206

[115] Komsuoglu B, Göldeli O, Kulan K, Komsuoglu SS, Tosun M, Kaya C, Tuncer C. Doppler evaluation of left ventricular diastolic filling in Behçet's disease.International Journal of Cardiology. 1994 Dec;**47**(2):145–150

[116] Gemici K, Baran I, Güllülü S, Kazazoglu AR, Cordan J, Ozer Z. Evaluation of diastolic dysfunction and repolarization dispersion in Behcet's disease. International Journal of Cardiology. 2000 Apr 28;**73**(2):143–148

[117] Ando M, Kosakai Y, Okita Y, Nakano K, Kitamura S. Surgical treatment of Behçet's disease involving aortic regurgitation. Annals of Thoracic Surgery. 1999 Dec;**68**(6):2136–2140

[118] Okada K, Eishi K, Takamoto S, Ando M, Kosakai Y, Nakano K, Sasako Y, Kobayashi J. Surgical management of Behçet's aortitis: A report of eight patients.Annals of Thoracic Surgery. 1997 Jul;**64**(1):116–119

[119] Ozkan M, Emel O, Ozdemir M, Yurdakul S, Koçak H, Ozdoğan H, Hamuryudan V, Dirican A, Yazici H. M-mode, 2-D and Doppler echocardiographic study in 65 patients with Behçet's syndrome. European Heart Journal. 1992 May;**13**(5):638–641

[120] Saadoun D, Asli B, Wechsler B, Houman H, Geri G, Desseaux K, Piette JC, Huong du LT, Amoura Z, Salem TB, Cluzel P, Koskas F, Resche-Rigon M, Cacoub P. Long-term outcome of arterial lesions in Behçet disease: A series of 101 patients. Medicine (Baltimore). 2012 Jan;**91**(1):18–24. DOI: 10.1097/MD.0b013e3182428126

[121] Hatemi G, Silman A, Bang D, Bodaghi B, Chamberlain AM, Gul A, Houman MH, Kötter I, Olivieri I, Salvarani C, Sfikakis PP, Siva A, Stanford MR, Stübiger N, Yurdakul S, Yazici H. EULAR Expert Committee. EULAR recommendations for the management of Behçet disease. Annals of the Rheumatic Diseases. 2008 Dec;**67**(12):1656–1662. DOI: 10.1136/ard.2007.080432

[122] Katabathina VS, Restrepo CS. Infectious and noninfectious aortitis: Cross-sectional imaging findings. Seminars in Ultrasound, CT and MR. 2012 Jun;**33**(3):207–221. DOI: 10.1053/j.sult.2011.12.001. Review

[123] Morelli S, Perrone C, Ferrante L, Sgreccia A, Priori R, Voci P, Accorinti M, Pivetti-Pezzi P, Valesini G. Cardiac involvement in Behçet's disease. Cardiology. 1997 Nov-Dec;**88**(6):513–517

[124] Zhu YL, Wu QJ, Guo LL, Fang LG, Yan XW, Zhang FC, Zhang X. The clinical characteristics and outcome of intracardiac thrombus and aortic valvular involvement in Behçet's disease: An analysis of 20 cases. Clinical and Experimental Rheumatology. 2012 May-Jun;**30**(3 Suppl 72):S40-S45

[125] Cho SB, Yun M, Lee JH, Kim J, Shim WH, Bang D. Detection of cardiovascular system involvement in Behçet's disease using fluorodeoxyglucose positron emission tomography. Seminars in Arthritis and Rheumatism. 2011 Apr;**40**(5):461–466. DOI: 10.1016/j.semarthrit.2010.05.006

[126] Aksu T, Güler E, Arat N, Zorlu A, Yılmaz B, Güray Ü, Tüfekçioğlu O, Kısacık H. Cardiovascular involvement in Behçet's Disease. Archives of Rheumatology. 2015;**30**(2):109–115. DOI: 10.5606/ArchRheomatol.2015.5019

[127] Hatemi G, Seyahi E, Fresko I, Talarico R, Hamuryudan V. One year in review 2016: Behçet's syndrome. Clinical and Experimental Rheumatology. 2016 Sep-Oct;**34**(6 Suppl 102):10–22. Review

[128] Savey L, Resche-Rigon M, Wechsler B et al. Ethnicity and association with disease manifestations and mortality in Behçet's disease. Orphanet Journal of Rare Diseases. 2014;**9**:42

[129] Ben Ghorbel I, Belfeki N, Houman MH. Intracardiac thrombus in Behçet's disease. Reumatismo. 2016 Dec 16;**68**(3):148–153. DOI: 10.4081/reumatismo.2016.887

[130] Fok M, Bashir M, Goodson N, Oo A, Moots R. Thoracic aortic aneurysms in Behçet's disease. Rheumatology (Oxford). 2016 May 13. DOI: 10.1093/rheumatology/kew226

[131] Ilhan G, Bozok S, Uguz E, Karamustafa H, Karakisi SO, Sener E. Management of extensive venous thrombosis following cardiac surgery in a patient with Behcet's disease. VASA. 2012 Jul;**41**(4):301–305. DOI: 10.1024/0301-1526/a000208

[132] Bardakci H, Kervan U, Boysan E, Birincioglu L, Cobanoglu A. Aortic arch aneurysm, pseudocoarctation, and coronary artery disease in a patient with Behçet's syndrome. Texas Heart Institute Journal. 2007;**34**(3):363–365

[133] Cingoz F, Bingol H, Ozal E, Tatar H. Coronary subclavian steal syndrome in a patient with Behçet's disease. Thoracic and Cardiovascular Surgeon. 2010 Jun;**58**(4):244–346. DOI: 10.1055/s-2006-924699. Epub 2010 May 31

[134] 139.Tasar M, Eyileten Z, Arici B, Uysalel A. Coronary artery bypass grafting in a Behçet's disease patient. Cardiovascular Journal of Africa. 2014 Sep 23;**25**(5):e13-e14. DOI: 10.5830/CVJA-2014–052

[135] Kobayashi A, Sakata R, Kinjo T, Yotsumoto G, Matsumoto K, Iguro Y. Off-pump coronary artery bypass grafting in a patient with Behçet's disease. The Japanese Journal of Thoracic and Cardiovascular Surgery. 2004 Nov;**52**(11):527–529

[136] Rajakulasingam R, Omran M, Costopoulos C. Giant aneurysm of the left anterior descending artery in Behçet's disease. International Journal of Rheumatic Diseases. 2013 Dec;**16**(6):768–770. DOI: 10.1111/1756-185X.12051

[137] Desbois AC, Wechsler B, Resche-Rigon M, Piette JC, Huong Dle T, Amoura Z, Koskas F, Desseaux K, Cacoub P, Saadoun D. Immunosuppressants reduce venous thrombosis relapse in Behçet's disease. Arthritis and Rheumatism. 2012 Aug;**64**(8):2753–2760. DOI: 10.1002/art.34450

[138] Cantasdemir M, Kantarci F, Mihmanli I, Akman C, Numan F, Islak C, Bozkurt AK. Emergency endovascular management of pulmonary artery aneurysms in Behçet's disease: Report of two cases and a review of the literature. Cardiovascular and Interventional Radiology. 2002 Nov-Dec;**25**(6):533–537. Epub 2002 Jun 4

[139] Ianniello A, Carrafiello G, Nicotera P, Vaghi A, Cazzulani A. Endovascular treatment of a ruptured pulmonary artery aneurysm in a patient with Behçet's disease using the Amplatzer Vascular Plug 4. Korean Journal of Radiology. 2013 Mar-Apr;**14**(2):283–286. DOI: 10.3348/kjr.2013.14.2.283. Epub 2013 Feb 22

[140] Cil BE, Geyik S, Akmangit I, Cekirge S, Besbas N, Balkanci F. Embolization of a giant pulmonary artery aneurysm from Behcet disease with use of cyanoacrylate and the "bubble technique".Journal of Vascular and Interventional Radiology. 2005 Nov;**16**(11):1545–1549

[141] Lee CW, Lee J, Lee WK, Lee CH, Suh CH, Song CH. Aortic valve involvement in Behçet's disease. A clinical study of 9 patients. Korean Journal of Internal Medicine. 2002;**17**(1):51–56

[142] Jeong DS, Kim KH, Kim JS, Ahn H. Long-term experience of surgical treatment for aortic regurgitation attributable to Behçet's disease. Annals of Thoracic Surgery. 2009 Jun;**87**(6):1775–1782. DOI: 10.1016/j.athoracsurg.2009.03.008

[143] Koné-Paut I. Behçet's disease in children, an overview. Pediatric Rheumatology Online Journal. 2016 Feb 18;**14**(1):10. DOI: 10.1186/s12969-016-0070-z. Review

[144] Lang BA, Laxer RM, Thorner P, Greenberg M, Silverman ED. Pediatric onset of Behçet's syndrome with myositis: Case report and literature review illustrating unusual features. Arthritis and Rheumatism. 1990 Mar;**33**(3):418–425. Review

[145] Koné-Paut I, Shahram F, Darce-Bello M, Cantarini L, Cimaz R, Gattorno M, Anton J, Hofer M, Chkirate B, Bouayed K, Tugal-Tutkun I, Kuemmerle-Deschner J, Agostini H, Federici S, Arnoux A, Piedvache C, Ozen S; PEDBD group. Consensus classification criteria for paediatric Behçet's disease from a prospective observational cohort: PEDBD. Annals of the Rheumatic Diseases. 2016 Jun;**75**(6):958–964. DOI: 10.1136/annrheumdis-2015–208491

[146] Allali F, Benomar A, Karim A, Lazrak N, Mohcine Z, El Yahyaoui M, Chkili T, Hajjaj-Hassouni N. Behçet's disease in Moroccan children: A report of 12 cases. Scandinavian Journal of Rheumatology. 2004;**33**(5):362–363

[147] Krupa B, Cimaz R, Ozen S, Fischbach M, Cochat P, Koné-Paut I. Pediatric Behcet's disease and thromboses. Journal of Rheumatology. 2011 Feb;**38**(2):387–390. DOI: 10.3899/jrheum.100257. Epub 2010 Nov 15

[148] Koné-Paut I, Yurdakul S, Bahabri SA, Shafae N, Ozen S, Ozdogan H, Bernard JL. Clinical features of Behçet's disease in children: An international collaborative study of 86 cases. Journal of Pediatrics. 1998 Apr;**132**(4):721–725

[149] Ozen S, Bilginer Y, Besbas N, Ayaz NA, Bakkaloglu A. Behçet disease: Treatment of vascular involvement in children. European Journal of Pediatrics. 2010 Apr;**169**(4):427–430. DOI: 10.1007/s00431-009-1040-y

[150] Marsal S, Falga C, Simeon CP, Vilardell M, Bosch JA. Behçet's disease and pregnancy relationship study. British Journal of Rheumatology. 1997;**36**:234–238

[151] Mirfeizi Z, Memar B, Pourzand H, Molseghi MH, Shahmirzadi AR, Abdolahi N. Ventricular endomyocardial fibrosis in a pregnant female with Behçet's disease. Asian Cardiovascular & Thoracic Annals. 2017 Jan 1;**2017**:218492316687177. DOI: 10.1177/0218492316687177. [Epub ahead of print]

[152] İskender C, Yaşar Ö, Kaymak O, Yaman ST, Uygur D, Danışman N. Behçet's disease and pregnancy: A retrospective analysis of course of disease and pregnancy outcome. Journal of Obstetrics and Gynaecology. 2014;**40**(69):1598–1602

[153] McKay LI, Cidlowski JA. Molecular control of immune/inflammatory responses: Interactions between nuclear factor-kappa B and steroid receptor-signaling pathways. Endocrine Reviews. 1999 Aug;**20**(4):435–459. Review

[154] 159.Noel N, Wechsler B, Nizard J, Costedoat-Chalumeau N, Boutin du LT, Dommerques M, Vauthier-Brouzes D, Cacoub P, Saadoun D. Behçet's disease and pregnancy relationship study. Arthritis and Rheumatism. 2013;**65**:2450–2456

[155] Kanda N, Watanabe S. Regulatory roles of sex hormones in cutaneous biology and immunology. Journal of Dermatological Science. 2005;**38**:1–7

[156] Gungor AN, Kalkan G, Oguz S, Sen B, Ozoguz P, Takci Z, Sacar H, Dogan FB, Cicek D. Behçet disease and pregnancy. Clinical and Experimental Obstetrics & Gynecology. 2014;**41**(6):617–619

[157] Jadaon J, Shushan A, Ezra Y, Sela HY, Ozcan C, Rojansky N. Behçet's disease and pregnancy. Acta Obstetricia et Gynecologica Scandinavica. 2005;**84**:939–944

[158] Wilson WA, Gharavi AE, Koike T, Lockshin MD, Branch DW, Piette JC, et al. International consensus statement on preliminary classification criteria for definite antiphospholipid syndrome: Report of an international workshop. Arthritis and Rheumatism. 1999;**42**:1309–1311

[159] Xu C, Bao S. Behcet's disease and pregnancy-a case report and literature review. Am Reprod Immunol 2017;77(1).doi: 10.1111/aji.12530 Epub 2016 Jun 14.

[160] Bang D, Chun YS, Haam IB, Lee ES, Lee S. The influence of pregnancy on Behçet's disease. Yonsei Medical Journal. 1997;**38**:437–443

[161] Komaba H, Takeda Y, Fukagawa M. Extensive deep vein thrombosis in a postpartum woman with Behcçet's disease associated with nephrotic syndrome. Kidney International. 2007;**71**:6

[162] Kale A, Akyildiz L, Akdeniz N, Kale E. Pregnancy complicated by superior vena cava thrombosis and pulmonary embolism in a patient with Behcçet disease and the use of heparin for treatment. Saudi Medical Journal. 2006;**27**:95–97

[163] Wechsler B, Genereau T, Biousse V, Vauthier-Brouzes D, Seebacher J, Dormont D, et al. Pregnancy complicated by cerebral venous thrombosis in Behcçet's disease. American Journal of Obstetrics and Gynecology. 1995;**173**:1627–1629

[164] Hiwarkar P, Stasi R, Sutherland G, Shannon M. Deep vein and intracardiac thrombosis during the post-partum period in Behçet's disease. International Journal of Hematology. 2010;**91**:679–686

[165] Castelli P, Caronno R, Piffaretti G, Tozzi M, Lomazzi C, Laganà D, Carrafiello G, Cuffari S. Endovascular treatment for superior vena cava obstruction in Behçet disease. Journal of Vascular Surgery. 2005 Mar;**41**(3):548–551

[166] Diav-Citrin O, Shechtman S, Schwartz V, Avgil-Tsadok M, Finkel Pekarsky V, Wajnberg R, et al. Pregnancy outcome after in utero exposure to colchicine. American Journal of Obstetrics and Gynecology. 2010;**203**:144.e1–144.e6

[167] Mainini G, Di Donna MC, Esposito E, Ercolano S, Correa R, Stradella L, Della Gala A, De Franciscis P. Pregnancy management in Behçet's disease treated with uninterrupted infliximab. Report of a case with fetal growth restriction and mini-review of the literature. Clinical and Experimental Obstetrics and Gynecology. 2014;**41**(2):205–207. Review

Chapter 10

Surgical Treatment of Angio-Behçet

Genadi Georgiev Genadiev, Lorenzo Mortola,
Roberta Arzedi, Giuseppe Deiana,
Francesco Spanu and Stefano Camparini

Additional information is available at the end of the chapter

http://dx.doi.org/10.5772/intechopen.68664

Abstract

Patients with Behçet's disease are at risk for multiple vessel-related complications including thromboses, stenoses, occlusions, and aneurysms. Surgical treatment of Angio-Behçet brings numerous challenges due to the peculiarities of the disease process and the high rate of complications. Recurrent vascular episodes are also quite common and Behçet patients require rigorous follow-up. In this review, we focus on the manifestations of Behçet's disease involving the venous system and the systemic arterial vasculitis focusing on the indications, workup, and techniques for surgical treatment. Several case studies from our own experience are presented together with supporting diagnostic imaging and the decision process whether to intervene is discussed. Although open surgery remains a valid option, new endovascular techniques are rapidly advancing and offer excellent results with important decrease in morbidity and mortality even in highly compromised patients.

Keywords: vascular, arterial, venous, EVAR, TEVAR, aneurysm, thrombosis

1. Introduction

Patients with Behçet's disease (BD) are at risk for multiple vessel-related complications including thromboses, stenoses, occlusions, and aneurysms. Venous involvement is predominant in comparison with arterial involvement (4:1) [1]. Recurrent vascular episodes are quite common with incidence of up to 23% after 2 years and up to 40% at 5 years [2]. Calamia et al. have proposed a classification of the vascular lesions of the great vessels [3] (**Table 1**).

Vascular arterial manifestations of Behçet's disease are observed in 7–29% of patients affected from this disease and arterial lesions represent 15% of all vascular lesions in BD [4, 5]. Arterial

Systemic arterial vasculitis
Aneurysms
Stenoses/occlusions
Pulmonary arterial vasculitis
Aneurysms
Stenoses/occlusions
Venous occlusions
Superficial venous thrombosis
Deep venous thrombosis
Cerebral venous thrombosis
Budd-Chiari syndrome
Portal vein thrombosis
Right ventricular thrombosis
Pulmonary emboli
Varices

Table 1. Classification of the vascular lesions of the great vessels.

lesions pose a greater risk and are associated with a large impact on the prognosis due to the severity of complications [6]. Most common arterial lesions observed in BD are occlusions/stenosis and aneurysms/pseudoaneurysms. Though theoretically any arterial vessel can be affected by these lesions, most commonly affected segments are, in order of frequency, abdominal aorta, pulmonary, femoral, popliteal, and carotid arteries [7]. Clinical presentation varies and can include acute or chronic limb ischemia, aneurysmal thromboses or rupture, and stroke [4]. Rupture is the most frequent complication of aneurysms and the most common cause of vascular-related death in BD [8]. Arterial involvement can be recurrent and is often associated with venous involvement; aneurysms can develop at various sites simultaneously and may be associated to occlusive lesions even in the same patient [9, 10]. Pulmonary arterial lesions are most frequently associated to venous thrombosis [11].

Surgical treatment of arterial manifestations of BD bears many pitfalls, since the obliterative endarteritis of vasa vasorum causes thickening of the medial layer and splitting of elastin fibers. Therefore, anastomotic pseudoaneurysms are likely to form, as well as pseudoaneurysms at the site of puncture in case of angiography or endovascular treatment; furthermore, early graft occlusion may occur [4, 8, 12].

For these reasons, invasive treatment should not be performed in the acute and active phases of the disease when inflammation is at its peak. The evaluation of disease's activity is usually based on relapsing symptoms, ESR (erythrocyte sedimentation rate), and serum levels of CRP (C-reactive protein) [13, 14].

Endovascular treatment can be an effective and safe alternative to open surgery, with less postoperative complications, faster recovery time, and reduced need for intensive care, while offering patency rates and procedural success rates comparable with those of surgery [15, 16]. This notwithstanding, long-term results of endovascular treatment in BD are still to be determined.

2. Venous involvement

Superficial vein thrombosis (SVT) has been found by some to be the dominant lesion (up to 53% of the patients), whereas others have found deep vein thrombosis (DVT) to be more prevalent (up to 80%) although still highly correlating with SVT [16–18]. Duplex ultrasound (DUS) is the diagnostic modality of choice allowing for differentiation between a recent (hypoecoic) and old (hyperecoic in the context of wall thickening) thrombus. Treatment is mainly medical, although there is considerable debate as to the use of anticoagulants, antiplatelet, or fibrinolytic agents. The European League Against Rheumatism (EULAR) does not recommend their use as the thrombus usually adheres firmly to the vessel wall and does not result in emboli which would explain the low incidence of pulmonary embolism [19].

Superior vena cava thrombosis can be observed in about 2.5% of the cases and can also be secondary to axillary or subclavian vein thrombosis [3]. Superior vena cava syndrome, which results from complete or partial obstruction of venous return from the upper body, can be asymptomatic or can present with dyspnea, facial swelling, head fullness, cough, arm swelling, chest pain, dysphagia, and pleural effusions. Obstruction of venous flow can also be a result of lumen reduction due to thickening of the vessel wall without evidence of thrombosis. The preferred diagnostic modality is chest computed tomography (CT). Magnetic resonance imaging (MRI) has increased sensitivity in establishing the thrombus extension particularly toward the heart.

Case 1 (**Figure 1**)*: A 20-year-old male patient with BD presents with ill-defined abdominal pain. A CT scan is performed showing a partial filling defect in the suprahepatic portion of the inferior vena cava, just distal to the right atrium. The hepatic veins were patent and venous flow through the partially*

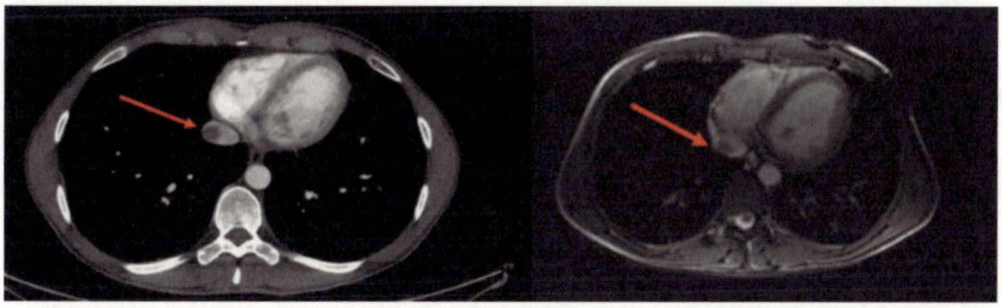

Figure 1. CT scan and Gd-DPTA MRI scan in a 20-year-old male BD patient showing inferior vena cava thrombosis in its supradiaphragmatic segment.

obstructed IVC was maintained. The patient was treated with oral anticoagulation therapy for 6 months, undergoes frequent follow-up visits, and is currently asymptomatic.

Inferior vena cava thrombosis can be found in up to a third of the patients with BD [3, 17]. Budd-Chiari syndrome is a complication resulting from the thrombosis of the retrohepatic portion of the IVC. DUS can be useful in the diagnosis and CT and MRI can help further define asymmetry in hepatic perfusion [20].

Portal vein thrombosis is another common finding in Behçet's syndrome occurring in approximately 9.2% of the patients and rapidly giving way to cavernous transformation characterized by numerous collaterals at the hepatic hilum and around the thrombosed portal branches [3, 21, 22]. Portal vein thromboses could present as ascites, splenomegaly, hepatomegaly, and hepatic infarction. Mesenteric ischemic involvement can also lead to infectious portal vein thromboses and liver abscesses.

Surgical treatment in venous thrombosis is limited to portocaval shunting in Budd-Chiari syndrome. Transjugular intrahepatic portocaval shunt (TIPS) can be performed if the vena cava is patent. Thrombolytic therapy can be considered in the acute phase involving the vena cava or portal vein with direct infusion of urokinase or tissue plasminogen activator (tPA) [23].

2.1. Abdominal aortic aneurysm

An abdominal aortic aneurysm (AAA) is defined as an abdominal aortic diameter of 3.0 cm or more in either anterior-posterior or transverse planes [24]. A pseudoaneurysm is defined as a tear through the layers of the arterial wall resulting in hematoma formation outside the vessel, circumscribed by periarterial tissue, with a persistent communication between the artery and the newly formed cavity.

While in atherosclerotic disease the indication to the treatment of AAA is dependent on the aneurysmal size because of the direct relationship between this parameter and the risk of rupture, in BD aneurysms should be repaired as soon as possible because of high rupture risk due to the underlying aortitis [13, 25]. Most frequently, the aneurysm is located below the emergency of renal arteries, but every segment of the aorta can be affected, and the shape is usually saccular [13].

AAAs are usually asymptomatic and may go unnoticed until symptoms develop in the late stages of the disease, such as compression of nearby structures, back pain, erosion of vertebral bodies, and hydronephrosis. At physical examination, a mesogastric pulsatile swelling can be observed.

The most dangerous complication of AAAs is rupture, defined as bleeding outside the adventitia of a dilated aortic wall, rapidly leading to death of the patient if a repair is not performed quickly. Rupture can occur in retroperitoneal cavity, with peritoneal tissue providing tamponade and thus reducing the volume of blood loss. Symptoms of ruptured AAA include abdominal acute pain and abdominal swelling, femoral arteries pulselessness and acute lower limbs ischemia, embolic events, and signs of hemorrhagic shock [16, 26].

http://dx.doi.org/10.5772/intechopen.68664

2.2. Imaging

Diagnosis can be confirmed by DUS, which is noninvasive, is cheap, and has high sensitivity and specificity for the detection of AAAs. Ultrasound is limited in the definition of infra- and suprarenal borders of the aneurysm, presence of periaortic disease, and of evaluation of iliac arteries aneurysms. Angiography is not usually recommended as routine imaging modality for AAAs. Additionally, patients affected from BD are more prone to undergo postangiography complications like pseudoaneurysm formation at the site of puncture [4, 26]. Computed tomography angiography (CTA) is a fast, reliable, and reproducible method for preoperative study of abdominal aortic aneurysms, providing detailed anatomical information like aortic diameters and segment lengths, as well as three-dimensional (3D) reconstructions and post-processing. These parameters are particularly needed in case an endovascular aortic repair (EVAR) is being planned. Magnetic resonance angiography (MRA) is also a reliable imaging method, but is more expensive and time consuming compared to CTA [18, 26].

2.3. Preoperative assessment

Medical optimization according to best current evidence is mandatory before arterial surgery, and in BD it includes the pre- and postoperative administration of glucocorticoids and immunosuppressive agents in order to minimize postoperative complications like anastomotic pseudoaneurysm formation [12, 27]. All patients should have an evaluation of their respiratory function, and they should be referred to the specialist in order to optimize respiratory function prior to surgery if needed. In case of smokers, smoking cessation is mandatory. Ischemic cardiac events are a major cause of perioperative morbidity and mortality in aortic and peripheral surgery, accounting for 10–40% of perioperative death due to myocardial infarction. Cardiac risk assessment is crucial. Detailed patient's medical history should be collected, a resting ECG should be performed in all patients, and further investigations such as stress echo or coronary angiography should be performed if needed [26]. Renal function should also be assessed prior to surgery, whether open or endovascular. Serum creatinine has to be measured and glomerular filtration rate (eGFR) estimated. If needed, patients should be referred to a renal physician for optimization of medications and of renal function prior to surgery [26]. Preoperative assessment should include a specialist vascular anesthetist's evaluation for both general (require for open surgery) and local anesthesia (could be considered in EVAR) [26].

2.4. Open infrarenal AAA repair technique

Open aortic aneurysm repair is usually performed through transperitoneal or retroperitoneal approach, depending on the specific patient's needs, on the location of the aneurysm, and on the surgeon expertise. For infrarenal AAA repair, midline laparotomy is the most usual approach, consisting of a vertical incision from the xiphoid process to the pubic symphysis, the extension depending on the involvement of the iliac arteries. After viscera exploration and retraction, the retroperitoneum is incised on the left of the midline, identifying the left renal vein and the proximal aortic neck.

A cornerstone to the surgical treatment of arterial involvement in BD is to perform the anastomosis, whenever possible, in a macroscopically disease-free neck, as far as possible from the inflamed segment [25]. The dissection continues vertically toward the right iliac artery. For complete left iliac artery's exposure, the dissection of mesosigmoid ligament is required. Once the proximal and distal neck of the aneurysm are identified and dissected, heparin is administered and the aorta is clamped proximally and distally to the aneurysm, extending to the iliac arteries if needed. The aneurysm is incised longitudinally, the mural thrombus is removed, and lumbar arteries' ostiums are sutured if bleeding. Inferior mesenteric artery may be ligated or reimplanted, depending on the adequacy of collateral circulation. An adequate sized tubular or bifurcated graft is then sutured with a continuous nonabsorbable monofilament suture to the proximal neck (**Figure 2**). Prosthetic or omentum wrapping on the proximal aortic anastomotic site is described in order to prevent anastomotic false aneurysm formation, which occurs in 10–50% of the cases [13, 25].

2.5. Endovascular aortic repair

Case 2 (**Figure 3**)*: A 45-year-old male BD patient presents with pulsatile abdominal mass. Duplex ultrasound and a contrast CT scan reveal the presence of an infrarenal abdominal aortic aneurysm with bulging of the posterolateral wall at the iliac bifurcation. The patient is successfully treated with a modular aortobisiliac endograft.*

EVAR is reported to be an effective and safe alternative to open repair for aortic aneurysms in BD, since the absence of anastomosis prevents the formation of pseudoaneurysms at their sites [14, 25]. Patients affected from BD may be better candidates for endovascular treatment than patients affected from atherosclerotic disease: they usually are younger, have smaller aneurysms, fewer comorbidities, and better renal function [28]. These characteristics positively affect the outcomes of endovascular interventions in BD: technical success rate is high due to the nonatherosclerotic nature of the lesions that implies easier introduction and navigation of endovascular devices inside vessels, mortality rate is lower (0.6 vs. 3.5%), and postoperative hospital stay is shorter when compared to open repair [13, 16]. Preoperative imaging is essential to EVAR in order to evaluate if the anatomical requirements for the endovascular repair are met: proximal neck diameter ≤32 mm, proximal neck length ≥10 mm, proximal neck

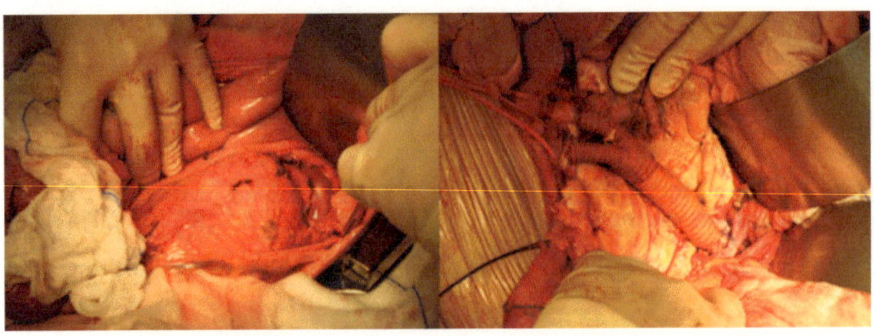

Figure 2. Open repair of a 78-mm abdominal aortic aneurysm (left) in a 42-year-old male BD patient with an aortobisiliac graft (right).

http://dx.doi.org/10.5772/intechopen.68664

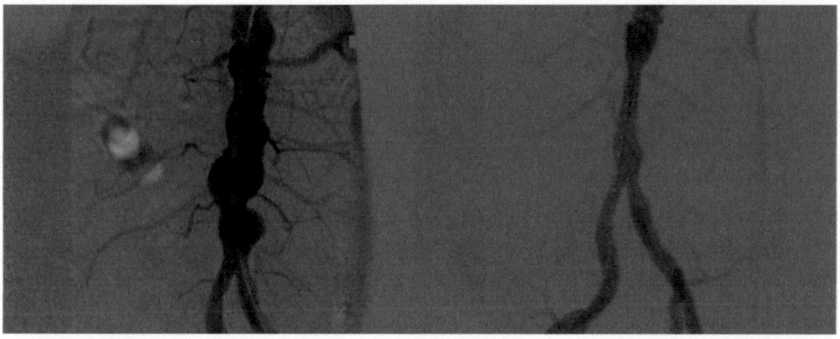

Figure 3. Endovascular repair (EVAR) of an infrarenal AAA (left) with an aortobisiliac endograft (right).

angulation ≤90° [29, 30]. Since the potential proximal progression of the disease, we suggest to consider a proximal neck length of at least 15 mm, thus preventing proximal leakage subsequent to the proximal expansion of the aneurysmatic sac. Anatomical features of iliac-femoral arteries are also to be evaluated. In BD, it is rare to find narrow, calcified, and tortuous arteries like in atherosclerosis; however, femoral arteries must be of adequate size since the endoprosthesis delivery system is introduced through these arteries. Nowadays, low-profile devices are available, with an outer diameter of 14F (1 F = 0.33 mm), allowing EVAR to be performed in a large percentage of patients [31].

2.5.1. Technique

The patient is placed in supine position. Bilateral femoral access can be obtained via surgical cutdown or percutaneous femoral artery puncture. The artery is punctured using Seldinger's technique after systemic heparinization. Under fluoroscopic guidance, an introducer is placed and a starter, hydrophilic guidewire, is advanced across the lesion and substituted with a stiff guidewire; the latter requires straightening tortuosity of the access vessel and improving the tracking capabilities of the introduced catheters and devices. On the contralateral access, an angiographic catheter is placed in aorta proximally to the aneurysm. Most of commercially available aortic endoprosthesis are modular, composed of a main bifurcated body, a contralateral branch, and in some cases an ipsilateral branch. Angiography is performed and renal arteries visualized. The main body of the endograft is then introduced and placed just below the emergency of the renal arteries; in cases of short proximal neck or juxta/suprarenal aneurysms, fenestrated and branched endografts are available. After placing the main body, the contralateral limb is progressed on a stiff guidewire through contralateral access and placed under fluoroscopic guidance. The aim of the endograft implantation is to exclude the aneurysmal sac from the blood flow, leading to its shrinkage.

2.5.2. Complications

Endoleaks are a primary complication of EVAR. Endoleaks can be defined as residual leakage of blood into the aneurysm and may lead to sac expansion and rupture. Endoleaks have been classified into five categories according to the site of leakage (**Table 2**). Type I endoleaks

I	Ineffective seal	IA	Proximal
		IB	Distal
		IC	Iliac occluder devices
II	Collateral flow inside the sac	IIA	Inferior mesenteric artery
		IIB	Lumbar arteries
III	Structural deficit	IIIA	Modular disconnect
		IIIB	Endograft rupture
IV			Graft porosity
V			Endotension

Table 2. Types of endoleak.

occur for incomplete sealing in the proximal- or distal-landing zone of the graft. The high-pressure flow seen in this complication exposes the patient to immediate risk of rupture and therefore should be treated promptly. Type II endoleaks occur as a result of collateral backflow into the aneurysm from branch vessels such as the inferior mesenteric or lumbar arteries. Type II low-flow endoleaks usually disappear on subsequent follow-up scans but as much as 25% require correction which can be performed with open, laparoscopic, or endovascular approach. Type III endoleaks occur in between the modular components of the endograft or through tears or defects in the graft and can usually be repaired by positioning additional cuffs or covered stents inside the graft. Type IV endoleaks occur through porosities in the graft fabric [32]. Type V endoleaks have unknown origin and are characterized by increased tension inside the aneurysmal sac (endotension). Although Type IV and V endoleaks are rare, they might lead to sac growth and if that is demonstrated during follow-up, open surgery for the removal of the endograft and substitution with a traditional prosthesis is necessary.

Case 3 (**Figure 4**)*: A 46-year-old male BD patient presents with pulsatile mass in the right groin, the site of a previous arterial access for positioning of an EVAR device for exclusion of abdominal aortic aneurism. DUS and contrast CT scan reveal the presence of a 41-mm pseudoaneurysm at the access site. The pseudoaneurysm is successfully treated with ultrasound-guided thrombin injection.*

Pseudoaneurysm formation at the site of puncture may occur, but these are easier to correct compared to pseudoaneurysms at the anastomotic site in the aortoiliac region [8, 14, 25]. In order to prevent this complication, it is recommendable to perform high-pressure compression at the site of puncture for 8 h after the procedure [7]. The use of closure devices may be an effective strategy to prevent this complication, though little information is available comparing closure devices to surgical cutdown in these patients [15].

Other rare complications in EVAR include peripheral or visceral embolization, acute renal failure, and graft migration [26, 32].

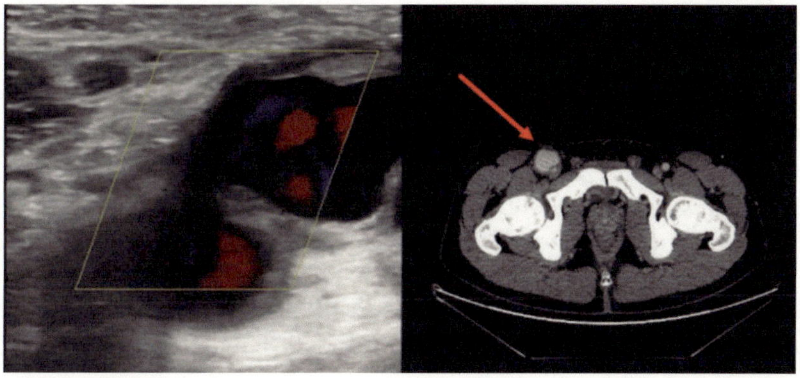

Figure 4. DUS and CT scan of a right common femoral artery pseudoaneurysm at a previous arterial access site in a BD patient.

2.6. Descending thoracic and thoracoabdominal aortic aneurysm

Descending thoracic aortic aneurysm (DTAA), defined as an aortic dilatation with at least a 50% increase in diameter located in any segment of the aorta between the left subclavian artery (LSA) origin and the diaphragm, is an uncommon finding in BD, though its rupture represents a catastrophic event and a major cause of death.

Crawford's classification, modified by Safi, of thoracic and thoracoabdominal aortic aneurysms (TAAAs) is based on the extension of the disease: type I extends from the origin of the left subclavian to the suprarenal abdominal aorta; type II TAA elongates from the left subclavian artery to the aortoiliac bifurcation; type III extends from the distal thoracic aorta to the aortoiliac bifurcation; type IV aneurysms are limited to the subdiaphragmatic aorta; type V, introduced by Safi, extends from the distal thoracic aorta to the abdominal aorta involving the celiac trunk and superior mesenteric artery origins, but not the renal arteries [33].

Chest and back pain are a common presentation of the disease, and physical examination can evidentiate signs of aortic regurgitation, cardiac tamponade, dyspnea, and dysphagia [33, 34].

Although several imaging techniques are available, such as MRI, positron emission tomography (PET), digital subtraction angiography, and intravascular ultrasonography, CTA scan is currently the gold standard for aortic imaging; it allows a conclusive study of thoracic aorta, showing an increased size of thoracic or thoracoabdominal aorta, and it can distinguish different aortic diseases like acute aortic syndromes (AASs) with a sensitivity up to 100% [18, 35].

AASs are defined as lesions involving disruption of the media of the aorta, with blood flow between the layers of the vessel or transmurally in the case of rupture [35].

According to Svensson, AASs are distinguished into five classes: class I is the classic aortic dissection, with a flap between true and false lumen; class II is the intramural hematoma;

class III is a limited intimal tear with an eccentric bulge at the tear site; class IV is a penetrating atherosclerotic ulcer with surrounding hematoma, usually subadventitial; and class V is represented by an iatrogenic or traumatic dissection [36].

The most dangerous complications of the invasive treatment of DTAAs are spinal cord ischemia (SCI), resulting in paraparesis or paraplegia (2–6% of the cases), and stroke (up to 8%). SCI is due to reperfusion injury to the spinal cord caused by the sudden interruption of blood flow and its subsequent restoration. Methods like somatosensory-evoked potentials (SSEPs) and motor-evoked potentials (MEPs) are employed to monitor the spinal cord function; cerebrospinal fluid drainage, left heart bypass, and cardiopulmonary extracorporeal circulation with induced systemic hypothermia reduce the risk of SCI [35].

2.7. Open repair

Open surgical repair should be reserved to patients unsuitable for thoracic endovascular aortic repair (TEVAR) in patients affected from DTAA, while remaining the recommended treatment of choice for patients affected from TAAA [35].

The location and extension of the aneurysm determine the site of incision; common approaches are left thoracotomy at V, VI, VII, or VIII intercostal space (ICS), allowing the exposure of the descending thoracic aorta from the origin of the LSA to the suprarenal abdominal aorta; left thoracophrenotomy at VII, IX, or X ICS, with the section of diaphragm, grants access to the distal thoracic aorta and suprarenal abdominal aorta; midline, paramedian, or bilateral subcostal laparotomy are indicated to obtain a transperitoneal access to the suprarenal aorta, the celiac trunk, and the superior mesenteric artery, while left transverse lateral laparotomy allows extraperitoneal access to the same segment; thoracophrenolaparotomy permits complete exposure of the whole aorta, from the origin of the LSA to the iliac bifurcation [37].

After exposure and clamping of the aorta, the aneurysmatic sac is incised and, after reimplantation of intercostal arteries distal to T8–T9 and visceral vessels if involved, a Dacron graft is implanted using the same suturing technique described in the section about open repair of abdominal aortic aneurysms.

2.8. Thoracic endovascular aortic repair and hybrid surgery

Case 4 (**Figure 5**): *A 26-year-old female BD patient presents with chest pain. After cardiac involvement is ruled out, a contrast CT scan reveals the presence of a pseudoaneurysm of the descending thoracic aorta. MRI and PET scans are also performed as evidence of aortitis is present (elevated ESR and CRP). The patient is successfully treated with a tubular endograft.*

TEVAR has become the first-choice treatment for suitable patients affected by DTAAs; when compared to open repair, TEVAR has lower mortality and morbidity rates and shorter length of hospital stay. In TAAAs, endovascular repair is reserved to those unfit for surgery.

Patients with a distal-landing zone of less than 15-mm length and a proximal neck diameter of >40 mm are unsuitable for treatment with currently available devices [35].

http://dx.doi.org/10.5772/intechopen.68664

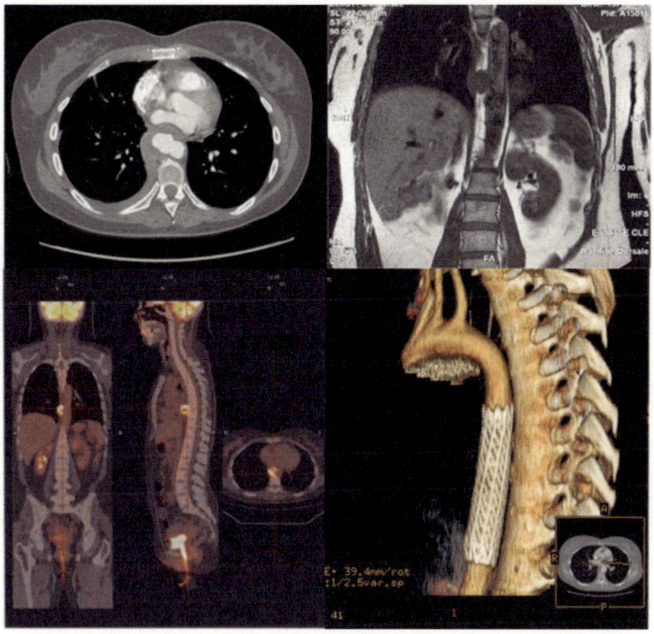

Figure 5. CT, MR, and PET scans in a 26-year-old female patient presenting with a descending thoracic aorta pseudoaneurysm. Lower-right image: exclusion of the pseudoaneurysm with a tubular thoracic endograft (3D reconstruction).

After gaining mono- or bilateral surgical or percutaneous access to the common femoral artery, the latter is punctured using Seldinger's technique after systemic heparinization.

Under fluoroscopic guidance, an introducer is placed and a Pig-Tail is progressed over a hydrophilic guidewire; a preliminary angiography and road mapping are performed; then the endoprosthesis' device is inserted over a super stiff guidewire, progressed to the aortic valve and retracted under fluoroscopic guidance. Angiography is performed to verify the correct positioning of the stent graft. Arterial blood pressure is lowered to 70–80 mmHg and momentary asystole is provoked in order to prevent the wind-shock effect, then the tube-shaped endoprosthesis is opened.

If one or more sovraortic trunks or visceral arteries are covered by the implantation of the stent graft, preliminary surgical debranching of these vessels is required. Debranching can be performed with a previous operation or during the same procedure, prior to the endovascular stage [12, 35].

Scallop designed, fenestrated, and branched custom-made endografts, with openings in the fabric or branches in correspondence to the origin of visceral arteries, are currently available [38].

Periscope and chimney/snorkel techniques, requiring antegrade catheterization from a trans-brachial access, consist in the placement of a stent graft into one or more branch vessels in a parallel path alongside the aortic endograft; these techniques are promising, though supported by little clinical evidence [35].

2.9. Pulmonary artery aneurysms

Pulmonary artery aneurysms (PAAs), true or false, are the most lethal complication of BD; it has been reported that about 50% of these patients die within a year after the onset of hemoptysis although more recent data show survival rates of up to 80% at 5 years, mainly due to earlier diagnosis and treatment [39, 40]. Emergency surgery for aneurysm rupture carries high risk and uncertain results [8].

Hemoptysis, due to arterial-bronchial fistulization, is the most common presentation of these aneurysms, appearing as polinodular opacities and hilar or mediastinal enlargements on chest X-ray scan [41].

CTA scan, as stated before, is an important imaging method in BD, allowing detailed analysis of the aorta and other arterial and venous vessels; compared to MRI, it also shows lung parenchyma in greater detail [41]. PAA has strong association with DVT, caval, or intracardiac thrombus formation [11, 40].

Medical treatment with immunosuppressive therapy is the main treatment for PAAs [19]. Invasive treatment of PAA should be performed only in case of massive, life-threatening bleeding. Surgical techniques consisting in lobectomy or pneumonectomy of the involved structure have been reported, but aneurysmectomy with direct suturing of the wall defect has shown to have better long-term patency rates; additionally, endoaneurysmorraphy seems to be coherent with the morphology of the false and saccular aneurysms of BD [41, 42]. As in the other arterial districts, even PAA surgery is burdened with recurrency at the site of suture or anastomosis.

Endovascular embolization techniques have been described and endovascular treatment seems to be a safe option: Amplatzer duct occluder and coils have been successfully used to thrombose PAAs, though some limitations as aneurysmal sac size and complications like caval embolization have been reported.

Transhepatic embolization of PAA with N-butyl cyanoacrylate glue and coils has recently been successfully attempted [43].

2.10. Peripheral aneurysms

Case 5 (**Figure 6**)*: A 22-year-old female BD patient in corticosteroid and azathioprine treatment is referred to the vascular surgery department with an accidental finding on a CT scan of a 23-mm aneurysm at the origin of the right subclavian artery. Due to the location and characteristics of the lesion and the young age of the patient, a strict follow-up protocol with DUS every 6 months and annual CT scans is recommended. The aneurysm has maintained a stable diameter after 6 years of follow-up visits.*

Peripheral aneurysmal degeneration is a common finding among patients with vasculo-Behçet.

http://dx.doi.org/10.5772/intechopen.68664

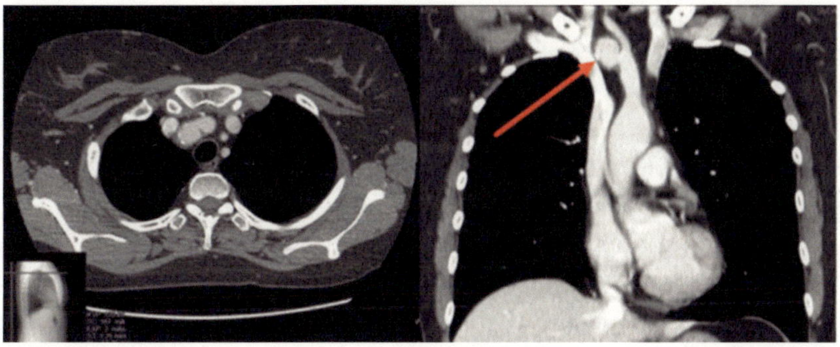

Figure 6. CT scan of a 22-year-old BD patient presenting with a right subclavian artery aneurysm.

Physical examination could reveal the presence of a pulsatile, hyperemic, and tender swelling in correspondence of a peripheral vessel, and all arterial segments should be explored and/or studied with CTA scan since multiple aneurysms in the same patient have been reported [10, 15].

Immunosuppressive therapy should be administered immediately, because early diagnosis and early administration of therapy will help in preventing the formation and progression of the arterial lesions [10, 20].

Case 6 (**Figure 7**): *A 43-year-old male BD patient presents with pain in the right groin area. Physical examination reveals a large pulsatile mass. DUS confirms the presence of a 50-mm common femoral artery aneurysm. The patient undergoes aneurysmectomy with Dacron graft interposition.*

Like the other arterial segments, peripheral arterial repair may be complicated by recurrency, anastomotic pseudoaneurysms, graft occlusion, and distal embolization [12, 44].

Surgical peripheral bypasses of affected arteries have been reported; the use of autologous saphenous vein is to be avoided, because the vein could be affected by vasculitis or previous superficial vein thrombosis, and synthetic grafts are to be preferred in these patients [44]. The choice of a disease-free segment for reconstruction is crucial.

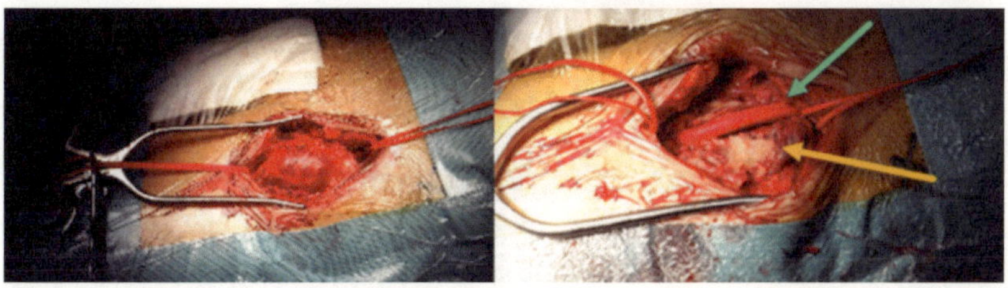

Figure 7. Open repair of a left common femoral artery aneurysm.

Case 7 (**Figure 8**)*: A 30-year-old male patient affected with BD was admitted at our division with a pulsatile, painful swelling in the right popliteal fossa. DUS showed partially thrombosed popliteal artery aneurysm. The patient underwent a femoral-popliteal bypass graft using a cryopreserved femoral superficial artery as an allograft. The procedure was uneventful, and short-term (6-month) follow-up showed graft patency, no detachment nor aneurysmatic degeneration at the anastomotic site.*

The use of allografts has been reported in the case of aortic substitution to be an appropriate therapy in patients affected from noninfectious inflammatory diseases including BD with uneventful mid-term follow-up [45, 46]. Allografts, if available, could be a valid alternative for peripheral procedures in BD patients where due to the ongoing vasculitis it might be undesirable to employ venous segments.

In cases where surgical peripheral revascularization is not feasible for the absence of a disease-free arterial segment, ligation after stump pressure measurement has been reported to be an alternative treatment; successful ligation of carotid, subclavian, iliac, superficial femoral, popliteal, and posterior tibial artery have been reported [12, 47]. The presence of collateral circulation allows arterial ligation without disabling ischemia in a large number of patients; furthermore, peripheral graft occlusion often results in a mild claudication, requiring no additional revascularization procedure [8].

Endovascular treatment of peripheral aneurysms includes stent graft implantation, with patency rate of 89% at 2 years, and coil/plug embolization [4, 15, 48].

2.11. Carotid and vertebral artery aneurysm

Case 8 (**Figure 9**)*: A 40-year-old male BD patient in immunosuppressive therapy presents with a pulsatile mass in the neck and a recent transient ischemic episode characterized by a dyspraxia involving the right upper limb. DUS is performed showing high tortuosity of the left carotid artery with a 40-mm partially thrombosed aneurysm just distal to the bifurcation. The finding is confirmed by a contrast CT scan. The patient is referred to surgery. Extensive neck dissection was required for the repair. After the aneurysmectomy, direct anastomosis between the internal carotid and the common carotid and reconstruction of a neobifurcation was possible. Patient was discharged on the third postoperative day with no neurological deficits.*

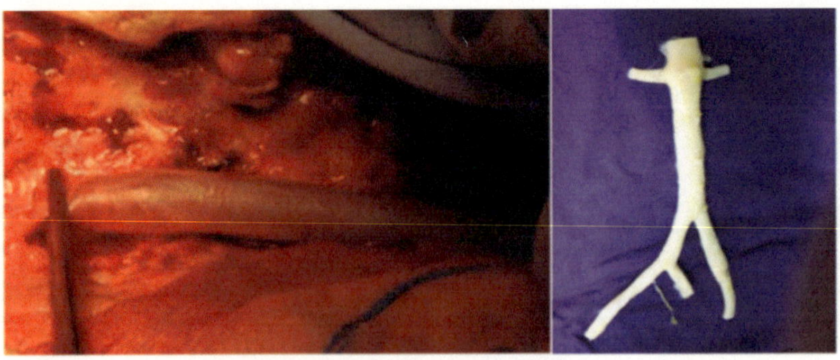

Figure 8. Femoropopliteal bypass grafting utilizing an allograft (left). Right image: aortobisiliac homograft prior to an implantation.

http://dx.doi.org/10.5772/intechopen.68664

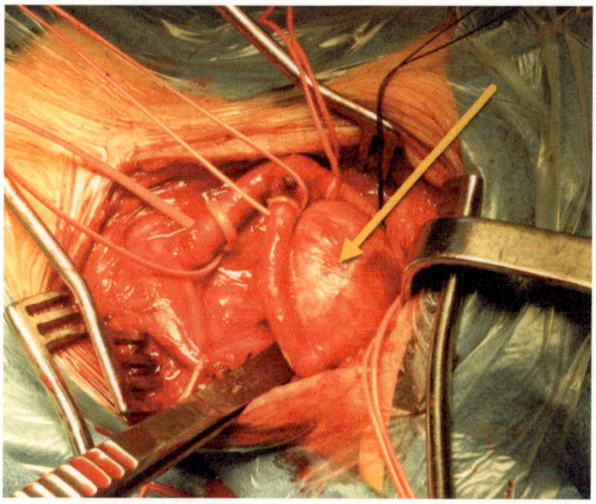

Figure 9. Open repair of a symptomatic left internal carotid aneurysm in a BD patient.

Few cases of extracranial carotid artery and vertebral artery aneurysms in BD have been reported [49–51]. Common carotid artery appears to be the most frequent location. Symptoms can derive from compression of nearby structures or from cerebral embolization from the aneurysmatic sac, resulting in neck pain, voice alterations, dyspnea, transient ischemic attacks, and ictus cerebri [47]. Rupture of these aneurysms is rare but has been reported [8].

Surgical treatment includes aneurysmectomy and synthetic graft bypass and, in case of emergency and impossibility to perform reconstruction, carotid or vertebral artery ligation [49, 51].

Endovascular treatment of carotid artery aneurysms is an option in cases where the aneurysm is surgically inaccessible, and it includes stent graft implantation and coil embolization. However, long-term results of endovascular treatment of carotid and vertebral arteries involvement in BD are still lacking.

3. Conclusion

Angio-Behçet's patients are challenging from a surgical standpoint. Both venous and arterial circulations are involved, even in the same patient, with a high rate of recurrence and postoperative complications. Though venous involvement is more frequent than arterial lesions, the latter account for the majority of deaths.

The need for a comprehensive vascular physical and radiological examination in BD patients presenting features of vascular involvement cannot be stressed enough.

Perioperative immunosuppressive and corticosteroid medications are the key to the success of any vascular surgical procedure in these patients.

New endovascular techniques are showing promising results for the treatment of arterial lesions with lower mortality rates and faster recovery time when compared to open repair. Technical success rate is close to 100%. Even though graft occlusions are not infrequent, they could be managed through endovascular-assisted patency procedures.

Open repair entails a high risk of pseudoaneurysm formation at the anastomotic site, and should therefore be reserved to cases unsuitable for endovascular procedures or where the latter have failed. Allografts could be a valid alternative to the use of autologous saphenous vein or prosthetic grafts for arterial substitution, though further studies are needed.

The management of venous lesions is mainly medical, and endovascular stents for the treatment of venous vessels are not yet available in a clinical setting.

The evolution of minimally invasive techniques is tracing new paths in the surgical management of Angio-Behçet's patients, broadening the array of tools available to the vascular surgeon and enabling him/her to tailor the treatment based on each patient's peculiar characteristics.

Author details

Genadi Georgiev Genadiev*, Lorenzo Mortola, Roberta Arzedi, Giuseppe Deiana, Francesco Spanu and Stefano Camparini

*Address all correspondence to: ggenadiev@gmail.com

AO "G. Brotzu", Cagliari, Italy

References

[1] El-Ramahi KM, Al-Dalaan A, Al-Balaa S, et al. Vascular involvement in Behçet's disease. In: Wechsler B, Godeau P, editors. Behçet's Disease. Amsterdam: Excerpta Medica; 1993. p. 531

[2] Melikoglu M, Kural-Seyahi E, Tascilar K, et al. The unique features of vasculitis in Behçet's syndrome. Clinical Reviews in Allergy & Immunology. 2008;**35**:40–46. DOI: 10.1007/s12016-007-8064-8

[3] Calamia KT, Schirmer M, Melikoglu M. Major vessel involvement in Behçet's disease: An update. Current Opinion in Rheumatology. 2011;**23**(1):24-31. DOI: 10.1097/BOR.0b013e3283410088

[4] Alpagut U, Ugurlucan M, Dayioglu E. Major arterial involvement and review of Behçet's disease. Annals of Vascular Surgery. 2007;**21**:232–239. DOI: 10.1016/j.avsg.2006.12.004

[5] Duzgun N, Ates A. Characteristics of vascular involvement in Behçet's disease. Scandinavian Journal of Rheumathology, 2006;**35**(1):65–68 DOI: 10.1080/03009740500255761

[6] Saadoun D, Wechsler B, Desseaux K, Le Thi Huong D, Amoura Z, Resche-Rigon M, Cacoub P. Mortality in Behçet's disease. Arthritis & Rheumatism. 2010;**62**:2806–2812. DOI: 10.1002/art.27568

[7] Balcioglu O, Ertugay S, Bozkaya H, Parildar M, Posacioglu H. Endovascular repair and adjunctive immunosuppressive therapy of aortic involvement in Behçet's disease. European Journal of Vascular and Endovascular Surgery. 2015;**50**:593–598. DOI: 10.1016/j.ejvs.2015.07.011

[8] Tüzün H, et al. Management of aneurysms in Behçet's syndrome: An analysis of 24 patients. Surgery. 1997;**121**:150–156. DOI: 10.1016/j.jvs.2011.07.049

[9] Sherif A, Stewart P, Mendes DM. The repetitive vascular catastrophes of Behçet's disease: A case report with review of the literature. Annals in Vascular Surgery. 1992;**6**:85–89. DOI: 10.1007/BF02000674

[10] Jayachandran NV, Rajasekhar L, Chandrasekhara PKS, Kanchinadham S, Narsimulu G. Multiple peripheral arterial and aortic aneurysms in Behçet's syndrome—A case report. Clinical Rheumatology. 2008;**27**:265–267. DOI: 10.1007/s10067-007-0713-z

[11] Hamuryudan V, et al. Pulmonary arterial aneurysms in Behçet's syndrome: A report of 24 cases. British Journal of Rheumatology. 1994;**33**:48–51. DOI: 10.1093/rheumatology/33.1.48

[12] Hosaka A, et al. Long-term outcome after surgical treatment of arterial lesions in Behçet disease. Journal of Vascular Surgery. 2005;**42**:116–121. DOI: 10.1016/j.jvs.2005.03.019

[13] Kwon TW, et al. Surgical treatment result of abdominal aortic aneurysm in Behçet's disease. European Journal of Vascular and Endovascular Surgery. 2008 Feb;**35**(2):173–180. DOI: 10.1016/j. ejvs.2007.08.013[P3]

[14] Liu CW, et al. Endovascular treatment of aortic pseudoaneurysm in Behçet disease. Journal of Vascular Surgery. 2009;**50**(5):1025–1030

[15] Kim WH, et al. Effectiveness and safety of endovascular aneurysm treatment in patients with vasculo-Behçet disease. Journal of Endovascular Therapy. 2009;**16**:631–636. DOI: 10.1583/09-2812.1

[16] Nitecki SS, et al. Abdominal aortic aneurysm in Behçet's disease: New treatment options for an old and challenging problem. The Israel Medicine Association Journal. 2004;**6**(3): 152-155. PMID: 15055270

[17] Düzgün N, Ates A, Aydintug OT, Demir Ö, Ölmez Ü. Characteristics of vascular involvement in Behçet's disease. Scandinavian Journal of Rheumatology. 2006;**35**(1):65–68. DOI: 10.1080/03009740500255761

[18] Ko GY, Byun JY, Choi BG, et al. The vascular manifestations of Behçet's disease: Angiographic and CT findings. British Journal of Radiology. 2000;**73**:1270–1274. DOI: 10.1259/bjr.73.876.11205670

[19] Hatemi G, Silman A, Bang D, Bodaghi B, Chamberlain AM, Gul A, Houman MH, Kötter I, Olivieri I, Salvarani C, Sfikakis PP, Siva A, Stanford MR, Stübiger N, Yurdakul S, Yazici H.

EULAR recommendations for the management of Behçet disease. Annals of the Rheumatic Diseases. 2008;**67**:12, 1656–1662. DOI: 10.1136/ard.2007.080432

[20] Hendaoui L, et al. Imaging features of Behçet's disease. Systemic Vasculitis. Medical Radiology. 2012;**1**:137–173

[21] Bayraktar Y, Balkanci F, Bayraktar M et al. Budd-Chiari syndrome: A common complication of Behçet's disease. American Journal of Gastroenterology. 1997;**92**:858–862. PMID: 9149201

[22] Chae EJ, Do KH, Seo JB, et al. Radiologic and clinical findings of Behçet disease: Comprehensive review of multisystemic involvement. Radio Graphics. 2008 Sep-Oct;28 (5):e31. DOI: 10.1148/rg.e31

[23] Emmi L, editor. Behçet Syndrome: From Pathogenesis to Treatment. Italia: Springer-Verlag; 2014. pp. 217–225. DOI: 10.1007/978-88-470-5477-6_20

[24] Wanhainen A, et al. Thoracic and abdominal aortic dimension in 70-year-old men and women – A population-based whole-body magnetic resonance imaging (MRI) study. Journal of Vascular Surgery. 2008;Mar;**47**(3):504–12. DOI: 10.1016/j.jvs.2007.10.043

[25] Vasseur M. Endovascular treatment of abdominal aneurysmal aortitis in Behçet's disease. Journal of Vascular Surgery. 1998; May;**27**(5):974–6. DOI: 10.1016/S0741-5214(98)70281-2

[26] Moll FL, et al. Management of abdominal aortic aneurysms clinical practice guidelines of the European society for vascular surgery. European Journal of Vascular and Endovascular Surgery. 2011;41 Suppl 1:S1-S58. DOI: 10.1016/j.ejvs.2010.09.011

[27] Park MC, Hong BK, Kwon HM, Hong YS. Surgical outcomes and risk factors for postoperative complications in patients with Behçet's disease. Clinical Rheumatology. 2007;**26**:1475–1480. DOI: 10.1007/s10067-006-0530-9

[28] Robenshtok E. Arterial involvement in Behçet's disease—The search for new strategies. The Israel Medicine Association Journal. 2004 Mar;**6**(3):162–3. PMID: 15055273

[29] AbuRahma AF, et al. Aortic neck anatomic features and predictors of outcomes in endovascular repair of abdominal aortic aneurysms following vs not following instructions for use. Journal of the American College of Surgeons. 2016;**222**:579–589. DOI: 10.1016/j.jamcollsurg.2015.12.037

[30] Simons JP. Exploring EVAR instructions for use in 2016. Endovascular Today. 2016; 15:48–52.

[31] Clough RE. Low-profile EVAR. Endovascular Today. 2016;**15**:72–75.

[32] Greenhalgh RM, Powell JT. Endovascular repair of abdominal aortic aneurysm the clinical problem. New England Journal of Medicine. 2008;**358**:494–501. DOI: 10.1056/NEJMcp1513724

[33] Safi HJ, Miller CC. Spinal cord protection in descending thoracic and dominal aortic repair. Annals in Thoracic Surgery. 1999;**67**:1937–9. DOI: 10.1016/ S1043-0679(98)70016-4

[34] Ohira S, Masuda S, Matsushita T. Nine-year experience of recurrent anastomotic pseudoaneurysms after thoracoabdominal aneurysm graft replacement in a patient with Behçet disease. Heart, Lung and Circulation. 2014;**23**:210–213. DOI: 10.1016/j.hlc.2014.05.009

[35] Riambau V, et al. Editor's choice—Management of descending thoracic aorta diseases. European Journal of Vascular and Endovascular Surgery. 2017;**53**:4–52. DOI: 10.1016/j.ejvs.2016.06.005

[36] Svensson LG. Intimal tear without hematoma. Circulation. 1999;99:1331. DOI: 10.1161/01.CIR.99.10.1331

[37] Rutherford RB. Atlas of vascular surgery: Basic techniques and exposures. Saunders. 1993;**1**:120–133. DOI: 10.1002/bjs.1800801151

[38] Frederick JR, Woo YJ. Thoracoabdominal aortic aneurysm. Annals in Cardiothoracic Surgery. 2012;**1**:277–285. DOI: 10.3978/j.issn.2225-319X.2012.09.01

[39] Kural-Seyahi E, et al. The long-term mortality and morbidity of Behçet syndrome. Medicine (Baltimore). 2013;**82**:60–76. DOI: 10.1097/00005792-200301000-00006

[40] Hamuryudan V, et al. Pulmonary artery aneurysms in Behçet syndrome. American Journal of Medicine. 2004;**117**:867–870. DOI: 10.1093/rheumatology/33.1.48

[41] Ceylan N, Bayraktaroglu S, Erturk SM, Savas R, Alper H. Pulmonary and vascular manifestations of Behçet disease: Imaging findings. American Journal of Roentgenology. 2010;**194**:158–164. DOI: 10.2214/AJR.09.2763

[42] Aroussi AA, Redai M, Ouardi FEl, Mehadji B-E, Casablanca M. Bilateral pulmonary artery aneurysm in Behçet syndrome: Report of two operative cases. 2005:1170–1171. DOI: 10.1016/j.jtcvs.2004.08.038

[43] Seizem NG, et al. Transhepatic embolization of bilateral pulmonary artery aneurysm with N-butyl cyanoacrylate and coils in Behçet disease. Journal of Vascular and Interventional Radiology. 2016;**27**:293–295. DOI: 10.1016/j.jvir.2015.10.012

[44] Iscan ZH, Vural KM, Bayazit M. Compelling nature of arterial manifestations in Behçet Disease. Journal of Vascular Surgery. 2005; **41**(1):53–8. DOI: 10.1016/j.jvs.2004.09.018

[45] Umehara N, Saito S, Ishii H, Aomi S, Kurosawa H. Rupture of thoracoabdominal aortic aneurysm associated with Behçet's disease. Annals in Thoracic Surgery. 2007;**84**:1394–1396. DOI: 10.1016/j.athoracsur.2007.04.110

[46] Sakuma K, Akimoto H, Yokoyama H, Iguchi A, Tabayashi, K. Cryopreserved aortic homograft replacement in 3 patients with noninfectious inflammatory vascular disease. Japanese Journal of Thoracic and Cardiovascular Surgery. 2001;**49**:652–655. DOI: 10.1007/BF02912473

[47] Goz M, Cakir O. Huge popliteal arterial aneurysms in Behçet's syndrome: Is ligation an alternative treatment? Vascular. 2007;**15**:46–48. DOI: 10.2310/6670.2007.00010

[48] Silistreli E, et al. Behçet's disease: Treatment of popliteal pseudoaneurysm by an endovascular stent graft implantation. Annals in Vascular Surgery. 2004;**18**:118–120. DOI: 10.1007/s10016-003-0107-x

[49] Bouarhroum A, et al. Extracranial carotid aneurysm in Behçet disease: Report of two new cases. Journal of Vascular Surgery. 2006;**43**:627–630. DOI: 10.1016/j.jvs.2005.09.049

[50] Posacioglu H, Apaydin AZ, Parildar M, Buket S. Large pseudoaneurysm of the carotid artery in Behçet's disease. Texas Heart Institute Journal. 2005;**32**:95–98. PMCID: PMC555835

[51] Gürer O, Yapici F, Enç Y, Çinar B, Özler A. Spontaneous pseudoaneurysm of the vertebral artery in Behçet's disease. Annals in Vascular Surgery. 2005;**19**:280–283. DOI: 10.1007/s10016-004-0147-x